Praise for *Sovereign Self*

"With warmth, clarity, wisdom, engaging boldness, and unswerving dedication, Acharya Shunya guides the reader through the mind's maze of maya-illusion straight to the liberating goal of Self-knowledge. This book is soul medicine—read it carefully, study it deeply, apply the practices, and discover its life-transforming promise for yourself. It is a modern treasure trove of Vedic wisdom so necessary and relevant for our times."

YOGACHARYA ELLEN GRACE O'BRIAN,
spiritual director of the Center for Spiritual Enlightenment
and author of *The Jewel of Abundance*

"*Sovereign Self* is a beautifully written and masterful guidebook that eloquently shows us how to recognize and embody our essential wholeness amidst our everyday life. Profound and practical, this seminal work reveals in-depth yogic wisdom teachings and practices we can easily engage to attain our full potential as authentic human beings. Acharya Shunya articulately and persuasively elucidates the timeless teachings that enable us to achieve the fullness of our human capacity. A must-read!"

RICHARD MILLER, PhD, author of *iRest Meditation, Yoga
Nidra*, and *The iRest Program for Healing PTSD*

"The essence of yoga is Self-knowledge, the realization of our true nature as pure consciousness. Acharya Shunya has shared that core Vedic teaching in a clear and understandable presentation that is accessible to all, reminding us of our real identity, eternal purpose, and the ultimate source of our healing: happiness and harmony."

DAVID FRAWLEY (VAMADEVA SHASTRI), DLitt, Padma
Bhushan recipient, author of *The Yoga of Consciousness*, and director
of the American Institute of Vedic Studies

"What depth of wisdom combined with remarkably useful practical advice, and what an honor to learn from a teacher trained in and practicing a living spiritual tradition. And, for a change, a master who truly understands the feminine. There are many spiritual guides in the world today—some authentically wise and awakened—but few who embody the wisdom, techniques, and secrets of a tradition developed over centuries by practicing masters. Please enjoy and benefit from this gift of the deepest heart and spirit."

ALLAN COMBS, PhD, author of *Consciousness Explained Better*
and California Institute of Integral Studies professor
of consciousness studies

"The highest form of dispersing Vedic wisdom is by example. If you have the privilege of meeting Acharya Shunya, you will experience her heartfelt transmission firsthand, as I have. When you read her book, you will observe that she has found a way to share this ancient wisdom with all true seekers. Highly recommended."

LARRY PAYNE, PhD, C-IAYT, author of AARP's *Yoga After 50 for Dummies* and founding director of the Yoga Therapy Rx and Yoga After 50/Prime of Life Yoga programs at Loyola Marymount University

"This book is a masterpiece written from the heart by a Vedic scholar, a step-by-step teaching that brought Acharya Shunya from darkness to light, from bondage to freedom. It should be essential reading for every person who is looking for answers to questions arising on their spiritual path."

DILIP SARKAR, MD, FACS, DLitt, faculty member at Vivekananda Yoga University and chairman at the Center for Integrative Medicine and Yoga, Taksha Institute

"This contemplative gem encapsulates the best of spiritual reflection. Each chapter starts with a pithy quote from a primary text, followed by words from the author's teacher and examples drawn from the insights and experiences of Acharya Shunya and her students. Instructive without being didactic, honest yet never trite, *Sovereign Self* provides beacons of light and wisdom for every spiritual seeker."

CHRISTOPHER KEY CHAPPLE, Doshi professor of Indic and comparative theology and director of the Master of Arts in Yoga Studies program at Loyola Marymount University

"Freedom, happiness, and peace are my three highest values—the same values that every human being aspires for. How do you find them? Fortunately, the operating manual is available to us. Humans who have gone before us have thought about this topic and researched it through their own life experiences. They have left behind their learnings in the form of ancient sacred texts and wisdom traditions. But such 'operating manuals' are written in ancient Sanskrit and can be dense and inaccessible. Acharya Shunya has done an excellent job unlocking the wisdom for us in a deftly and lucidly written book, in a language accessible to a global audience today."

GOPI KALLAYIL, chief evangelist of digital transformation and strategy at Google, author of *The Internet to the Inner-net* and *The Happy Human*, and creator of the Kirtan Lounge series

"The Vedic idea of the sovereign and blissful Self, and the psychic discipline to recover it from oblivion while living our everyday life, is powerfully presented in this book. It is an antidote to the postmodern concept of a fragile and anguished self that lives in mortal fear of choosing between Tweedledee and Tweedledum."

SWAMI BODHANANDA SARASVATI, chairman of the
Sambodh Foundation (India) and the Sambodh Society, Inc. (USA)

"The power and beauty of storytelling is such that one can impart complex concepts to a child or a scientist alike. By weaving together basic principles of ancient scriptures, Acharya Shunya leads one to declutter the mind step-by-step and be a witness to attaining the holistic Self. She anchors inner awareness by offering meditation pearls to transition from self-pity, to empathy, to self-freedom. Ultimately, story merges into *sadhana* to cultivate a lifestyle by sheer daily practice of Patanjali's eternal foundations—personal and societal ethics (*yamas* and *niyamas*)."

MATRA RAJ, OTR/L, C-IAYT, president of the International
Association of Yoga Therapists

"Acharya Shunya's book arrives in an age when people are thirsting for an authentic path to lead from darkness to light. This very practical, straightforward book is the dip of cool water needed to slake that thirst."

DIANE FINLAYSON, MA, editor of *Yoga Therapy Foundations,
Tools, and Practice* and department chair of the Master of Science in
Yoga Therapy program at Maryland University of Integrative Health

"In this elegant offering, Acharya Shunya distills the most ancient of the world's wisdom teachings to their luminous essence. The result is a potent elixir for our times. With a special gift for embodied feminine knowing, Acharya Shunya dissolves the obstacles that have prevented free access to these treasures and invites everyone to the table of liberation and joy."

MIRABAI STARR, author of *Caravan of No Despair* and *Wild Mercy*

"*Sovereign Self* is an integral guide to psycho-spiritual well-being based on the wisdom traditions of India . . . a concise compendium of yoga for well-being."

DEBASHISH BANERJI, Haridas Chaudhuri professor of
Indian philosophies and cultures and Doshi professor of Asian
art; program chair for the East–West Psychology Department at
the California Institute of Integral Studies

"*Sovereign Self* is a most welcome addition to the burgeoning shelves of books that apply India's ancient spiritual wisdom to modern life. It is welcome because Acharya Shunya is the real deal. A lineage holder immersed in the tradition from a young age, she is grounded in the full breadth of Vedic wisdom and well-acquainted with its depth. She is also a pragmatic teacher, and her book guides us in the everyday application of precepts and practices that will enhance anyone's life regardless of their beliefs or background."

PHILIP GOLDBERG, author of *American Veda*
and *Spiritual Practice for Crazy Times*

"Shunya is a master storyteller, and throughout this book, she relates incidents from her own life with a sensitivity and candor that instantly illuminate the relevance of ancient Vedic wisdom to the modern reader. The chapter in which Shunya movingly relates her childhood confrontation with death is particularly infused with pathos, grace, and the ring of spiritual truth. This book is a radiant gem and a must-read for those on the path to growth, transformation, and self-awareness."

SUDHA PRATHIKANTI, MD

"Acharya Shunya's fearlessly straightforward yet nurturing voice manages to illustrate our obstacles of ego without an ounce of shame or blame, but rather provides encouragement and the recognition that the struggle is real—indeed, that it is shared. It is rare to find wisdom imparted with such lightness and grace while carrying such mighty weight. I highly recommend this book to anyone seeking to live their best life and awaken to joy."

HEATHER SHEREÉ TITUS, cofounder of Yoga Unify
and director of the Sedona Yoga Festival

"This beautiful work is a treasury of Vedic knowledge and wisdom that is both practical and inspiring. It is a warm invitation to experience for yourself that your mind is a reflector of the divine powers of your soul."

HEMA PATANKAR, author and teacher at Living Sanskrit,
Ayurveda program advisor at Vedika Global, and former executive
director of Muktabodha Indological Research Institute

SOVEREIGN SELF

SOVEREIGN SELF

Claim Your Inner Joy and Freedom
with the Empowering Wisdom
of the Vedas, Upanishads,
and Bhagavad Gita

ACHARYA SHUNYA

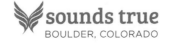

sounds true
BOULDER, COLORADO

Sounds True
Boulder, CO 80306

This book is not intended as a substitute for the medical recommendations of physicians, mental health professionals, or other health-care providers. Rather, it is intended to offer information to help the reader cooperate with physicians, mental health professionals, and health-care providers in a mutual quest for optimal well-being. We advise readers to carefully review and understand the ideas presented and to seek the advice of a qualified professional before attempting to use them. Some names and identifying details have been changed to protect the privacy of individuals.

Published 2020

Book design by Happenstance Type-O-Rama

Printed in the United States of America

Library of Congress Cataloging-in-Publication Data

Names: Shunya, Acharya, author.
Title: Sovereign self: claim your inner joy and freedom with the
    empowering wisdom of the Vedas, Upanishads, and Bhagavad Gita / Acharya
    Shunya.
Description: Boulder: Sounds True, 2020. | Includes bibliographical
    references and index.
Identifiers: LCCN 2020017829 (print) | LCCN 2020017830 (ebook) | ISBN
    9781683645818 (hardcover) | ISBN 9781683645825 (ebook)
Subjects: LCSH: Self-realization—Religious aspects—Hinduism. | Spiritual
    life—Hinduism. | Spiritual exercises. | Self-realization in literature.
Classification: LCC BL1238.34 .S58 2020 (print) | LCC BL1238.34 (ebook) |
    DDC 294.5/44—dc23

LC record available at https://lccn.loc.gov/2020017829

LC ebook record available at https://lccn.loc.gov/2020017830

10 9 8 7 6 5 4 3 2 1

"O My Mind,
  Lead me from falsehood to truth.
  Lead me from darkness to light.
  Lead me from mortality to immortality."

BRIHADARANYAKA UPANISHAD, 1.3.28

"Your mind will be released from all bondages
  upon realizing the sovereign truth within."

SHVETASHVATARA UPANISHAD, 6.13

CONTENTS

Contents

PART III
EMBRACE THE JOY OF YOUR SOVEREIGN LIFE

Contents

INTRODUCTION
AN INVITATION TO
THE SOVEREIGN SELF

We humans have accepted a shackled existence. Many of us feel our life is simply a jail sentence. We disappoint ourselves. We don't necessarily even like ourselves. We go about life imprisoned in our false beliefs, confirming our imagined personal limitations. We beg for freedom, recognition, and love from others, forgetting that our happiness, acceptance, and worth are up to us, that they are achieved through an inward journey toward the Self, never outward. We don't recognize the truth that we are the ruler of our own lives, in full command of our own experience.

Absolute authority over your inner world is your spiritual birthright. This book will give you the tools to reclaim a sovereign life.

No matter what set of limitations and restrictions you currently face, self-imposed or societally imposed, they will fall away. Your mind will become fearless, bold, and unassailable. You will begin leading a powerful and unbounded life from within. You will greet your same old life as if you were meeting it for the first time.

The enlightening wisdom contained herein will help unshackle your mind from any false or disempowering beliefs that are holding you back. You will begin to enjoy freedom from fear, freedom from wants, and freedom to reinvent yourself, rewrite your destiny, and lead your life the way you have always wanted to lead it. You will awaken to a secret spiritual dimension hidden inside of you: "Self" with a capital S. This Self is known as *Atman* in ancient Sanskrit, which means "the boundless one."

Once you begin living in the world not simply as a powerless individual but as Self, you will live in the same body and with the same relationships but no longer operate in the world from the same mind, with its attachments and

1

numbing obligations to social roles. You may look the same outside, but you will experience a wholly different, boundless presence inside the same body.

When you begin to make choices from your inner freedom, you will no longer search the world and your relationships for crumbs of happiness. Something deeply powerful, abidingly abundant, forever free, and expansive inside you will begin to bless you from within. Then everything, even a tired, old life circumstance, will take on a new splendor as an opportunity to express your sovereignty.

Bondage to Suffering Has Always Been Optional

My life was not always sovereign. For a while, my mind was plunged in the depths of darkness, devastated from sorrowful relationships, despairing from the sudden deaths of people I loved, and disheartened by the shocking curve balls that life can throw our way. Yet despite everything—even losing my sense of worth for a short time along the way—here I am. I feel the power, wholeness, and joy of being alive! These are not mere words. This is my visceral experience of my own self-worth after I regained the sovereignty to write my life script anew. I don't regret my learning curve, my mistakes in the past. I am proud to be mentally and spiritually sovereign today, and you can be too.

As you journey through this book, a beautiful, light-filled, powerful, and awakened state of mind, free of cravings and of fears, awaits you on the other side. You, too, can be the master of your destiny, just like the thousands of people I have helped awaken to sovereignty worldwide. You too can experience significant mental and spiritual autonomy. With the aid of the Vedas' timeless wisdom, you can play a role in shaping and awakening planetary consciousness. Take this opportunity to reexamine your assumptions about yourself and awaken to what lies within us all.

The Gift of the Ancient Vedas

Sovereign Self embodies awakening teachings and practices from ancient, enlightened men and women of India, known as the Vedic seers. Their wisdom was preserved in a body of sacred literature known as the Vedas (*VAY-duhs*). These texts provide access to their original understanding of *advaita*, or "nondual consciousness"; yoga, the practices that enable a still mind; Ayurveda, the first holistic system of health and healing; and *moksha*, the path to self-actualization and self-realization through union with a transcendent state of pure being.

Hindus revere the Vedas, although the Vedas—which are more a way of conscious living and thinking than religion—precede Hinduism. All subsequent religions that emerged in India were influenced by the Vedas, to a larger or lesser degree. The Vedas attempt to seek answers to the age-old questions, "Who am I?" "Why do I suffer?" "What happens after death?" "Why am I never fulfilled?" "What am I made up of?" "What is the purpose of my life?" The Vedas dare to ask, "What intelligence existed before the big bang?" and "Who or what existed before the so-called creator existed?"

Once exclusively transmitted orally from a lofty master to a trusted disciple in Vedic spiritual lineages, the great wisdom of the Vedas can be found easily today, published as four big books called the *Rig-Veda, Sama-Veda, Yajur-Veda,* and finally the *Atharva-Veda.* They are rare among sacred texts in that they have contributions not only from male seers known as *rishis,* but from twenty-seven female seers known as *rishikas,* who have also contributed their channeled wisdom in the form of hymns and knowledge-packed verse. But the seers are only channels of a greater cosmic intelligence that is formless and nameless. The Vedas are called *apaurusheya*—having no human author, as such. This transcendental wisdom was simply revealed in the depths of the awakened consciousness of the rishis and rishikas, in meditation. Therefore, Vedas impart wisdom for the true being, never dogma.

Each book, or Veda, can be divided into two parts. The first part is known as the *Samhita* section. It teaches *dharma,* or universal ethics, and reverence of nature and her forces, a sacred way of life aligned with universal laws and in celebration of a great universal intelligence. The second part of each of the Vedas, known as the *Upanishad* section, is of special significance. These 108 major and minor texts (in total) contain pure nondual wisdom—mystical teachings on the true Self beyond the mind and body. The Upanishads try to answer the question, "Who am I?" They show the way out of the magical show that is this universe through *jnana,* or "knowledge" yoga, leading to a final liberation or complete spiritual freedom from the wheel of birth and death, known as *moksha* or *mukti.*

The Upanishads define the Self, or *Atman,* as the innermost imperishable essence of all living beings, a consciousness that transcends the perishable personality. The Self is awareness itself, forever self-aware, sovereign, awake, unbounded.

And when this Self expresses itself as consciousness underlying every particle of this universe, from a blade of grass to human soul, then it is called *Brahman*.

> *"The Self of the individual [Atman] is identical to the Self of the universe [Brahman]."*
>
> BRIHADARANYAKA UPANISHAD, 1.4.10

Self is not a theoretical concept alone, but the ultimate reality that the Upanishads advise each one of us realize. In the *Brihadaranyaka Upanishad*, a famous Vedic seer gives his last teachings to his student, who happens to be his wife: "Self alone is worthy of seeing, hearing, contemplating, and realizing, because Self alone is the supreme Truth."[1] This quest for the Self is the profound teaching of the Upanishads and the heart of this book.

The Bhagavad Gita is also an Upanishad—a later addition to the canon and perhaps the most popular one of them all. It contains the quintessence of all the remaining Upanishads. "Bhagavad Gita" literally translates into English as "Song of God." It was spoken on a battlefield by the god Krishna, considered an incarnation of Supreme Reality, to Arjuna, a warrior confused in the midst of a war. In a metaphoric representation of life as a battle of conflicting choices, Krishna, the teacher, summarizes to Arjuna, the disciple, an entire gamut of Vedic teachings that ultimately lead Arjuna to realize the Self, in a mere seven hundred verses. These include the nondual wisdom (*Advaita Vedanta*), the many interconnected paths to yoga, and the timeless and universal Vedic principles of right values (*dharma*), right action (*karma*), and right knowledge (*jnanam*) that are so useful for a successful worldly and spiritual life. These wisdom lessons that transcend cultural boundaries address how to overcome existential suffering and offer a way to live life intelligently, heartfully, and gracefully to gain perfect self-knowledge and mastery of the Self. As a result, the Gita, as it is commonly called, is one of the most popular scriptures worldwide and has been widely translated and commentated on in almost every language of the world.

When I refer to "the Vedas" collectively, I am referring to this entire family of texts. Though will I elucidate many concepts from the first part of the Vedas in this book, I will rely more frequently on the Upanishads and the Bhagavad Gita. I have put forth my own translation of the ancient verses, unless explicitly stated.

The philosophical wisdom of the Vedas pervades not only Hinduism, Buddhism, Sikhism, and Jainism; their universal and timeless knowledge has influenced civilizations across the centuries. The Vedas are the foundation of both yoga and meditation—the most beautiful contributions of ancient India to humanity—and of Ayurveda, the world's first truly holistic and comprehensive system of mind-body-soul health, now popular worldwide. They have made a lasting impression on influential historical figures, such as Gandhi, Rudolf Steiner, Carl Jung, Aldous Huxley, Huston Smith, Joseph Campbell, and Immanuel Kant.[2]

Henry David Thoreau wrote: "What extracts from the Vedas I have read fall on me the light of a higher and purer luminary . . . simpler and universal."[3] Celebrated Indian poet and Nobel Laureate Rabrindranath Tagore referred to the Upanishads as "an eternal source of light."[4] Ralph Waldo Emerson noted most eloquently: "It was as if an empire spoke to us, nothing small or unworthy, but large, serene, consistent, the voice of an old intelligence, which in another age and climate had pondered and thus disposed of the questions that exercise us."[5] The Austrian physicist Erwin Schrödinger discussed the universal nature of knowledge and the universal nature of consciousness found in the Upanishads. He said: "There is no kind of framework within which we can find consciousness in the plural; insofar as any is available to us at all lies in the ancient wisdom of the Upanishad."[6] His contemporary, Nobel Prize–winning Danish physicist Niels Bohr, said, "I go into the Upanishads to ask questions."[7] And influenced by Schopenhauer, the German scholar Paul Deussen translated the Upanishads and said, "On the tree of wisdom there is no fairer flower than the Upanishads and no finer fruit than the Vedanta philosophy."[8] Nuclear physicist Robert Oppenheimer learned Sanskrit to study the Bhagavad Gita and said, "The Vedas are the greatest privilege of this century."[9]

We also find references to the ancient wisdom of the Vedas in the writings of modern thought leaders and teachers, including Ram Dass, Eckhart Tolle, Deepak Chopra, and Michael A. Singer.[10]

The test of the truth of the knowledge in the Vedas is that it must remain uncontradicted. That something is experienced, universally believed, or of tremendous practical utility does not necessarily mean that the knowledge is true. For example, we all experience sunrise and sunset. Nevertheless, this fact does not mean that the rising and setting of the sun is true knowledge since it is contradicted by astronomical knowledge. Valid knowledge in the Vedic tradition, known as *pramana,* is that which is not contradicted. I invite you to hold the teachings of the Vedas up to this standard.

What is the essence of this philosophy that has proven to be so perennial? In truth, explain the Vedas, we are not simply mortal bodies made up of perishable matter, but rather pure, infinite, immortal, nondual consciousness encased in mortal matter-suits. We are all always sovereign, free, eternally peaceful, and whole. We have simply forgotten our spiritual truth. An infinite mindset is important if we are to recognize who we really are, if we are to lead a truly joyful and expansive, fearless, and sorrow-free life.

Until we have awakening and liberating wisdom by our side, we remain identified with our worldly smallness. We keep looking for happiness, wholeness, and fulfillment outside of ourselves. This forgetfulness is the root cause of sorrow and psychological bondage. Self-discovery and self-realization must be humanity's priority, even amid the many daily roles we play. We must recognize that we remain infinite, even while living out our finite stories.

In this book, I will help you end this forgetfulness, remind you of your latent powers, and transmit, from my soul to yours, the teachings and practices that have delivered me from darkness to light, from bondage to freedom.

I awakened to discover something beautiful inside me,
and now you will too.

How to Read *Sovereign Self*

I suggest you read this book in sequence as the concepts and guided practices build on each other. Part I explores in detail the pathology of our delusion and how our mental patterns hypnotize us into believing we are disempowered and enslaved to the world. When we understand the net of ignorant delusion that binds us, we are ready to learn a strategy to break free and embody a more sovereign state of mind.

Part II offers a wealth of practices that activate an illumined state of mind, one that is more discerning, judicious, and inherently wise. You will learn how you can convert your mind into your friend on your journey, rather than a dictator, distractor, or detractor. You will learn to engage and be in this world as a worldly being in relationship with others, with greater psychological self-determination and emotional coherence.

Part III reveals a code of universal ethics that empowers you to act in the world with the full power of evolved spiritual awareness. As you "pull yourself together" in this way, you develop the clarity and wisdom to set life goals that acknowledge your essential nature. Embodying your sacred purpose prepares you for awakening—the achievement of the sovereign Self—and a life of bold authenticity, abiding joy, and inner freedom.

As you encounter the original ancient verses of the Vedas, Upanishads, and Bhagavad Gita, try reading them out aloud. They are loaded with rich meaning and subtle symbolism. I suggest that you take notes, journal, or sketch as you go. Resist the urge to compare these teachings to any prior knowledge you may have encountered. Let them work on you. The more slowly you go and the more you contemplate what you have read, the more quickly your mind will decondition from its current state of bondage and open to true wisdom.

Your mind is very intelligent. It simply needs a few keys to unlock its thought padlocks. Even while holding jobs, paying bills, raising children—even with no time to meditate, chant, or sign up for a yoga class—if you contemplate these teachings in the privacy of your own mind, you will remember who you really are.

Under all the hurt, betrayal, anger, hatred, insanity, powerlessness, disillusionment, and sorrow of this worldly life, you are pure possibility. Know how infinitely whole, powerful, joyful, and ultimately free you are beyond your struggling personality. I invite you to meet your sovereign Self.

PART I

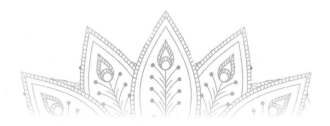

Recognize That
You Are Sovereign

1

Atman: The Self Awaits Your Discovery

"Aapnoti sarvam iti Atman . . . That which is boundless is who you are, Self."

ADI SHANKARACHARYA, *TATTVA BODHA*

The human mind is not an ordinary intelligence. You are not equipped with a mind merely to help you survive as an "evolved animal" as evolutionary biologists would have you believe. Mind is an extraordinary awareness-intelligence, a reflector of divine powers of your soul.

Behind the ordinary mind is the real power, a universally pervading intelligence, a transcendental, divine, all-knowing existence that I call the Self with a capital S. Self is akin to spirit in the trio of body, mind, and spirit; it is the divine power that illumines everything and everyone but is itself invisible.

In the poetic *Chandogya Upanishad*, we find a dialogue between a sage and his disciple son on who we truly are.[1]

The father beckons his son: "Bring me a fruit of that banyan tree."

"Here you go, Father."

"Break it."

"Okay, I have broken it, Father."

"What do you see there?"

"I see tiny seeds, Father."

"Break one seed open."

"Alright, I have broken a seed, Father."

"What do you see there?"

"I see nothing, Father."

His father said: "From that nothingness, my dear, grows this whole banyan tree. Believe me, my dear; all that exists comes from the Self, which is invisible (appears as no-thing). That is real. That is the Self. You are that, dear one."

The father continued: "You see nothing in the seed, but everything resides in that seed. This big banyan tree cannot emerge from nothingness. Only you cannot see that subtlest of subtle 'somethingness'—life-enabling Self!

"It is Self that resides inside the seed, from which has sprung forth this enormous tree. That invisible power pervades everywhere and everything. It is all of existence. It appears as nothing to you since it is subtle, so your senses and mind cannot grasp it, but that does not mean Self does not exist. Believe me, my dear; all that exists arises from Self, which is the invisible but ultimate reality. You are that Self, dear one."

Your Self, too, is hidden like the intrinsic emptiness buried inside the seed. Since your Self is not material, you are unaware of it. You cannot know it via your senses. Being spiritual, it is unavailable for gross or subtle perception. Yet it pervades your entire being as supremely intelligent self-awareness, so you can know it in your pure, self-aware mind.

When the seed is broken, it reveals an invisible fullness, a pregnant emptiness, the potent essence and life that in time can spawn an entire forest. As we recognize and work through the different layers covering the true Self, we will begin appreciating its presence, an all-powerful life-force within. Self is pure consciousness that animates and enlivens the body and mind, and yet it continues to survive and exist even after the body ends, just like an ocean continues to exist even if a wave ends. It is like how the substratum of clay continues to exist even if a pot fashioned from that clay breaks or how electricity continues to exist even if the bulb breaks.

If this is the first time you are encountering the teachings on soul as pure consciousness, you may be surprised by the sheer boldness of the Vedic vision in recognizing what is immortal, divine, all-powerful, and ever blissful inside you.

If you really think about it, however, all the wonderful attributes you assign to your mind, like intelligence, awareness, power, joy, wholeness, love, and clarity, don't originate in the mind. The mind only appears intelligent because there is a super-intelligent consciousness or "Self" behind it.

You use your mind, but you are not your mind, ego, or intellect.

The body is beautiful—a vessel of sexual, physical, and vital strength. It can move, digest, even reproduce, and enjoy itself through its five senses in the world of sensorial delights, yet the source of life behind this living body is the invisible Self.

You inhabit your body, but you are not your body.

The Self is self-luminous, self-revealing, and self-evident and endows the mind with its existence, powers, and function.

You are indeed *pure consciousness*—sinless, sparkling, ageless, timeless, immeasurable, pure-bliss consciousness that animates your body and mind, but is never circumscribed, defined, or confined by your body or mind.

Though in ordinary parlance we say we must awaken to who we are as if Self were a goal to be reached, you are already that beautiful, blissful, powerful, and eternally whole presence. You don't have to become anything new; you simply must remember who you (already) are. Upon rediscovering or reclaiming the forgotten Self, a deep sense of belonging, purpose, and well-being takes over.

This Self is called "Atman," a Sanskrit word meaning "that which is boundless."

Your true Self, the Vedas say, is boundless existence, unchanging consciousness, abiding bliss. It shines as the eternal light within your heart. In fact, your mind depends on the boundless Self for its intelligent awareness, and the body depends on it for life, as it is Self that makes the body sentient.

You are the Self.

You are eternal.

You are unchanging.

You are ever pure.

You are ever free.

The Self does not age, no matter what the age of the body. Self is never tired, worried, confused, or lost, even if your mind is tired and worried. Self is forever the possessor of complete wisdom and bliss, even if your mind is clouded temporarily or your happiness feels blocked.

Seemingly by default, we are disconnected from our own inner spiritual dimension and live submersed in the outer, material world as material bodies with material names and material addresses, enjoying our material objects (people and things) that we possess and covet. This is the root cause of human suffering.

Deep down in your mind, masked by your thoughts, lies your implicit identification with the Infinite.

> *But you have forgotten the infinite presence in you and*
> *are caught up in fretting over the finite.*

Yes, your mind, the gateway to the palace of your true, amazing, and infinite Self, has been overrun by myriad worldly details. Its walls are rotting with stuck feelings, its windows are sealed shut by sorrowful memories, and its every inch is taken over by your virtual possessions, relationships, losses, and fears. The slew of likes and dislikes, the glue of attachments and aversions, and the acid of rage and resentment have locked you out from meeting, knowing, and enjoying your own unbelievable destiny to be truly happy, truly peaceful, and truly sovereign! We lose our self-governance when our sense of identity remains fused with a changeable shadowy mind that picks up cues from society and follows its dictates. This forever-fluctuating and naturally fearful mind only knows bondage. It is not free in any sense, nor steadfast, and therefore neither fearless nor powerful.

> *Indeed, when identified with the mind, the Self appears other*
> *than what it is—finite. But know this: the Self is infinite.*

Here is the good news.

When you begin questioning and probing your mind—when you ask: "Is this it? Or is there more to find out about me?" when you lighten, cleanse, and purify your mind with the aid of the wisdom tools that I share in part II—you will be able to pierce the veils of the mind and enter the realm of a divine, transcendent, infinitely powerful, and beautiful Self, which is of the nature of Divine Consciousness. What up to now has been veiled from you will be unmasked. You will be blessed with wholeness from within!

The Self is worth pursuing, as the well-being that comes from aligning with it is incomparable to even the highest form of joy in the material universe.

A particle of its bliss supplies the bliss of the whole universe. It illuminates everything. The knower of the Self revels in an ecstasy that is indescribable, pure bliss, incomparable, transcending time, ever free, and beyond desire.

You Are the Happiness You Seek

Once a king built a palace of mirrors and kept a beautiful blooming rose at its center. The mirrors enhanced the beauty of the rose. Then he set a pigeon free in the palace. Seeing the numerous reflections of the rose, the pigeon was attracted to them and began pecking at each mirror. Crashing into the mirrors, it only hurt its beak each time. Instead of finding happiness, it became more sorrowful, since what it was seeking was only a mirage, not the truth. But it would not give up.

Finally, exhausted with the fluttering about, it lost desire to look for the rose and collapsed, landing on the real rose. At last it was satisfied.

Our search for happiness is the same. According to the Vedas, bliss is something we bring with us to this life and take forward with us to other lives we may have in future because bliss lives inside us. It is always within us because bliss is the true state of the Self (though our mental state in each moment determines whether we feel it or not). That is why the Bhagavad Gita says: "One who is happy within, who rejoices within, who is illuminated within, that seeker attains absolute freedom and achieves the Self."[2]

Although bliss is within, we keep searching for it in the enchanting mirage of external objects. However, our own blissful Self is the rose that we seek. A vast multitude of bliss is stored within us, known as *ananda* in Sanskrit. You can say Self and bliss are interchangeable. Pure bliss, ananda, will arise in the river of the Self because blissful is the nature of Self.

Ananda is beyond the realm of the senses and beyond the understanding of your mind or possession of your ego because this bliss is your own innermost nature. In fact, whenever the senses are turned inward through meditation or self-contemplation, ananda quietly reveals itself from within.

That is why ananda does not require any external pleasure-giving object for its existence. It can exist despite sorrowful circumstances too. It does not wane with time, unlike sensory pleasures. In fact, it keeps growing and expanding to overflow and fill our homes, communities, and the hearts of people we encounter. We are joyful in the company of people who are in touch with their inner ananda.

No wonder the ancient seers exclaim with conviction: "For Self alone causes abiding bliss."[3] And the Bhagavad Gita says, "An awakened one has become free from a self-ignorant mind, and as a result, enjoys contact with bliss of Self."[4]

We seem to prize happiness or joy over and above everything. Yet, we are rightly skeptical of people who say they can show the way to happiness. But here is what I want to tell you: when we stop chasing mirages outside of ourselves, bliss is self-revealing. A baby, free from desires after having fed at the breast of its mother, lies in bed enjoying its own natural bliss. Any time one of us is free of desires and happy with what is coming to us in natural course, we become bliss personified. Bliss is the very nature of Self. Ananda and Atman are never apart from each other. A continuous state of joy emerges from spiritual existence.

Bliss of Self is not attached to an object or experience, as in, "When I eat chocolate cake, I am in bliss," or "When my lover says they love me, I feel happy." What will happen when the cake is finished and the lover decides that they do not love me after all?

Vedic scripture informs us that we are the source of the happiness that we seek, that our very nature is *boundless happiness, fullness, peace, and bliss.* When one's basic nature is of happiness, having a *desire* to be happy is itself ignorance and the beginning of *un*happiness. When the desire to be happy ends, that is where happiness lies.

The only problem is that we do not know we have forgotten our inner treasures!

The Misguided Search Outside

Being part of a sleepwalking or unconscious society populated with non-sovereign minds conditions us, from childhood, to seek happiness outside of ourselves.

You see, ever since you forgot your nature, which is self-fulfilled, self-content, and radically happy, and became solely identified with your perishable body and ephemeral pleasures in a world marked by impermanence, you have looked for yourself and your happiness in ice-cream cones, orgasms, hugs, handbags and pretty clothes, approval and positive strokes, classy furniture and cutlery, diamond necklaces, promotions, relationships, pets, and pretty much anything that can give even an iota of happiness.

Have you found your happiness yet?

I think not. Sadly, we all feel that our happiness is one partner, one job, or one more well-completed project away. Therefore, the enslaved, sleepwalking mind seeks drugs, alcohol, sex, relationships, et cetera, to get that happiness. The temporary happiness the mind experiences with each of these eventually fades. Then our mind experiences its opposite, sorrow and insecurity.

Naturally, these misperceptions only arise in a mind that has not been exposed to the truth of its inherent happy nature and how to internally align with it. So, egged on by our own ignorant minds, off we go, chasing yet more ephemeral happiness . . . and losing touch with our inner happiness along the way.

But Vedic wisdom reassures us that the Self is always there. This never changes, and it alone is our source for abiding security, wholeness, and happiness. In fact, it is the only constant.

A sovereign mind is always happy because happiness is a state of Self. A mind that is no longer seeking fulfillment and happiness in the world but sources them from within, by knowledge of its divine origins and its connection with Universal Intelligence, is a sovereign mind because it is established in its own fullness. Such a mind feels radically content, even while we live our routine lives.

Once we are convinced beyond a shadow of a doubt that happiness and wholeness are our own essential nature, then we make the search of this inner treasure the primary focus of our lives.

In the meantime, I hope my words will help you see yourself in a true sovereign light. That is the real victory of light over darkness—when you can clearly discern the ignorance within. One day soon, you will also discover what is enlightened and shining within you. You will awaken to your own incredible Self.

2

Maya: The Illusion That Conceals Your True Self

"Forgetting our divine truth,
We become enmeshed in the world of change
And bewail our bondage.
But when we see Self in all its glory,
cheered by all, we achieve lasting sovereignty."

SHVETASHVATARA UPANISHAD, 1.6

Although mental and spiritual sovereignty are our true nature, humanity has tragically forgotten its inner spiritual core. Therefore, we need wisdom reminders.

All beings are afflicted with a spiritual forgetfulness that keeps our minds from grasping the amazingly boundless and bountiful nature of our Self. Our minds become identified with and then engaged and entangled with whatever they encounter through the senses. This clutters the mind and leads to sorrow. Rather than unbounded expansive awareness of our potential to be or become what we want, we think bounded thoughts and are proscribed by our thinking.

My spiritual teacher, Baba, who was my also my paternal grandfather, explained this to me once in poetic terms:

"This world is an enchanted show, Shunya. A spell has spread from mind to mind throughout this world, so that the One appears as many. This spell is called maya.

For the duration of the phantasmal life we lead through the maya-filled mind, we believe adamantly in the roles we play, the relations we have, and the goals we hold dear. None of this is true—just like the cities we visit and the people we meet in our nightly dreams who appear real enough within the dream but disappear upon waking up in the morning.

One more final waking up is pending, the awakening from the dreams of maya that occur to us even when we are apparently awake and engaged, with alert senses, in the world of experiences. Even then, we are asleep, cosmically asleep to the Ultimate Reality."

Our forgetfulness of our inner truth has other consequences too. It induces a confused consciousness that does not permit us to discern between appearances and reality. When I asked Baba why we forget that we are always sovereign in matters of fullness, fulfillment, and joy, he responded that no one knows. The Vedic tradition does not claim to know either. It is not a know-it-all tradition that makes up stories to justify what it does not know. It simply sticks with what it observes to be universally true.

This cosmic forgetfulness, maya, is like a spell of bewilderment and spiritual blindness cast over our minds that causes a metaphysical ignorance of our true Self. Simply put, maya causes self-ignorance.

Maya prevents us from seeing what is there and makes us see what is not there. It has two characteristics: concealment (of what is) and projection (of what is not).

Through concealment, maya veils our consciousness and prevents it from knowing what is there. Through projection, maya compels the ego to know, perceive, or deduce something that is not there. People who are under the spell of maya suffer a double tragedy: they do not know what is there, but they believe firmly in the projections of the mind, or what is not there.

Thanks to this spell in our mind, a nonexistent ghost can terrify us if we simply believe it to be real. We might create images and stories (appearances) of the ghost, perhaps living in the attic or under the bed. Even a nonexistent snake can cause panic. We literally can die of a heart attack even if the snake is just a rope or a garden hose, coiled up in a dark corner. If a rope *appears* as a snake, it can elicit a deluded, panicked response in our mind. Such mirages flourish in the maya-sponsored collective unconsciousness.

At some point, you—the birth-less, death-less, disease-less Self—begin identifying with the body mirage and think of yourself as only a physical entity, one that can be broken, ruptured, or bled to death with ease. You naturally begin to fear disease, aging, and death. Biological, emotional, and social potency—health in every dimension—is your true nature, yet you subscribe to limitations wholeheartedly. This is due to maya.

When you identify with the mind mirage and its fluctuations, you identify with ceaseless changing states of mind: agitated, dull, depressed, and morbid. You *become* dark emotions and morbid thoughts, consumed by countless distractions and ceaseless worries. Your mind is naturally an instrument of abundance, yet by the mind's false associations, you experience the opposite. Despite material wealth in your life, you feel nonabundant. This is due to maya.

When you identify with the impermanence and mutability of the world mirage, you become a sleepwalker. You accept this "house of change" as your only and final home, and you forget that you are *dreaming* this shifting, morphing universe. Your true home is not some impermanent sandcastle, but you don't think to look somewhere else when you believe you are limited to living in a mirage called "the world."

Maya is fundamentally unknowable. We don't know why it exists or when it began, but like any form of ignorance, maya will only cease to exist when sacred instruction and right knowledge—knowledge of the Self—arise in the mind. With such knowledge, we slowly remember our own inner nature and begin to live from inwardly validated and experienced mental and spiritual sovereignty. We live as rulers of our own lives.

Until then, the spell of maya first conceals who you are—the ever-present, formless Self—and then projects what you are *not*: body, mind, and intellect, the *not-Self*. Similarly, the bewitched mind conceals your state of inner fullness, peace, and bliss, and it projects a struggling you, a collapsed you, and even a time-bound, space-bound, diseased you. Ignorant of our true nature, we feel ourselves to be powerless, helpless, existentially frightened, and separate—from each other and from everything. And, at the deepest level, despite being in relationships, we feel gut-wrenchingly lonely, once again thanks to maya!

Therefore, no mind is free from the spell that makes it fall asleep, metaphysically speaking. Maya is not just lack of correct knowledge. It is opposed to knowledge as it not only conceals the true nature but also presents the false in its place. The Bhagavad Gita puts it aptly: "Soul's wisdom is veiled by ignorance. Hence, human beings are deluded."[1]

Ralph Waldo Emerson, the American literary figure and lover of the Bhagavad Gita, wrote this poem called "Maia":[2]

> Illusion works impenetrable,
> Weaving webs innumerable,
> Her gay pictures never fail,
> Crowds each other, veil on veil,
> Charmer who will be believed,
> By man who thirsts to be deceived.

Thanks to our forgetting who we are, we are often imprisoned by what others think we are and what others want us to become for them. When we run out of roles to be played, a maya-drunk society hands us yet more well-worn scripts — and off we go again, creating all-new, but old, narratives that never seem to get us closer to our innermost truth. No role celebrates our genuine greatness. No wonder we never feel enough! Instead, we experience only more alienation from our true Self.

A spiritual fog envelops my mind and yours, dear reader, and envelops all creatures of this universe, collectively and individually.

We humans appear to be awake, with our eyes open, but spiritually speaking, we are fast asleep, even comatose under the maya fog. Therefore, animals and plants appear more in touch with who they are, their inner nature, than we do — for them, ignorance is bliss.

Forgetfulness Has Consequences

The degree to which we believe in the illusion of maya makes all the difference between self-acceptance and self-nonacceptance.

Spiritual sleepwalkers continue to look outward, never inward, and remain in bondage to fulfillment-promising objects and relationships. They are always busy trying to control the uncontrollable; rearranging their life circumstances; manipulating or pleasing people; or hoarding, selling, worshipping, or serenading money, sex, partnerships, while all along their relationship with their own inner potential remains unexplored. Infinite wholeness and fullness cannot be attained through the impermanent things of this world.

It is as if, in the bright sunshine of Self, a shadow on the wall notices its monochromatic color and bewails its grey limitation. What kind of color—material or spiritual—can address this fundamental lack?

Can anything worldly (wealth, fame, sex, a loving partner, a beautiful home, loving pets, health, or stamina) or otherworldly (visions, angels, meditative trance, mantras, rituals, or pilgrimage) color the shadow? The sense of inadequacy at the core of the shadow can only be overcome by connecting with its source, the sun, which is a bouquet of colors unto itself.

Shadow must recognize that it has no essence, reality, or validity apart from the light. Ego has no substance, apart from the Self. It all depends on how you choose to view yourself . . . as ego with limited power or Self with unlimited soul power.

Ignorance of your identity is at the root of your powerlessness. You were never at any time the shadow. You are the magnificent sun. You must remember that our true nature is Self, which is unimaginably powerful.

If not for the illusions of maya, you would see yourself as free, a truly sovereign being in this very moment. You have pure freedom to define, redefine, or undefine yourself and your life script as you please. Total freedom allows you to simply be yourself as you are right now or to change your mind, despite any goal-driven pressures, distractions, successes, or failures that conceal your higher truth. You cannot become free by doing or not doing any specific thing, by holding onto some relationships, or by letting go of others. You are free, right now. If all paths have led you to this moment, then your freedom is *right here* inside the good, bad, or ugly circumstances in your life, *right here* in the challenge facing you *right now.*

Welcome to the Sleepwalker's Club

Under maya's spell, we all fall asleep or, at best, are sleepwalkers. As creatures ensnared in maya's trap, we forget the nature of our Self, which is inherently joyful, infinitely playful, and creative. Instead, our mass-hypnotized mind experiences ignorance of its true nature and feels powerless, helpless, existentially frightened, and condemned to suffer sorrow.

Maya strikes universally. In everyone's mind, it creates delusion and feeds the sense of a separate, limited *identity maker* known as ego, or *ahamkara*. The ego is an aspect of your self-ignorant mind, and I will use "ego" and "mind" interchangeably going forward.

Your Ego Is Your True Self's Poor Cousin

". . . for the ego gropes in darkness while the Self lives in light . . ."

A well-developed theory of the ego was brought forward by the Upanishads thousands of years before Freud and his student Jung.[3] In his seminal work, *The Collected Works of Carl Jung* (*Symbols of Transformation, Volume 5*), Jung brings up the Upanishads and quotes from them several times.

In the Upanishads, the ego is known as ahamkara. "Aham" means "I," and "kara," "maker." This "aham" is really nothing more than one singular "I" thought, at the core of your being. The ego is constructed from one dominant thought, *I am*.

Therefore, at your core, you are nothing more than a master thought (*I Am*) that is spinning and weaving your entire life experience in your awake world, your dreaming world, and your deep-sleep world. Your worldly persona is being constructed again and again through this one thought. And this thought continuously collects around it more thoughts, ideas, and beliefs, all of which are manufactured from thoughts. Therefore, in the final analysis, your ego is a "thought matrix." This thought matrix makes and unmakes you, every day, every moment of every day.

In Western psychology and thought, "ego" is often referred to in a negative way such as, "stop being egotistical." As if ego is an indulgence that others are free of. But the Upanishads tell us that we humans universally possess an ego. It is our original self-limitation, thanks to maya fogging our minds. And that is why we are confused about who we are in reality—pure spiritual existence—and what we appear to ourselves, which is the mere "thought matrix" of ahamkara. (Oh, maya!)

How beautifully a seer of the Vedas explains the coup accomplished by the ego: "As the formations of clouds generated by the sun's rays come to veil the very same sun, so too, the ego arisen from the Self covers the reality of the Self and shines itself."[4]

That is why ego in the Vedic sense can be described as the cause of the universal spiritual darkness, or shadow, that surrounds us humans. It has an effect of blocking us from our own truth of Self. As a result, we start believing the misconception *I am the body, mind, and intellect*. It is like the electricity saying, "I am the bulb." It is like the great river saying, "I am the glass of water." We forget that we are the independent, boundless, limitless, Self.

Despite the ever-fulfilled Self being your truth, you hang onto unfulfilled egoic illusions. You identify with the perishable, and you forget the imperishable. You identify with your ego's fleeting experiences and not with the truth of your immutable awareness. You identify with your mental modifications and don't look for the detached, tranquil, unmodified observer of the experiences, which is the Self.

When Ego Manifests a False Sense of Self

The term *jiva* refers to the illusionary self or false persona that emerges from the thought matrix that is the ego. Ego, born of illusion, collects its favorite strengths, traumas, joys, sorrows, and memories, and it builds an identity that it feels is unique and separate from every other sentient being on the planet, complete with zodiac signs, favorite colors, likes, and dislikes. No wonder the ancient Vedic seers went out of their way to emphasize the difference between Atman, the true being, and jiva, the false being, whose origins are the ego.

As the ancient nondual commentary *Vivekachudamani* by Shankaracharya explains, in the presence of light, shadow has no existence: "You are indeed the supreme Atman, but due to your association with maya [self-ignorance] you find yourself under the bondage of the not-Self [body, mind, worldly roles based on egoic-jiva]. . . . All the effects of self-ignorance, root and branch, are burnt down by the fire of self-knowledge, which arises from discrimination between these two—the Atman and the jiva."[5]

The ego-borne jiva believes and behaves according to a shifting sense of "I" in the mind, feeling worthy when applauded and dejected when criticized. A boy raised by wolves behaves like a wolf when his ego-mind believes he is one.

But once he discovers his identity, the wolf-boy's innate human propensities shine through. Similarly, our shadow self, raised by parental, cultural, and societal wolves, continues to operate through its belief systems. We are trained to describe ourselves as loser or achiever, good or bad, but such dualities produce only deep sorrow down the road. Powerless or powerful, confused or all-knowing, stupid or smart, these attributes belong only to the false self. Living life this way exhausts us since we constantly feel we must try to control everything. Yet nothing is in our control, and everything appears intense, unforgiving, and of paramount importance.

As an egoic personality (jiva), you borrow consciousness, intelligence, and power from your true nature and then forget where it all came from. You become a worldly defined and limited persona, estranged from your own source. As a worldly body, you live, eat, opine, dream, sleep, love, achieve, fail, compete, age, make love, complain, delight, suffer, or enjoy . . . but all along remain ignorant of your Self, which is inherently whole, powerful, joyful, and of the nature of unconditional love.

Essentially, the jiva is a limitation of consciousness. It is fated to be whatever the thoughts pertaining to it are about. Who we really are is the nondual Self, the Atman, but because of maya, the veil of ignorance, we believe ourselves to be limited to a separate soul, contained in a body and mind.

The jiva could be thought of as the Self (Atman) together with the *upadhi* (limitation) of *avidya* (maya-borne self-ignorance). An upadhi is something that appears to restrict or limit but that is transparent in the light of knowledge. A Vedic metaphor that is used to explain this is a jar being an upadhi, or boundary, for the space contained within it. But space is everywhere, unaffected by the presence of the jar. In the same way, the body, mind, intellect, and ego seemingly serve to limit the original Self, creating an egoic jiva, a jar full of consciousness that appears to be separate from all-pervading, unlimited consciousness, power, and bliss.

Fortunately, we can end self-ignorance, simply by choosing not to be ignorant. When the same shadowy consciousness (jiva) "decides" to undertake self-inquiry and ask the ultimate question, *Who am I?* no one can prevent you from knowing the truth of whether you are only a jar of space or all-pervading space, a mere wave or an entire ocean. Life is a game we are playing, a game of hide-and-seek, a game that is often costly to us, but in the end, only a game.

This is described poetically in the *Mundaka Upanishad* where the ego and Self are compared to two birds, both dwelling in the same tree (your being).

One of them eats the bitter and sweet fruits eagerly (the ego experiences bitter joy and sweet sorrow) while the other simply looks on at the busy bird, calmly, as pure awareness (Self).

> *"Two birds are seated on the same tree. One of them [the ego], sunk in igno-rance [maya] and deluded, grieves its impotence, is busy tasting sweet and bitter fruits. The other simply looks on, peacefully. But when the sorrowful bird chances upon the serene, self-possessed bird, it realizes its own glory (I am that peaceful one!) and becomes free from sorrow and lamentations."*
>
> MUNDAKA UPANISHAD, 3.1.1–3

The Shadow Jiva Is Set Up for Sorrow

For the loss of connection with our true Self, we pay a heavy price in emotional and existential sorrow. We think, *I am a biologically determined, socially and culturally defined "being,"* and embrace limitations as our destiny. The jiva, unfortunately, is never satisfied, nor content, since it is a rootless, soulless, shadow self and spiritually estranged, unaware of its own truth.

While the basis of our true being is a sovereign spiritual reality, the nature of our jiva is the ego's illusions, impermanence, and bondage. Aren't you too carrying around your own saga of sorrows and gains, losses and victories? Well, all of this is visualized, composed, edited, and narrated by your ego.

This is the mischief of maya. Its illusions convince you to settle for a much less powerful and limited version of yourself. All of this is happening in your nonawakened mind alone, but it is still enough to imprison you in a deluge of suffering-generating limiting beliefs, unless and until the mind awakens to its potential. Under maya's influence, your mind is unconscious of this potential, despite your divinely blissful nature still shining in the background.

Indeed, the jiva is the ultimate clutter (upadhi) covering your Self while falsely posing as the Self. It is a mere reflection, an illusion, a mental projection, born from your past sensory experiences and accumulation of memories, ideas, and thoughts. While the spiritual reality, your Self, is permanence and abiding joy, your jiva deals with illusions, impermanence, and dissatisfaction that invariably lead to suffering.

Your inner light is reflected outward via the mind, but self-ignorance in the form of misperceptions and false beliefs, such as *My fulfillment, wholeness, happiness, and satisfaction lie outside me*, block that light. Instead of radiating the light in sublime inner self-contentment, you radiate the egoic shadow, jiva. In this state of darkness, we often self-sabotage our inner knowingness and instead create for ourselves fear, rage, sorrow, and unimaginable suffering.

When our minds are blocked, cluttered, and self-ignorant, it is as if the divine, supremely powerful, blissful, and limitless Self has been reduced to a mere shadow.

Let Go of the False Self by Reclaiming the True Self

As Self, you are a sovereign emperor. But as a mere worldly individual, you are a beggar for transient happiness, chasing after crumbs of existentially costly and tragically ephemeral worldly pleasures. And then, any happiness from external sources may come with a high price: a lover who gives great sexual pleasure but is emotionally unavailable, a job that pays well but imparts killer stress, a necklace that looks beautiful but puts you in heavy debt to credit card companies.

And the saddest part is that you have forgotten that happiness is so close all along. The nature of the Self is unalloyed, everlasting bliss. Our unhappiness is directly related to our mental perception of limitedness. It is a mere belief, no more than a thought, and not necessarily a reality.

Your Self is infinite, complete, and ever full and doesn't need something, someone, or some life situation to go a certain way so you can feel fulfilled. If life conditions are going in our favor, that is great. But if they are not, believe it or not, you can still feel good. Many people can feel quite all right in a situation that might break another's heart. All happiness is already present within you. Simply pause long enough to learn to find it within. You are enough.

My guru Baba used to ask me, "Are you really limited, or do you just 'think' you are limited?" He reminded me:

"As long as you keep believing in the maya-based shadow—that is, the 'little person jiva' who is born in and operates from the mind, overwhelmed by

its erroneous notions, attached to its handful of obsessions and cravings and desires—it will continue to exist, always with an accompanying sense of lack. The jiva is unaware that it is a mere construct of thoughts, a shadowy reflection of the ultimate bigness, fullness, and abidingly joyful nature of Self, the true you. If you keep believing in the validity of the shadow and doubting the light itself, you will also keep believing in the inadequacies, sorrows, and disappointments it experiences nonstop."

The Sanskrit word *atmavaan* means "mindfulness," in the sense of staying consciously aware of Atman. It entails choosing to remain alert in our life by remembering, *I am pure awareness with a body and mind; I am not merely a struggling body- and mind-based individual ego. I am Spirit Divine.* It entails not getting carried away by external circumstances and not leading an automated, scripted, entirely unexamined life.

Let your life be a deliberate one so you can be deliberate in your every goal, not simply a clone of the rest of sleepwalking humanity. Only then can your speech and your actions be deliberate and truly representative of the unique you.

The Vedas say the Self is joyful, free, whole, and powerful. When I use such words to describe your Self, understand that they are not add-on qualities, which may increase, decrease, or vary from person to person. Just as wetness is inherent to water and heat is the inherent quality of fire, wholeness, knowingness, abundance, power, fullness, and infinite joyfulness are the inherent qualities of your true Self. When its light shines within you, it spreads outward to illumine and enlighten your mind, intellect, and relationships. Then you experience infinite joy, love, peace, wholeness, happiness, creativity, satisfaction, and even personal miracles.

You have already begun the journey to reclaiming true Self by picking up this book. As you turn your attention toward your sovereign Self, the darkness, slowly yet steadily, disappears. The light within will begin to glow brighter and brighter, shining from your more translucent mind. Knowledge of Self lays bare the secrets of life and removes the screen of spiritual self-ignorance to reveal the underlying truth! Finally, our imperfect knowledge and our bloated egos are washed away, and we can lead our life from reality. Just as darkness is banished when the sun appears, the truth of your real nature arises when you are exposed to enlightening wisdom.

It is possible to create a life more wonderful than anything you can imagine, but it takes looking at who you are in a very different way.

> *By remembering who you are, the Self, the whole*
> *world of appearances will fade from view.*

The Maya of Spiritual Bypassing

"Just as yoga has undergone many distortions in the West, which has reduced it largely to a physical asana practice, so too Advaita is often getting reduced to an instant enlightenment fad, to another system of personal empowerment, or to another type of pop psychology."

DAVID FRAWLEY, VEDIC SCHOLAR[6]

You must remember that the journey from jiva-shadow to Self is not accomplished simply by ignoring the shadow and instead imagining a new "light-filled personality" that has emerged overnight! It is easy enough to put the mind in an imaginary state of "spiritual perfection and transcendence" using nondual meditations and abstract beliefs like "Oneness" so the confused, self-ignorant, and often-wounded ego-mind believes itself "awakened." The mind can certainly be expanded by inner work, but is the inner work complete? Hardly.

We can't simply put on new shiny clothes over old tattered ones. Atman, the spiritual Self hidden within, cannot be superimposed on a cluttered, maya-drunk mind. This would simply be *spiritual bypassing*, putting forth a compensatory personality in the same old maya-filled mind, albeit outfitted with spiritual ideas and untested beliefs to cover our deficiencies. Rather, the mind must be purified with self-knowledge. As self-ignorance is slowly shed, the hidden portal of the boundless Self shines increasingly from within, until one day the same old mind is blessed with it.

Spiritual bypassing is the tendency to use spiritual ideas and practices to sidestep or avoid facing unresolved emotional issues, psychological wounds, or unfinished developmental tasks. The term was coined in the early 1980s by John Welwood, a Buddhist teacher and psychotherapist, who observed it among members of his Buddhist community.

"Aspects of spiritual bypassing include exaggerated detachment, emotional numbing and repression, overemphasis on the positive, anger-phobia, blind or overly tolerant compassion, weak or too porous boundaries, lopsided development (cognitive intelligence often being far ahead of emotional and moral intelligence), debilitating judgment about one's negativity or shadow elements, devaluation of the personal relative to the spiritual, and delusions of having arrived at a higher level of being," wrote Robert Augustus Masters in his book *Spiritual Bypassing*.[7]

Such bypassing happens in every spiritual community, including Neo-Advaita. Neo-Advaita is a recent and somewhat simplistic version of Vedic nondual teachings.

The original Vedic tradition and its teachers, like myself, place an explicit emphasis on instructing the sleepwalking ego step by step to help it shed its typical darkness, or self-ignorance. We don't want to bypass ego. We just wish to lovingly instruct it and help it poke its head above the ocean of maya.

An uninstructed ego-mind is unable to shine forth the light of Self from within, just as a dirty mirror cannot properly reflect your face. In the same way, a purified and instructed ego can be a friend in your spiritual quest, capable of reflecting the true Self. It will have remembered what it had forgotten! A person who once behaved in selfish and self-destructive ways, for example, might start behaving in truly inspiring, selfless ways, guided from within.

Understand this: there never are two selves, but only one Self. The shadow self is a mere mental projection. The egoic self lasts only if self-ignorance lasts. Then, with self-knowledge, when ignorance ends, so does the shadow self. The small self (jiva) never really existed, except as a shadow in the ego-mind. Upon awakening, you begin operating from your sovereign nature.

A burnt rope cannot be used to tie anything; the moment it is touched, it disintegrates into burnt ash particles. Similarly, if you have metaphorically burnt your ego to radiant ashes with the fire of knowledge, if you have purified it with self-disciplining practices, a burnt ego-rope cannot tie you to this world and its false cravings and identities, can it? Then, ego-free, you will continue living in the world, enjoying the world, but as if freed from bondage to this world and free from your identity in it as a struggling, time-bound body.

This awakening, albeit not instantaneous or spontaneous but earned gradually, is permanent, since the joy and wholeness are not borrowed or imagined but intrinsic to your inner or true nature that had been concealed. When you uncover the greater truth through dedicated practice, what you reveal is *you*, the real, sovereign you! After all, Self is always present. *Isn't this beautiful?*

To access the Self, it is necessary to unclutter the mind from its false beliefs and attitudes, from maya. To do that, we undertake conscious disciplines and cognitive practices that purify the ego-mind (such as those in part II of this book), along with ensuring the ego's moral growth and spiritual maturity via instruction in right values (which we'll get to in part III).

Neo-Advaita practitioners and teachers of nonduality often recognize no such qualifying prerequisites. While recommending that we see through the ego and dismiss the ego as our identity, many modern teachers dismiss cultivating preparatory mental disciplines. In my mind, this is intellectual conceit. There is a penchant to enjoy the tasty fruit of a hallowed tradition, but not bother with watering its roots, by dismissing its requirements. No wonder the vulnerable aspirants become high on the Neo-Vedanta drug of denying the ego as a complete illusion! When everything we feel, including our pain and our doubts, can be dismissed as mere illusion, naturally one feels a temporary relief from life itself. The trance-like bubble is temporary escapism from reality, but it sure creates thousands of idolizing fans for the *checked-out* teachers, who get away with throwing snippets of a great tradition at the idolizing crowds. The leader and the led operate from spiritual delusion.

In contrast, the original Vedic nondual tradition holds that the ordinary, ignorant self must be methodically prepared and qualified to receive knowledge of the nondual Self. The seeker, to be considered mature and ready for awakening knowledge, must cultivate the following four disciplines:

- *Viveka*: Spiritual discernment: to be able to tell the real from the unreal.

- *Vairagyam*: Nonattachment: letting go of unreal thoughts, desires, and attachments.

- *Shadsampat*: Six cognitive virtues: thought-control, sense-control, lifestyle-stability, forbearance, faith, and inner tranquility.

- *Mumukshutvam*: Intense yearning for awakening for self-realization.

As you can see, the Vedas set the bar quite high. It's important that we take the time to embody ego-deconditioning disciplines, see through the illusion of the small self, and awaken to the real Self. As you proceed through this book, you will gain the knowledge and tools to apply these four disciplines to spiritual maturation. I will go into more detail on this traditional approach to preventing the undesirable detour of spiritual bypassing in chapter 23.

Misdirected Cravings for True Self

We are all searching for our Self but in truth we are never separated from it. Deep down, a part of the ego remembers who it really is on a profound, though unconscious, level. We have only forgotten about it—that is maya. Therefore, with right knowledge, we can reclaim it.

This deep memory of the Self manifests even in the case of someone who steals. On the surface, it may not seem like a thief would have any memory of their true nature as a sovereign being. If the thief remembered, then why would they steal for crumbs of happiness?

When we dig deeper into the thief's motivation however, we see that they stole in order to become happy, whole, or complete. The thief's real nature is *radical fullness*. And the thief's ego remembers this in a twisted way—by trying to take someone else's stuff!

All the different examples of how our egoic persona acts out—by lying, stealing, cheating, manipulating, overeating, gossiping, and even committing crimes like murder—are distorted ways the ego expresses a craving to experience its essential nature, the full, complete, and eternal Self.

We often lie to ensure our (essential) security. We break others down by gossiping to feel a sense of our own (internal) perfection. We overeat to feel the satisfaction of our (inner) fullness. We cheat and manipulate to grab power from others to experience our own (inherent spiritual) power. We cheat and betray within our sexual relationships to feel greater moments of (inner) joy. We kill others to not only get someone out of the way of our own happiness, but to experience a sense of our own power or sense of immortality. In this way, even our wrongdoing points to the truth about who we really are.

The first role of the ego is to associate with experiences and spin an "I" and "mine" narrative. Its second role, however, is to act as the portal to infinite happiness and knowledge. This must be accomplished by effort, reflection, and discrimination aided by wisdom of the Vedas. Our journey of awakening to our Self depends on how we reconcile our ego with our Self and bringing the ego into greater alignment through sacred instruction.

Accept the Ego to Realize the Self

Unfortunately, we often betray and abandon ourselves, again due to maya. We are subconsciously searching for the real deal (Self), but we keep ending up with shadow self (jiva)! No wonder we keep criticizing ourselves, disliking ourselves, and even scolding ourselves without really knowing how to reclaim our inner fullness.

True self-acceptance lies in realizing the fact that we must stop trying to fix ourselves. After some time and reasonable effort, we simply must see through it. Perhaps it is time to stop criticizing the clingy, attached, fearful, and dependent jiva that lives inside maya sandcastles. Instead it is time to be free and to act from that freedom because you have been the Self all along! Who you think you are will determine how you act.

I ask my students never to be embarrassed or ashamed by a split between who they are today, the sorrowful egoic jiva, and the Self, which is their true nature. My student Joanne writes:

> *"Sitting with my teacher, listening to her words on these teachings pierces through my beliefs, habits, and judgments, and opens me up. This hasn't happened all at once. No, it takes many times, over and over, to really see who I am beyond the clothing my body, mind, and intellect wear, and that I am not dependent on others for my sense of being okay. I do forget and get caught up in everyday situations, but then I remember again to pause, soften my heart, or contemplate my teacher's words. It's all a process, a transformation, a coming home to the freedom and fullness within . . . the beautiful, amazing, sovereign, and joyful Self."*

Through self-ignorance, we identify with our ego and its thoughts, attachments, emotions, attitudes, and ideas (the thought matrix) and inadvertently believe them. But self-knowledge enables us to ascend into superconscious states, where our ego-hood can flower into true Self-hood. We can learn to constantly remember that any emotion or attitude we experience — like anger or defiance — may temporarily color the ego-mind, but it is not our real nature as Self.

The word for achieving liberation or sovereignty in the Vedas, "moksha," also means "free of all wrong notions." We attain it when our mind finds freedom through self-knowledge. Freedom from what? From our own ignorance that hypnotizes us to seek fullness and fulfillment outside of ourselves in the world of transient pleasures and promises! You are enough, the Vedic scriptures tell us repeatedly. Freedom is obtained, then, not from the world or from bad people or even from running away from the devil. The liberation we seek is freedom from our own emotional delusions and false dependencies upon the world.

Guided Practice: The One Truth

The Vedas say that you become what you believe. Therefore, I have provided some thought suggestions to help deconstruct illusion and guide your ego toward constructing an identity that is closer to your sovereign truth. As you meditate on these words, your mind will become what you believe. The veil of limitations and illusions will begin to thin. Every time you remember, *I am Atman, the boundless one*, you will experience inner expansiveness. Why? Because expansiveness, not limitation, is your deepest truth. Limitation is maya.

Meditate on any one of these thoughts to reconnect with your sovereign Self:

I am Self, the Ultimate Reality.

I am enough unto myself.

My bliss lies inside me.

I am beautiful as I am.

I am divine.

I am made of sunshine, moonlight, and starlight.

I am enough as I am.

I am sovereign.

It bears repeating: under all the hurt, betrayal, anger, hatred, insanity, disillusion, and sorrow, the ancient Vedas say you are pure joy, pure love, pure creation, and pure possibility. As Baba used to say to me, the knower of the Self becomes free in every sense and sets others free too!

> O Shunya,
> Your soul is such a truth teller,
> It never lies to you.
> Maya deceives you,
> forces you to chase mirages nonstop,
> until you become empty inside out.
> The soul says, "Oh stop, oh please stop
> Come turn inward and rest
> And drink from my cup,
> the cup of my Self.
>
> When the guru spoke,
> I remembered.
>
> I remembered I am made of the tapestry of God,
> I shine from the same light the stars shine forth,
> I am of the softness and gentleness of flowers,
> And the peace that abounds in the morning dawn.
> I wish to be one, one with the Divine
> I seek rest, restfulness in my own Self.

3

Samsara: The Virtual Prison
of the Suffering Mind

"For release from bondage of the delusional mind, cultivate assiduously the knowledge of reality."

ADI SHANKARACHARYA, *VIVEKACHUDAMANI*, 149

There are two kinds of worlds: one is the objective world in which we all transact, called *jagat*. This world is commonly shared by all beings and objects, including you and me. The second is the virtual or subjective world we create with our thoughts and beliefs, called *samsara*.

Our mind needs a reality check. We need a cognitive, knowledge-enabled way to guide our mechanical, conditioned, and scripted mind out of the woods of subjective reality and corroborate our thoughts, judgments, perceptions, and beliefs with what is transpiring in the objective world outside us.

Each one of us is building and dissolving samsara in each moment, through our personal subscription to myth-reality-based thoughts (wrong beliefs that increase a sense of separation, competition, and scarcity consciousness); likes and dislikes; ideas; and deep-seated mental tendencies, propensities, and established reflexive response patterns.

If there are seven billion people on this planet today, for example, then we also have seven billion subjective worlds present alongside the one, physical, tangible, objective world we all commonly share. In relationships, each of us is an "object" for the other, and when we communicate with each other, we elicit "subjective" responses (from each person's own perspective).

That is why under similar circumstances, two people can have entirely different responses. A simple example might be two people, both pretty much in the same economic situation, laid off from work. One might be relatively fine about the situation and take it as a "sign from the universe" to try something new, perhaps even change their life path; the other may feel a sense of failure or shame or that they were a victim of management and feel the need to get on antidepressants.

Samsara is then, quite literally, our "suffering mind." It consists of projected myth-realties since it has no true existence in the objective reality. It is simply our individual assumptions about the world, people, self, and God at a given moment in time.

The Vedas talk about two kinds of samsara: the personal, which is the frothing and fuming in our personal minds, and the universal, which refers to the collective delusions and spiritual ignorance held by humanity, causing untold existential suffering and bondage to the material world. Bound to the ceaseless wheel of birth and death, we are mandated to come back repeatedly in new and varied bodies to play out the same sleepwalking scripts, unless we awaken to who we really are.

The Hindu, Buddhist, Jain, and Sikh traditions, all influenced by the Vedas to some degree, expound beautifully on the universal samsara and put forward their own methods to claim freedom from it. But in this book, I am choosing to focus on the mini-samsaras that each one of us is nurturing in our own mind.

The objective world is neither full of pain nor joy. The world is simply an invitation to respond to it. The world becomes different things to different people depending upon what is going on inside their personal samsara. Without liberating self-knowledge, we remain trapped in our suffering mind.

And if we are trapped in our own hypnotized mind, can we ever be free, either spiritually or psychologically? Can we ever hope to awaken spiritually or even grow up emotionally? On a regular basis, something or other will trigger our mind, be it an election, boredom, our spouse drinking one extra glass of wine, an unexpected fever, a traffic jam, or a random memory. Bam! Our myth-reality gets skewed, and our suffering mind starts ruminating on out-of-control thoughts. We no sooner manage to free ourselves from one issue when the next one crops up. On some pretext or another, the suffering continues.

For example, in the situation above, even if both people get a new job, one or the other may become preoccupied with getting promoted. Their employment issue may be resolved, but they are still not happy because the money, status, title, et cetera become new cravings in the hypnotized mind.

Is there no end to this cycle?

Emotional and existential suffering sprouts within our own mind in response to the circumstances outside of us, but it doesn't come from the outside, per se. It is reassuring to know this at one level because then we can hope to cultivate the wisdom to train our mind to respond differently. We can hope to find the strength within to do something about the suffering. We can hope to become free of suffering if we so desire, and why not? Sovereignty is your true nature: Find it. Live it. Share it.

Let us now understand what our suffering mind is made of, what triggers suffering, and what we can do to train our mind differently.

How We Manufacture Samsara

The suffering mind is a subjective world of our own creation that is cyclic in nature. It is made up of our thoughts, emotions, and feelings. Naturally, the contents of our subjective state have the power to make us happy or unhappy, satisfied with ourselves, or chronically discontent. Since our happiness is tied to our subjectivity, let us explore this facet of the mind to understand how we can be happy, as the ancient seers promise we are meant to be—since happiness is our true nature.

We gather and carefully nurture our suffering mind using our own free will. We feather this private emotional nest with plumes of our individual myth-reality: likes and dislikes, attachments and aversions, grief and anger, opinions and judgments, obsessions and fetishes, misapprehensions, mirages, and delusions that are peculiar to us alone. Our cherished memories, precious resentments, deep-seated pride, private forbidden cravings, and dysfunctional tendencies form a virtual kingdom that the ego proudly claims as its own and thrives within, calling it "my world."

The suffering mind starts early on, when we are still toddlers and our ego is still unfolding. We walk into this setup. The anguish a child feels at the loss of a preferred toy or teddy bear is almost as intense as the anguish a CEO may experience upon being fired from a coveted company. We cannot say to the two-year-old, "Your anguish does not matter." All anguish is qualitatively the same—and it comes from the same place: the suffering mind!

Wherever a cluttered mind exists, there exists subjective suffering, which breeds alienation from the Self. Some of us manage to hide, rationalize, or medicate the anguish, but none of us can deny that every day we are smothered by untold pain arising from our own inner world. Until we awaken spiritually and see through its circuitous hold on us, we are all victims of our own suffering mind. It doesn't really matter that in the objective world. Mom would have bought us another teddy bear soon enough or that the job ending was really an opportunity to take a well-deserved vacation. The suffering tends to continue on one pretext or another.

Samsara, or our suffering mind, is also the home of our egoic personas. It is here that the roles we play and the stories of struggle, separation, and sorrow that we act out are all manufactured. Samsara is the castle of our ego. Its towers and turrets of misperceived notions in duality are far removed from the nondual reality of our true Self.

The very fact that we have authored the suffering mind is good news. Self-ignorance feeds the suffering mind, but self-knowledge dismantles it. We can hit the delete button on it!

My student Jamie loves knowing she has this power. She writes:

"The idea that samsara (and suffering) is not a condition of the external world, but is in fact an internal fantasy world of my own creating, is a new idea for me. It's empowering because if I'm solely responsible for my samsara, I can also take responsibility for dismantling it, and my ability to do this is not dependent on others or what is happening in the external world. What great news!

Of course, it's one thing to know and another to do! As I've contemplated and tried to practice this in my own life, I've observed how strongly my ego wants to keep shirking that responsibility—blaming my suffering on outside forces or fixating on how to change the external situation even as I know intellectually that this only serves to strengthen my suffering mind.

But even if I haven't been able to conquer my ego in the moment, I have found that just the increased awareness of the types of stories that populate my suffering mind has been helpful. I've started to notice recurring types of thoughts and beliefs I'm likely to lose myself in, for example the 'you don't belong here' or the 'he doesn't appreciate you enough' story. This has helped me stay vigilant of when I may be going down a self-created suffering rabbit hole!"

Samsara is considered a spiritually diseased state of our mind. Our subjective conclusions, illusions, and projections eat away at us from the inside out, affecting our emotional well-being, thinking ability, and capacity for making proper judgments. The false constructs of samsara prevent us from knowing who we really are: the Self.

The Slippery Slope of Unconscious Attachments

Our suffering mind tends to dwell upon one thing or another in the world. When we constantly focus upon any object outside us as our source of happiness, we begin to think about that object nonstop. It takes the form of a desire—it can be a living object, as in a person; a nonliving object, like a car or necklace; or a preferred situation in the world or a desired outcome, like a promotion. We continue to think about it, desire arising like waves, initially feeble, then strong with the wish to get what we want. In our imagination, that object becomes a source of our potential happiness. We must use our discernment to determine if it is worthwhile to dwell upon that object, asking ourselves, *Will this person really complete me and fulfill me? Will I really be happy if I buy a new car?*

It is easy to distract the mind when it first lands on a new object of desire, but most of us do not think to quell this growing sensory fascination. Instead, we go on dreaming about the lover we pine for or the bigger car that our neighbor is driving, whether the lover is available to reciprocate our affection or whether the new car is affordable. Initially, the attraction is like a weak disturbance, but over time that minor ripple becomes a huge wave that overcomes us. Given time and our indulgence, any passing thought can become a powerful want! We must make it a point to examine whether it is healthy to think of the specific object constantly, to fantasize and obsess in this manner. If we are alert and intelligent, we can nip the growing samsara in the bud. This first stage of attachment is known as *abhilasha*. It simply means "to desire."

Instead, we often develop strong opinions of how we want things to flow for us, little realizing that we can rarely control such cosmic equations. We like anything that we think brings us closer to our goal of desire fulfillment, and we dislike whatever we feel obstructs us. We become like teenagers who favor friends who lead them astray or introduce them to bad habits while rejecting parents who institute boundaries for their safety and well-being. This escalates our experiences to the next stage of desire, known as *lolupa*, which means "eager or intensified desire."

When our mind is filled with likes and dislikes, we lose our capacity to be cheerful or even neutral. We cannot weigh pros and cons, choose wisely, or act with unbiased intelligence. Rather we respond from our raging emotions because samsara is fastidiously cherry-picking every day, seeking out activities, ideas, and people it likes and actively avoiding others.

Our "liking" can grow into a full-fledged attachment known as *raga*. It denotes an addictive, almost pathological state of desiring. And then the problems begin since now, due to raga, we feel we cannot live without what we desire. We sign away our inner joy to the object we desire. Raga is also often accompanied by equally powerful aversion, known as *dwesha*. We become attached to whatever we think will bring us closer to our goals of desire fulfillment, and we have aversion toward whatever we think is an actual or perceived threat to attaining that desire.

Often our desires are not fulfilled. Unfulfilled or thwarted desire gets converted, first into grief, anxiety, or self-pity, known as *shoka*, and then anger in the form of frustration, irritation, and finally rage. This is known as *krodha*, an umbrella term for aggressive emotions directed toward self or others.

In fact, anger is the same as desire, only in a different form. Anger is caused when we experience obstacles to getting what we want or when we fear the loss of what we want, such as wealth or relationships. Therefore, desire invariably leads to anger.

When the mind is in the grip of anger, we lose our ability to discern or judge between what is appropriate and what is not. Anger makes people more likely to take risks and to minimize how dangerous those risks will be. We might find that we emotionally explode in response to our own parents, to whom we otherwise always show regard. Or, in a state of stress over a lost promotion, for example, we could slap our child. We forget who we are and lose our sense of decency.

We might fail in our usual treatment of our parents, our children, or others we respect, and hurt those we hold dear, those whom we wish to protect and shower with love.

Anger gives birth to a temporary insanity called delusion, or *moha*. Delusion is a mistake, a confusion, arising from a false notion. Thanks to delusion, we forget what is expected of us when we interact with the world of other people. We slam doors, curse, say things we will regret, vindictively backbite, damage property, and emotionally, verbally, or physically abuse others. At a minimum, we trash our own diet and lifestyle, destroying our own mood, health, and well-being. This kind of acting out almost always follows anger. When we are in this delusional state, we can forget our values, our prior learning, our prior resolutions. This is the stage of "spiritual forgetfulness," or *smriti-nasha*.

Delusional and forgetful of our spiritual nature, we make wrong judgments that may hurt us and our loved ones, and ultimately, humanity. Nondiscernment can become our default mode, leading us to make erroneous judgments all the time. We may decide that it is okay to have an affair, to take too much sleep or pain medication, to steal from our parents or friends, to shoplift, to drink every night and maybe one or two glasses in the morning, or to speak inappropriately to people. And we feel justified in our actions.

For example, sometimes attachment and aversion causes parents to fight a lot. At this point, they have already reached the advanced stage of forgetfulness. They may scream at their kids for trivial matters or try to "put them in their place." They completely forget their prior beliefs and values about raising children with love and providing them with an emotionally safe home. The parents may have regrets later, but in that moment when they took out their anger on their beloved kids, they were not themselves. They forgot what they stood for and who they were in a kind of temporary insanity. We have all been there. We all know what it feels like. We inwardly bewail, "How could I do that? What was I thinking? Where was my mind?"

The final stage is that of corrupted wisdom, or *buddhi nasha*, when our inner judgment between right and wrong action is chronically bewildered. We don't think that our mind is muddled or that we need to reexamine our beliefs. In fact, we may even think everyone else is stupid, crazy, or simply misinformed, incapable of understanding where we are coming from. In this advanced stage, our faculty for distinguishing between what is acceptable or unacceptable, what will serve us and what will sabotage us, gets corrupted and begins to give us wrong inner guidance. Our own mind becomes our enemy, pretending to be our friend but leading us astray. We imagine ourselves very wise, but we act in stupid ways! People may laugh at us behind our back or mock us, and our loved ones pity us, yet we go about feeling smart and full of ourselves. Alas, our wisdom has grown muddy and grimy with misperceptions.

In this final stage of attachment, we are convinced of our perceptions and judgments. We never stop to consider if we may be biased. We only take in information that confirms our preexisting beliefs. We like to think we are being objective, even logical and clever, when making judgments and decisions about the world and our relationships. But sadly, our biases are so entrenched and corrupted that our faculties of discernment are out of order, and we can't help making poor decisions.

Interestingly, modern cognitive psychology confirms what the Bhagavad Gita taught humanity thousands of years ago. A cognitive bias is a systematic error in thinking that affects our decisions and judgments. Cognitive biases are rooted in thought-processing errors that often arise from problems with memory. The way we remember an event or what we choose to remember about it may be distorted in a way that in turn can lead to biased thinking and decision making. Additionally, with a strong cognitive bias, we only legitimize sources of information, thoughts, and ideas that confirm what we already know or want to believe. If we never examine our beliefs in the light of rationality, a self-perpetuating cycle of ignorance results.

All these myth-based biases can also lead to justifications. We think, *Yes, it is all right to drink alcohol to make up for the "I am not good enough" feelings; Yes, it is okay to lie on my résumé since getting ahead is important in this dog-eat-dog world; Yes, it is okay to show those people who is boss; Yes, it is okay to have an affair if my partner can't or won't meet my needs.*

When the mind is taken over by myth-reality, access to knowledge is obstructed to the point that it is useless even to pursue a wisdom teacher like myself or Baba; the false beliefs have metastasized. At this stage, not even the Self within can crack a new idea into the mind. Without self-reflection, no guru-like figure or mentor can, from outside, introduce new wisdom. Where before there was some hope, now there is none. This is a point of no return; even the intellect and its wisdom does not function for such a person.

In the state of corrupted wisdom or loss of the inner faculty to discern between a right or wrong path of action, the criminal may become hardened; the luster, a molester; the inadequate parent, a raging monster; the lover, a sex addict; and the devotee of god, a scary zealot. An honest employee may steal from their employer and justify it in their own mind; the upright citizen may perform treason against the nation; a guru may have sex with their own disciple; a parent may slap an innocent toddler due to work stress; a friend may gossip about another despite not wanting to; an email that should never have been sent might go out "reply all"; a call that may best not have been made is made anyway; an extra slice of cheesecake must be eaten.

I think you get the idea.

The Bhagavad Gita says that with the loss of discrimination comes the potential loss of human life because from this point forward, our mind becomes a self-sabotaging and self-destroying entity. It confuses and blinds us. Such a person, forever in the misdirected search for wholeness, power, peace, and happiness, can only reap more and more sorrow.

The disease of the subjective mind, samsara, is indeed cyclical in nature. But don't worry. You can get off the samsara roller coaster in your mind at any time. Becoming aware of what is going on in your mind is half the battle won. You can begin untangling yourself when you see how you are cornered by your own attachments. The knowledge I am sharing with you is a key to the padlocks of your own mental prison. In fact, this liberating knowledge is already freeing you, right now, as you are reading my words. Cultivating and enjoying a healthy mind and reconnecting with your inner sovereign nature is entirely up to you. I will show you how to break free from samsara in the coming chapters.

4

❖◇»»»»▸•◀«««««◇❖

Raga: Breaking the Cycle of Attachment

"Attachment alone is the main cause for unhappiness."

MAHABHARATA, 3.2.27

The world and its objects, things, and people are neither good nor bad. Nor is desire a bad thing if it is kept in perspective. It is we who ascribe our highly subjective meanings to the world and then lose ourselves in our mental samsaras, in chasing the people and objects we have developed a fondness for and running away or hiding from things to which we are averse.

The Bhagavad Gita describes the ladder of the human fall, from consciousness to unconsciousness, liberty to bondage, happiness to suffering in two verses in chapter 2: "When a person dwells with the mind on sense objects, the person experiences attachment to them. From attachment springs desire, and from desire (if thwarted), comes anger. Anger clouds the judgment and gives rise to delusion; delusion causes loss of memory, one can no longer learn from past mistakes; we lose the power to choose between the wise and the unwise, and this loss of discrimination leads to untold suffering."[1]

I spent many years contemplating this verse. I was surprised that everywhere I turned for greater explanation, all I came across was a basic word-by-word translation. I wanted to know, how can this verse help me?

I therefore developed a psychological process that addresses this seven-stage pathology (samsara karnam) that universally afflicts the human psyche. I have been using this process to help my students.

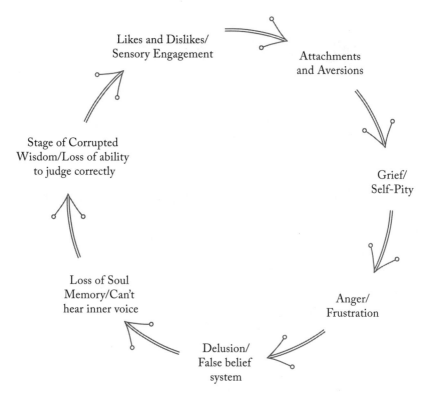

Figure 4.1: Samsara Karnam: The Wheel of Samsara

As discussed in the previous chapter, our fascination with objects outside us occurs because we wrongly attribute our happiness to these objects rather than knowing that our inner joy is our true source of happiness and that external things and people can only give us temporary pleasure. Blindly dwelling upon any object leads to attachment, grief, anger, memory loss, and finally full-blown delusion. Therefore, the ancient wisdom seers ask us to know our mind and its conscious and unconscious patterns and to master them.

Let me give you a few real-life examples to help you sidestep this pathology rather than get up caught in it.

The Man Who Wanted Silence

I once had a student who liked silence. His sense of hearing preferred silence and disliked noise. This corresponds to the first stage of the cycle of samsara, *sensory engagement / likes and dislikes.* Our senses are free to roam the world of objects. When our senses are arrested by specific objects, be they material or virtual, our preferences arise. This is entirely a sense-driven behavior at this early stage. We prefer some tastes to others, favor one color over another, without much thought behind our preferences.

Soon, the student started expressing a liking for certain spiritual protocols, such as maintaining silence. He disliked students who did not follow the practice. Initially, he was viewed by everyone as an "evolved" soul, and he was cheerful at that stage. But I was concerned about his intensity for "things spiritual." His preference for silence had grown into an attachment. He refused to answer even a basic question like, "Did you turn on the heat?" He began policing others, his aversion translating to a barely restrained scowl if people spoke, even in whispers. He had now reached the stage of *attachments and aversions*—this is raga, which is translated as "becoming colored," and refers to excessive or obsessive attachments that confuse the mind.

The student went through a short phase of not feeling heard or supported. He could not find the atmosphere he needed to go inward or like-minded students who would understand his heartfelt request. He felt like a victim, and though he stopped asking people to be silent, he was not content. He appeared distressed. This corresponds to the stage of *grief/self-pity.*

Then, when caring students approached him with genuine smiles or offers of help, he would reject them. He was simmering with unexpressed rage. His anger showed in his eyes; he pointedly sat apart from everyone during dinnertime. Often my students sit alone, as solitude is something we all cultivate at my school. But his solitude had invisible daggers around him; the more sensitive students felt afraid to approach him. His self-pitying grief had moved on to the stage of *anger/frustration.*

One day, he "lost it." He screamed at the top of his voice at the students, when I was not present, about their "disrespect" toward the teacher and the depravity of their souls. He demanded higher spiritual standards and silence. When some students pointed that someone demanding silence should not raise his voice, he began to throw things. By then, he had lost his ability to discern Any wisdom he had gleaned from his study was of no avail to him as he ranted and raved away. He was asked to leave the school. Anger had tipped over into the stage of *delusion.*

Many years later, he wrote a letter begging to meet me. I agreed, but in the half-hour we spent together, I saw that he had passed into chronic delusion, disconnected from the inner guidance of his true Self. His mind was swarming with mythical beliefs. The sages call this stage *loss of soul memory*.

He then flitted from teacher to teacher, path to path, quickly finding fault in each of them. He found himself in conflict with his family and neighbors and was generally upset that the world was not going according to his view of how it should proceed. He told me that he meditated a lot and asked me if I needed his services as a meditation teacher (he wanted to recruit himself as my teaching assistant). He did not have an iota of self-doubt and never entertained the thought that he might be, to any degree, responsible for the "bad stuff" happening to him. He had reached the stage of *corrupted inner wisdom*, in which we lose the ability to make correct judgments.

The student looked ordinary on the surface. He spoke eloquently and with self-confidence, and he had a pleasant demeanor. But his suffering mind was seething with poisonous thought-snakes crawling all over his mind's myth-reality and hurting him greatly. His life was out of control because his suffering mind was out of touch with any semblance of a greater interconnected reality. All he had was his subjective world to go by; what was happening in the objective world was beyond his ability to conceive.

In one sense, his screams for silence were really his mind's misplaced need to find solace in his Self, but with lack of self-knowledge, he was looking for that spiritual peace and silence outside him in the world. His mistaken beliefs were that he must fight for everything, including peace, and he continued to do that.

When I last saw this student, I could feel his sorrow, his aloneness, his suffering. His retreating figure looked so vulnerable that my heart went out to him. I sincerely hope he finds his way to a greater understanding. If I could offer him one teaching, it is this: our myth-reality remains real and can exert sorrow upon us only so long as we believe it is real.

Delusions in the suffering mind are of many kinds. You could have a delusion that your marriage is healthy when you know your spouse lies to you. You might have a deluded belief about your family, such as the idea that you are all fair and respectful to each other, even when they are in fact mean and disrespectful to you. Delusion can be about how we treat ourselves. For example, the addict who cannot acknowledge how overeating or overindulging in alcohol is slowly killing them. Or it could be about allowing ourselves to wallow in self-pity without taking ownership or accountability for our part in our problems. Whatever form the delusions take, they are all caused by our unwillingness to face reality because we are attached to our own version of reality—one in which we float along in a pleasant relationship, are supported by a loving family, and can indulge in the temporary relief intoxicants or "comfort food" can bring without any repercussions to our health.

When we are blindsided by the delusions arising from our attachments, we may find ourselves participating in "urgent" life events, such as entering relationships or leaving them, starting businesses or ending them, and so forth, without adequate planning, deliberation, or justification, and often to our own disadvantage. All such mindless actions cloud our inner joy, while our outer search for morsels of happiness intensifies. Though externally we may look successful or pious and manage to hold a job, raise babies, drive a car, vote, or even run for the presidency of the greatest nation on Earth, many of us are living from a deluded state of mind.

The Man Who Wanted Harmony

Now let me lead you through another case, one that was not so outwardly dramatic, but inwardly delusional, nevertheless.

Sensory engagement / likes and dislikes. In this case, the person highly values the idea of family. His eyes and ears enjoy the sights and sounds of a happy family being together, engaging in chitchat together.

This person is an ultra-sincere human being to the point of being a bit overconscientious. One of his preferences is a harmonious home environment for himself and his children from a previous marriage. However, despite his best efforts, there is friction between his teenage kids and his second wife, and sometimes he gets caught in the middle—a situation he seriously "dislikes."

Attachments and aversions. His liking for a harmonious home environment has gone beyond a mild preference into a serious attachment, or raga. It must be this way, no other. He'll do anything to keep things smooth and "happy." He will take his wife or kids out for movies separately if he feels there is even a remote chance they may lock horns. He talks nonstop at the dining table in case an uncomfortable silence arises. He will make love to his wife, even if he does not want to, simply to keep the peace.

Grief. When, despite his efforts, the family atmosphere gets unstable, he is overcome with sorrow even if it is not a big deal—as if it *is* a big deal. Given that he puts so much (unasked for) energy into keeping things stable, any slight variation in the emotional scale of his home life is a personal tragedy for him. He weeps privately, his heart and head hurt, but ever the harmonizer, he packs away his own sorrow and reminds his wife how much the kids care for her and how much he needs her to be there for him as he parents them. Sometimes he begins crying as he convinces each belligerent party to kiss and make up, never once questioning his own attachments.

Anger. After many failed attempts at perfect harmony, *he* is angry. But he never vocalizes it. He is angry with his wife and kids. He has private thoughts of getting out of the marriage, of leaving wife and kids behind, but he snaps out of such thoughts quickly and goes back to radiating warmth. For the most part, he is good at swallowing his anger. But his health is declining, and recently his body has been full of rashes, unexplained inflammation. He is in a rage. And he does not even know it.

Delusion. One day, his eldest teenage daughter comes home way beyond the curfew hour. His wife answers the door, and the two have a showdown—a nasty exchange. Operating under the delusion that this is all somehow "his fault" and "there was no hope," the man gets seriously sad. That night he drinks himself to bed and takes an extra sleeping pill. The samsara snakes in his mind hissing, *You have failed, you are a bad dad, a bad husband, a bad human, life is unfair.* However, the next morning when he wakes up (albeit very late), he is back to being the harmonizer, pleaser, and everyone's rescuer, while his wife and daughter remain belligerently unapologetic, blaming each other.

Memory loss. Under the force of mighty delusions, now chronic, this person simply cannot accept that his family life does not live up to his self-imposed expectations. He feels terrible inside, having forgotten that he can turn to his sovereign Self within for guidance in any situation. More and more he turns to numbing the pain with alcohol, not realizing that it has become a harmful addiction. But what he cannot let go of, at any cost, is his addiction to seeing harmony in his family.

Corrupted wisdom.   Outwardly, he is such a nice dad, a good husband, a kind neighbor; he is cool, smiling, ever helpful—but delusional. At this advanced stage, his private samsara is ridden with shame, blame, and untold sorrow, giving birth to yet more attachments and aversions. His liver-enzyme readings are also alarming. The suffering mind, samsara, goes around and around, relentlessly. He is now on antidepressants, several of them, and drinks regularly, though he has been warned not to mix drinks and psychiatric drugs. He never once questions the expectations and attachments that are driving him toward slow emotional suicide. The person who once showed up at work cheerful and ready to accomplish anything has now been passed over for promotions twice. At home, he often lies curled up in one spot instead of gardening, walking the dog, or exercising like he used to. His demeanor is still kind and caring, and he tries to help his family members when they ask him, but his will feels weak and his eyes look numb. He lacks conviction and joy at every level. Privately, he wants to die.

His delusions have killed his joy.

If this man had been my student and listened deeply, he would have known that there was one thing he could control and harmonize and feel good about: his own inner universe. But his sovereign domain, unfortunately, was overrun by the illegitimate crop of desires, borne of his unexamined attachments.

Internally, he was completely divided, unaware of his true needs, physical, emotional, and spiritual. But had he examined one enslaving belief at a time, he could have come to understand that his need for outer harmony in his home and family life was really an inverted need of his bewildered ego to look within and ensure his *inner* harmony was in place. He might have begun to listen to his soul's voice rather than simply rattling on and on at the dinner table, talking for everyone else. But we do that; we forget ourselves for our attachments, our ragas, be it for a "perfect" family or a lover, for a child, for wealth or for professional success, or even for one perfect orgasm. We sell ourselves short, way too often.

What unique purpose had he come to manifest in this divine body, that he had seemingly forgotten, while he walked on eggshells, minding other people's moods and rescuing them from discomfort? Caring for others' emotional needs while neglecting his own? He was "fixing" outside, while inside he succumbed to the poison of delusional mistaken notions.

So many happier and healthier options could have been carved out, including accepting the fact that harmony is not always possible when we want it! He could have suggested family therapy or perhaps embraced family arguments as part of a normal process of resistance that leads to bonding. He and his loved ones might have had enough of a meltdown to at last begin to talk and communicate naturally with each other. Or they might have agreed to disagree, but at least they would have faced what they needed to face. However, in the name of having a perfect "happy family," he kept pushing the conflicts under the rug. His dependency on alcohol and sedatives continued to grow. His delusory attachments reduced him to a very sorry version of himself.

Authoring Our Sorrow—One Attachment at a Time

I have shared some dark examples above, but I hope they illustrate how far humanity has strayed from our inherent and childlike wholeness, believing the tales of our ego, its myth-reality, and the lie that our happiness is to be found outside of us.

We create our own psychological bondage, *one attachment at a time*—whether it be to an object, a person, or a preferred set of circumstances—which prevents us from exploring a bigger universe of more easeful, worldly, and spiritual choices that can set us free, including the ultimate choice of letting go and seeing what stays and what goes in the great flow of pure consciousness.

You need not fall down the seven-step ladder of unconsciousness. In fact, through reading the case studies and the description of each stage, your own bulbs may light up. You always have free will to not allow any object, living or nonliving, to colonize your samsara through attachments. The rest of this chapter and the rest of this book will help you proactively avoid becoming unconscious. That is my whole purpose in sharing this Vedic wisdom with you!

Don't Seek Meaning in What You Value

To come fully back to our Self, a deep understanding of a knowledge-enabled spiritual teaching is critical. Enlightenment is required if we are to dismember the delusional suffering mind and realize the true Self; we must recognize that we all are looking for stability—permanence in a realm of impermanence.

Believing we are made complete by what is "out there," an author thinks that without writing daily and getting books published on a regular basis, being read by more and more people, his life is meaningless. A painter obsessed with painting, which is her muse and inspiration (understandably so) thinks that without her art and its appreciators, life is meaningless. Our family man thought, *Without my happy family dream come true, my life is meaningless.*

We may not go to this extreme, but if we are suffering and psychologically enslaved to the need for our expectations to be met, then we still are emotionally imprisoned and deluded to a greater or lesser extent. We each are identified with and even addicted to certain objects, people, and outcomes, and we believe that our life will be meaningless and empty without those ducks lining up exactly as we think will please us. That rarely happens in this realm of impermanence, so we're all coping with private disappointments and sometimes even depression.

And this is where I affirm that *our life is meaningful.* Period. Nothing can make or give meaning to your life; you, who are pure existence, give life to everything else. It is you who lend meaning to everything through your thoughts. If you were to change your thoughts right now, you could also change that meaning. But *after* we have imparted meaning to things, we think it is the objects that impart meanings to *us,* and we become emotionally dependent upon them. This is the delusion or muddling up of meaning in myth-reality. For example, the man who valued silence (that is, he imparted meaning to silence) became dependent on circumstances that provided him with that silence. It became the factor that determined his value. And the man who imparted so much meaning to the dynamics of his family wanted to earn back his life's meaning through the family.

I want to tell you that your true Self is a momentous, blissful, and unimaginably powerful existence. Your life is meaningful, worthwhile, and supremely valuable unto itself. *You* add meaning to your life; nothing in your life adds meaning to your life because in your essence, *you* are pure existence. Let the whole world come to you; *your* life is meaningful. Let the whole world go away from you; *your* life is meaningful. Therefore, do not connect the purpose, meaning, or value of *your* life to anything else at all.

Our minds must be trained with the kind of contemplations and self-knowledge I am introducing to you here so you will know without an iota of doubt that your life is meaningful because you are you. Period.

Relationships and Attachment

Humans come together to engage in relationship through darkness and light, through hatred and love, through laughter and pain. Ultimately, the various rubbing of our shadows awakens us to something else that lies beyond our shadows . . . our sovereign truth.

No body, no object, no experience belongs to you exclusively. All beings, objects, and experiences will come and go through the revolving doors of your vast consciousness, and your egoic persona awakens to realize the false grounds it is building for its ephemeral happiness. In your pure state, you have relationships with all beings and with no beings at the same time since nonduality is the truth. There is no other, just one Self.

The grieving, lonely, hurt self is your false egoic self who has a sense of ownership and thereby a sense of expectation, lack, loss, grief. This false self is a projection of your mind and not your reality. The Self has no superficial ownership and yet always has everything and everyone within its fold of consciousness. So, there is no point in insisting upon specific relationship outcomes or in losing our mind or spiritual joy in the process.

I teach my students to love themselves unconditionally because our true nature is unconditional love and joy. So, we must stop searching for happiness. Simply give it a break and see what emerges from within.

We are sorrowful because we forget who we are. We are not simply the wife, husband, son, daughter, seeker, provider, friend, or lover. We are the divine Self. We need not beg for morsels nor live in constant deprivation. We can simply let go of attachments, our ragas, and the mindless scripts that bind us, and then take steps that align with our sovereign birthright.

Guided Practice: Practicing Wholeness, Reducing Attachment

Any time you feel anxious or needy, any time you find yourself fixated on things outside of yourself for fulfillment, put both hands on your heart, one on top of the other, and repeat, with self-acknowledged feelings, the following words:

My wholeness lives inside me; my joy is right here in my own heart; my fullness lies right here. I can feel it. My Self is unconditional love; love is flowing through my heart.

This is the wholeness mudra, or the hand-heart gesture. It gets you in touch with your own indwelling Self. This gesture with the accompanying words instantly reawakens soul-memory. When we make contact gently, the splendid inner Self contacts us back and gives us gifts untold!

Things begin changing when we remember who we truly are, beyond the mind and egoic personality. That is why a respected Vedic text observes this: "Desire and anger are objects of the mind, but the mind is not you, nor ever has been you. You are Self, pure awareness itself and unchanging—so live happily."[2]

Self-Knowledge Is Critical to Overcome Attachments

If you are feeling unworthy or unwanted or needing to prove yourself, you have been thinking delusionary thoughts that are contrary to the reality of your own true Self. You are authoring your own sorrow. When our mind is under the spell of desire-related attachments and anger, grief, or disappointment, it has no perspective of its own. There is no room to breathe or change scenery in this mind. This mind is bound to the external world of objects and its preferred outcomes.

Thoughts such as *I must drink coffee, I must be successful, I must have a bestseller,* and *I must be married before I am thirty-five* are all sorrow-giving raga that color our mind. To want coffee is normal. But to want it desperately is an attachment. To want success is normal. But to insist upon success is an attachment. To want to write a book that does well is normal. But to be devastated if one does not write the next bestseller is an attachment. To want a loving partner is normal. But to become desperate if it does not happen or if we end up married to an incompatible person for the sake of being partnered, the attachment has gone too far.

As I have said, ignorance of our sovereign nature leads to misperceptions of our situation and a false belief that our happiness lies in the people and objects that surround us. We begin experiencing internal conversations about what we like and what we dislike. It is our desire to and inability to control these things that lead to our suffering. It arises from *within us*, not from the outside world, causing the inside world of emotions to fall apart.

It is with knowledge of our Self that we can tackle our emotional problems. Holding in mind the truth of our own nature, we receive the practical benefits of greater inner poise, such as a more serene state of mind and a greater sense of discernment in exercising our choices. This includes knowing that *I can change my samsara's propensity for suffering to joy by exercising my higher will—and what I cannot change (the outer circumstance), I can accept without undue suffering, again by exercising my free will.*

Our five senses are like five pet dogs that we must train and discipline—they must know you, the Self, is the master, not them. The Self must take the sensory dogs for a walk in the direction you want them to head and not allow them to take you wherever they want to go.

This can happen for you too. Once you remember who you are, even if at first only intellectually, suddenly your universe will no longer remain a collapsed, single myth-belief hanging you by a thread between staying alive or choosing death. Your mind can be an awakened mind—a vast expanse of pure potential to be or to become by intention; to change your beliefs at will; to spiritually unmold, shape-shift, and allow innumerable permutations and combinations that transpire joyously!

All we must do is stop trying to control this magical existence and simply let it be. And then be in it with personal sovereignty as our most superior value.

The "I Am Enough" Affirmation

"From inner contentment, the highest happiness is attained."

YOGA SUTRAS, 2.42

Meditate on this positive affirmation to help break attachment:

*I am enough (because my joy, power, wholeness,
and love lie inside me).*

This affirmation often helps us center in the truth of Self, instead of being tossed about in the waves of our samsara ocean.

I encourage you, too, to make this your primary belief by repeating it to yourself often. It will change your life for the better. Your neediness will end. You will no longer give away your power in search of morsels of happiness from others. If it is flowing, good, but if it is not, you are still good because you are enough.

Breaking through the cycle of hypnotic joy-seeking in the world is life-changing. Think *I am enough* thoughts and you will be fulfilled because you become what you believe. Try it, and it will set you free.

5

⋘⋙⋙⋙⋘⋘⋘⋙⋙⋘⋘⋘

Vasana: Healing Our Restless
Relationship with Desire

*"The turbulent senses do violently carry away the mind of a wise person,
though one may be striving to control them."*

BHAGAVAD GITA, 2.60

We've just explored the seven-step mental process that can quickly transform a calm mind into a self-created monster of suffering, grief, anger, and delusional projections. This suffering mind not only can cause emotional distress in the moment, but it can imprison us for an entire lifetime, our whole being colored by mental self-afflictions. Trapped in the jail of attachments and aversions, our mind is our worst enemy, never allowing us to relax into the greater flow of the Self.

To become free of the suffering mind, let us look below it, into the deepest unconscious layers of the mind. Why are we so consumed with likes and dislikes? What compulsions allow samsara to steal our peace? Desire. Our desires fuel our likes and dislikes. Shall we then stop desiring altogether? No, say the Vedas. Desires are completely natural and legitimate.

The Vedas are practical. They simply want us to be mindful and ensure that we do not satisfy our desires from an unconscious or attached place. Let me share insights on how you can manage your desires, satisfy your needs, meet your goals, and have some fun in the process too—without activating your suffering mind every time a desire is not fulfilled. We begin with identifying two kinds of desires: healthy and unhealthy, or *purushartha* and *vasana*.

Purushartha: The Criteria for Healthy Desires

To ensure your desires do not create unconscious attachments and aversions, they should be:

- nonbinding
- equitable (balanced)
- universal
- pure
- reciprocal

Let us explore each of these five criteria, one by one.

Nonbinding

Binding desires agitate the mind, trapping us in an endless cycle of suffering. Nonbinding desires can be pursued with self-restraint and mindfulness. They do not trap us in a cycle of generating even more desires. If we can stop ourselves from blindly satisfying a desire, it is nonbinding. For example, I love chai. If thinking of chai makes me crave it to the point that I am distraught if I cannot locate a chai shop, then it is binding. If it does not, then it is nonbinding, and I can continue enjoying it.

The object is to convert all our binding desires into nonbinding ones. You are the Self, an all-powerful entity. You can actively alter cravings by not permitting your mind to indulge them or by doing something completely different, something that is contrary to the desire. For example, I enjoy taking short naps. But then I realized that my desire to nap was holding me hostage. On the days I could not nap, I felt irritated and peeved. I also felt resentful with whatever thing or person kept me from taking my nap, say a visiting friend or a chore that I had to accomplish. All in all, my well-being was no longer being served by napping. It was being usurped by my addiction to napping. Therefore, next time the desire arose in my mind, I used my willpower to instead go outside in the sunshine, read a book in the backyard, work in my vegetable garden, or take my dog for a lovely walk. Soon, the nap's binding nature went away, and now I nap when I want to and not because I must.

Equitable (Balanced)

We are comprised partly of matter and partly of spirit. In fact, the entire universe is pervaded by matter and spirit. But, if all our desires are material in nature, then our whole personality will be imbalanced. Despite our material possessions, we may feel empty. The Vedas tell us that it is important to spend time daily pursuing our spiritual well-being, too.

Conversely, if you are operating under the belief that to be spiritual or god-loving, you must be poor, single, sexless, and only employed in the nonprofit or humanitarian sector, then your desires are not balanced. Spiritual pursuits can include meditation, worship, taking spiritual classes, offering selfless service, reading spiritual books, and being a part of a spiritual community. Ethically earned money and material assets can be a great force for doing good in the world. To be truly abundant in every sense, both material and spiritual, try not to entertain extreme desires with an either-or mentality.

Universal

The Vedas explain that all humans must recognize and fulfill desires pertaining to the four universal goals of life. These are the desire to ensure material survival and abundance (*artha*); experience happiness through healthy pleasures, including sex (*kama*); cultivate mindfulness, virtues, and a higher code of personal values (*dharma*); and seek spiritual freedom and personal awakening through cultivating self-knowledge (*moksha*).

By promoting these four macro-goals, namely, of desiring wealth, pleasure, values, and awakening, the Vedas are suggesting that no human should omit any one of these desires or think they can bypass one or another.

This is precisely why these desires are called universal—they are universally relevant. Within this class of human goals that are shared by all, we can look to fulfill our own desires, boldly, without doubts or guilt. For example, certain religions view sexual pleasures with a suspicious eye. Some suggest embracing poverty to find God. But the Vedic tradition is truly holistic and recommends fulfilling our desires for sex or money proactively and of course ethically, since they are *universal*. In fact, denying ourselves our universally mandated goals can lead to psychosomatic disorders or perversions and complexes. I simply love this expansive, inclusive, 360-degree holistic worldview of the Vedas. (See more on these universal desires in chapter 17.)

Pure

We tend to be selfish in matters of our own happiness, especially when we believe that our happiness must somehow be captured from outside us—through landing that dream job, business deal, marriage proposal, or what have you. We feel anger, greed, jealousy, rivalry, anxiety, tension, stress, worry, frustration, and depression when our egos operate from scarcity consciousness. Then, turf wars, intimidation, manipulation, lying, scheming, and even crime cannot be ruled out. When we are ignorant of the infinite wellspring of happiness that lies within, our ego will go to any length to fulfill it desires.

We need never feel desperate for anything or anyone outside us. In fact, true happiness often lies in walking away from what our ego seems to be lusting for and losing our emotional sovereignty in the process. But our ego continues to operate from a scarcity, competitive, struggling mindset, which gives birth to a self-serving and self-absorbed attitude.

If our actions are tainted with egotism, entitlement, and sheer mindless greed, then our desires are "impure." It is great to be happy, but our happiness should not come at the expense of another. When we fulfill our desires ethically, strategically, and pure-heartedly through peaceful collaborations and harmonious processes, we not only acquire our goals outwardly, but we feel internally validated by our soul. We experience joy, power, and peace from within since our conscience, that part of our ego that still remembers deep down that it is part of something greater, approves.

Reciprocal

The Vedas are clear that our desire to receive must be balanced with a desire to give back. The desire for acquisition is natural. However, the desire to give back must be cultivated. The entire cosmos gives generously to us, sustaining our life. We must not hesitate to reciprocate in kind. If we do not give back, we remain in the selfish mode of our ego. Reciprocal desires are the best kind since they are selfless and therefore do not generate any karmic bondage.

When we give, help, and share, instead of merely receiving and enjoying, our mind fills with new thoughts of interconnectedness and compassion— noble ideals that transcend the default, sorrow-causing, egoic mode of self-absorption. Our daily choices then naturally align with a giving consciousness. It makes us wonder, *How can I, too, be a gift to the universe? How can I give back in my own unique way?* When we maintain this balance, we help maintain the very cosmos.

Our true nature is cooperation, not competition, because we are not our individuated egos but rather the interconnected and commonly shared Self. Therefore, it is easier and more natural to cooperate than to compete. Discernment, however, as to *whom* we cooperate with is important—healthy boundaries may be needed with individuals acting in non-dharmic ways, or who are filled with baser motivations.

The importance of reciprocity in our desires, the emphasis on cooperation over competition, and the acknowledgement of our cosmic interdependence taught by the Vedic sages differs from the individualistic, self-centered approach to life taught in modern times. And it contrasts with the current world trend toward entitlements and expectations, which create a culture of blame, compensation, and irresponsibility.

Vasana: Unhealthy Desires and Cravings

All desires besides the four purusharthas are regarded as unhealthy. These desires are unconscious compulsions that arise in the mind due to self-ignorance. They are not simple, mundane desires, but powerful hankerings that hypnotize you. They carry unconscious power, sweeping aside conscious resolutions and ambushing your inner peace. A compulsive desire is known as a *vasana*.

Vedic literature understands these to be unfulfilled desires, seeds, or imprints carried over from previous lifetimes. Impressions deposited in our subconscious mind at random times outside of our control, they surface in the conscious mind, exerting a compulsion to be fulfilled that is hard to overcome with ordinary willpower. The mind tries to satisfy these urges blindly, greedily, almost as if under the influence of a force greater than it. The result is often yet greater suffering and greater loss of soul-memory and soul-wisdom.

The urges can be dark or light, good or bad. The darker desires lead us from pillar to post and activate our suffering mind. I call these dark, unconscious vasanas *obsessions*. They enslave us to be fulfilled, and when we do fulfill them, they still leave us high and dry, addicted to crave more! This kind of unhealthy desire, which arises in all of us at times, must be recognized and then set aside. What are these obsessions? Let us explore them in depth.

Vasanas are not mundane desires for food, basic comfort, sleep, and companionship, but carry an addictive, enslaving charge. Each obsession, when fulfilled, gives rise to more obsessions. It is a trap. Irrationally hooked to the obsession, we believe it will make us a more acceptable, likeable, expanded, indestructible version of ourselves in the world. Vasanas, in general, matter to us because they promise to make us appear cosmically bigger or more powerful—even if we do not feel expanded and worthy inside. But obsessions are merely illusions, chains that imprison us in our suffering minds. Obsessions invariably create bondage, not freedom. They lure us, and then they trap us. Only a vasana-free mind can be a sovereign mind. None other.

My Baba used to say that suffering mind arises when the mind becomes active with these obsessions:

"This worthless samsara is born of one's vasanas and disappears in the absence of vasanas."

Vasanas Cause Restlessness

Obsessions are the root cause of mental restlessness and psychological burdens. When an obsession manifests—say, an obsession for ice cream versus an ordinary healthy desire for ice cream—the mind will activate and refuse to quit until it attains the object of desire. All thoughts, overt and covert, will flow toward the imagined happiness from eating ice cream until it is obtained. Replace ice cream with any object that makes you blindly want it—your lover, a promotion, a certain car, or an afternoon nap!

Most human beings cannot resist or suppress these super-charged obsessions. Our egoic will alone is too weak. Soon, we may have enjoyed one too many scoops of ice cream, one too many lovers, and one too many afternoon naps.

We may be reeling from the side effects, yet we do not stop due to the obsessive, restless nature of vasanas.

We are all slaves of our respective obsessions. They emerge, seemingly out of nowhere, and make us needy. These addictive desires and powerful wants trap us and make us do their bidding until we become aware of them and gain the wisdom to deal with them. Until then, we are hypnotized chasers of crazy-making desires.

"The person who stirs up his lusts and vasanas can never know peace.
But the one who has gone beyond vasanas knows peace.

The peaceful one lives unagitated by cravings;

Free from ego and free from pride."

BHAGAVAD GITA, 2.71

Vasanas are like super-sophisticated illusions. We could even say that they *form* the mind when it is ignorant. Gaining true knowledge, we come to recognize their lack of worth and can consciously give up trying to fulfill obsessions. Then the seed of unconsciousness will dissolve, and the true Self, unfettered, will shine forth in a conscious, free, obsession-free mind.

Vasanas Bind Us by Fulfillment

Since vasanas are unconscious and binding, we are a slave to whichever obsession is expressing itself in the moment. With increasing desperation, we try to fulfill that obsessive desire. Look around; everyone is scrambling to fulfill their silent obsessions—be it for love, sex, god, wealth, fame, or knowledge—without pausing to ask themselves: "Why am I chasing what I am chasing? When and what is enough?"

We are forever striving to fulfill the needs of the fragile egoic persona, which will always remain empty and unfulfilled. The waves of time make this ever-changing "I" even more insecure. It reels with crazy desires to gain security, compliments, and strokes at any cost, fueling even more desires and related attachments and aversions. However, for the ego, security, peace, and happiness are always one more desire away. Often people lie on their deathbed and tell their loved ones their "last wish"—their final, leftover obsession that the suffering mind is still suffering about. According to Vedic understanding, if left unfulfilled, such a desire will carry over to the next lifetime or life story.

Three Universal Vasana Types
That Afflict Human Minds

Vasanas are born from false beliefs about the Self. The Vedas identify three of these. The first false belief—*This world is real*—causes us to fixate on the world; to try to make a place in it to earn approval, fame, or other worldly accolades; and to seek recognition at any cost. We are crushed if the world ignores us, as it feels like abandonment. It never dawns upon us that what we observe must be different from our Self, the observer. Desires born of this belief are known as *loka vasana*.

The second false belief—*I am a body* that belongs to this world—causes us to fixate on the body and consider it to be our entire self. We are unaware of any spiritual component and deep inside doubt its existence, even if some teacher tells us that the body is only a container of the real invisible Self. Oh no, we insist. Our body is all we have, and we love it. We are devastated if it even gets a scratch, pimple, or wrinkle since in that case, the self is damaged. Desires arising from this belief are known as *sharira vasana*.

The third false belief—*My worldly knowledge is truth*—causes us to identify with what we know. Intellectual knowledge at one level feels like knowing our own self, and we die protecting our intellectual positions. Ego swords are quickly drawn to defend differing views on everything from child-rearing to when to fertilize the roses. We may even fight to the death to protect closely held truths in the form of religion. Surely, our Self is greater than what we know. But if we believe otherwise, we generate desires known as *shastra vasana*.

I urge you to reclaim your truth, which has nothing to do with the world, the body, or the bits and bytes of knowledge that your ego accumulates with such pride.

The question is: Who are you if you are not wearing these three pieces of egoic clothing? These three main types of unconscious obsessions have been compared to an iron chain. Body obsessions keep us occupied at the physical level, worldly obsessions trap us at the mind level, and knowledge obsessions keep us locked at the intellectual level. As the arrows indicate in the Three Vasanas diagram opposite, they feed each other. Let us examine the three types of vasanas in depth.

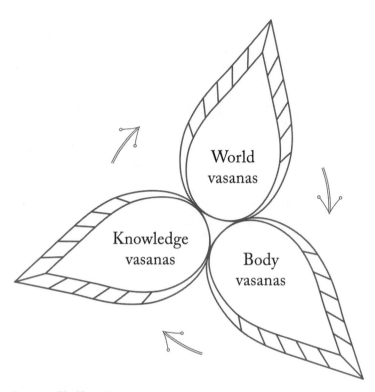

Figure 5.1: The Three Vasanas

World Vasana: Let Me Please, Possess, and Perform for the World!

When we are unconsciously bound to the world, we never really live out our true potential. In our ignorance, we give away our power and right to determine our life script to the world, spending our time, assets, and skills trying to win recognition, approval, and acceptance, all along remaining ignorant to the fact that sovereignty lies in not caring so much for the world, but instead turning inward to explore what lies within.

Until we are enlightened about our true nature, our ego feels powerless, overcome, and impressed by the world; certain family members or the society we live in may seem to possess an inexplicable power over us. You have world vasana if you fashion your life according to society's standards rather than discovering your own standards, beliefs, and values. You have world vasana if a family member's approval or disapproval still makes or unmakes you. The person's words, thoughts, and actions take on exaggerated importance. You struggle to gain the world's, your family's, or society's approval at the expense of following your own inner voice.

Unchecked, this vasana pathologically and obsessively enslaves you to others' expectations, to their approval or rejection of you, making you bend over backward to please. The world is a marketplace. If you are not alert, you may find you are selling yourself short, tossing away your talents, heart, skills, strengths, and hard work in the marketplace of this world.

In addition to relationships, you may blindly run after worldly objects, such as a bigger house, a better job, or more education. The Vedas say we must build our worldly stability, so there is nothing wrong with this per se. But your striving becomes an "unconscious obsession" when you value all this just because everyone else does. You never pause to wonder how *you* define "enough." The idea of "enough" is subjective and relates to your search for contentment. But when will you be content? Soon? At some point? Or maybe never?

"As fire is enveloped by smoke, as a mirror by dust, as an embryo by the womb, so the wisdom (of the blissful Self) is enveloped (concealed) by vasanas—this desire is hard to appease, like a fire.

Vasanas delude the embodied being [jiva], by concealing the true Self. Therefore, reining in first the senses, overcome the vasanas [see through them], [because] this vasana is the destroyer of Self-knowledge."

BHAGAVAD GITA, 3.38–41

Contentment, spiritual happiness, is called *santosha*. It means choosing to be happy with the few things that are obtained with one's own efforts in a natural way. It also means to be free of greed, to avoid hoarding, and to not be coveting others' wealth or luck. Santosha is the mental quality that helps fight greed and stops us from hoarding and instead allows us to enjoy inner bliss. The following story will help you understand the motivations that come from a sovereign mind versus a vasana-driven mind.

My guru Baba told me this story over forty-five years ago. It stayed with me. Incidentally, another name for Goddess Lakshmi, the Hindu goddess of wealth and prosperity, is Santoshi—the goddess who grants the treasure of inner contentment, as the ultimate wealth. When we have contentment, we think nothing of giving away diamonds.

One day, a poor person approached a sage, and said to him, "In my dreams God appeared and said, 'A great sage will let you out of your poverty by giving you something special.'"

The sage said, "I do not have anything. But let me rummage in this one bag I carry on my shoulder as I walk about the world." The sage found a huge stone. It was a giant diamond, which he happily gave to the person, saying, "Maybe this will help you?"

The villager was dumbfounded. He was happy initially, but he tossed and turned all night. The next morning, he trudged back to the sage.

"What do you want from me now?" asked the sage.

The person spoke his heart's desire: "I want that wealth which makes you so rich that you do not mind giving away a diamond to me!"

The sage replied, "That wealth is called santosha—contentment."

Worldly obsessions may also compel you to seek the respect of others by adopting their bad habits (for example employees who work late to please their boss, just like their colleagues). No one stops to consider if what they are doing serves them. The result is mass sleepwalking, the blind leading the blind. Our choices are truly not ours. We are completely influenced by worldly tendencies!

The first thing we must learn to do is to stop trying to keep up with the Joneses. A sovereignty seeker must first learn not to live according to others' opinions, but to accept both censure and praise and do the right thing, guided by their inner voice. This is the beginning of sovereign living, a life beyond unconscious compulsions, relations, and gratifications.

Nothing outside of you can *give* meaning to your life. Your life is inherently worthwhile. You are life—since you are that divine Self. Everything else is merely experience that comes and goes. You add meaning to life. Let the whole world exist or not, but your life is meaningful, period. Therefore, do not connect your purpose or meaning to anything else.

Initially, we must train our mind to be aware of our own worldly obsessions—the ways the world has made us identify with it and, in the process, forget or disregard ourselves, our needs, and our desires. Your life is complete unto itself, irrespective of any object that you temporarily possess. Without this understanding, your possessions become attachments. You cling to them and lapse into emotional suffering if you lose them.

Money plays a major role in the world, and often we begin to value it even more than our ethics, health, and family. Some of us stay in jobs where we are treated like slaves. Many women and men marry or stay in dysfunctional relationships for the sake of money, never questioning why, or how much is enough. It is all right to turn out creative projects that society acknowledges, acquire power to do good, and earn degrees if we love knowledge. But as we pursue these desires, we should ask ourselves, Why? What is our goal? Who decides what is enough?

Otherwise, your mind will be preoccupied with getting that promotion, becoming rich or thin, living in a certain neighborhood, or gaining a special credential. These comparison-causing, envy-generating, stress-arousing thoughts don't sound like a sovereign person's thoughts, do they?

In the aftermath of world vasanas, our peace is destroyed. This "worldly tendency" blocks our "spiritual tendencies." We may not even have the time or inclination to explore our spiritual sovereignty when we value only what society or family calls freedom: the financial "independence" of a large savings account, for example.

When we believe without questioning what the world says, we remain cut off from any deeper source of wisdom. We fall into the "never enough syndrome." Each desire, once fulfilled, gives birth to other desires. For example, say you got that promotion. Now you want a raise, the right work team, a nicer office, and so forth. Often, in pursuit of these false standards, we act unethically to earn appreciation and respect in the world. This hurts us inside and makes us vulnerable to external punishment as well. We sink deeper and deeper into bondage. . . so much for freedom.

All in all, the world is a great place to get lost in, and it gives birth to countless likes and dislikes at every step. Whether you conform or rebel, you still are pandering to the world, your ego trapped in delusional beliefs and activities. It takes courage to step back and say, "I will lead my own life, my way." This is where the real movement happens toward mental and spiritual sovereignty.

The Bhagavad Gita observes: "As enjoyments, born of contacts [with external objects], have a beginning and an end, they become the cause of unhappiness. The wise do not seek happiness in them."[1]

No experience—be it of untold riches, love of our beloved, respect and care from our children, or even fame and professional success—leaves us fully secure, neither wanting nor needing. In fact, each experience of so-called fulfillment in the world gives birth to a chain of desires. The boat of ephemeral security and a rosy future is capsized with fear of loss, abandonment, displeasure, loss of reputation, and disease. You see, happiness and sorrow come together into the world, one loudly, and the other quietly, through the back door. Baba used to say, *"This world is a bridge, enjoy while crossing, but don't build any castles."*

The greatest bliss of all-pervading reality is hidden inside every object of the world. It is that which shines and draws us toward it. But we can remember that our Self, too, is bliss incarnate. Then we need not chase objects on autopilot as if hypnotized by the world or be crushed if the world rejects us. The Bhagavad Gita says, "When the senses withdraw from seeking happiness outside and mind becomes engaged in the meditation on Self, it finds infinite happiness in the Self."[2]

Body Vasana: My Body Is My Fortune, Let Me Feed It, Fix It, Indulge It!

The body is the temple of your soul, a vehicle for your spiritual journey. No wonder you instinctively like it to be healthy. Naturally, it must be fed pure foods, exercised, and allowed to play. But you must understand that you are not the body alone.

In the misplaced search for Self, your ego can become unconsciously obsessed with your body as the ultimate reality and with the source of the myriad pleasures that belong to "my body." We get locked in a frantic pursuit to devour the world with the five senses, the body being the basis for all our delusions and decisions. We find more and more ways to pamper the body, give it more rest, feed it richer foods. The body is treated as a commodity to achieve an array of ends, our personal happiness dependent on its state.

Of course, the sages in Ayurveda (the Vedic system of holistic health) recommend that we provide sustenance, beautify, comfort and take personal pride in the physical body. We should value the body as the temple for the Self within because it has been given to us to perform certain actions—work, service, worship, laughter, meditation, and so forth. Nowhere, however, is it recommended to go into debt to wear the newest clothes, "perfect" the body through plastic surgery, or refuse to go outside with a pimple on our face. Even a person with a beautiful body can become emotionally deluded when others praise them or constantly court them as a celebrity. They may lose compassion, become unrealistic about who they are, or be devastated by aging.

You have body vasana if you are obsessed with your shape, looks, or health to the point of stress. What about incessant shopping syndrome, compulsive body building, punishing diet regimens, eating disorders, sex addiction, and zero tolerance of bodily discomforts such as summer heat or a tiny bug bite?

In body vasana, the senses call the shots. Food, rest, and sex take on outsized importance. The mind then starts to feel that sex must be acquired, whether by staying in a dysfunctional relationship only for the sex or through pornography, infidelity, or even sex crimes. Some people start, end, and stay in relationships for sexual reasons alone. Emotional devastation, body shame, jealousy, possessiveness, greed, lust, and sex crimes are not uncommon. If nothing else, the body's looks, disease, health, pleasures, rest, needs, age, and impending death color the samsara with a slew of uncontrolled likes and dislikes.

Any excessive sensual experience can cause suffering in our subjective mind. Bodily desires become needs, and needs become obsessions. Pleasure then leads to pain. We can also feel terrified by the process of aging: every gray hair, wrinkle, or loss of vitality can disturb our peace of mind, making our own body a prison. The body's attributes can also become the criteria for the way we may judge others: skin color, height, weight, gender, or age. And even as we are judging others, we feel vulnerable because of our own physical appearance.

Bodily obsessions also manifest as attachment to other bodies. This attachment is inherently selfish, as we become consumed by what we can get from others in our lives to the point that we may not even consider what is best for these other people and creatures. This can even include pets we claim to "love." Attachments can also manifest at the opposite end of the spectrum, as hatred. Body vasana can lead to jealousy, overeating, and even murder or suicide when the ego is lost in the insatiable, unconscious desires of the physical being.

Who are *you*, since you simply use your body? You are not your body. Think about it.

Knowledge Vasana: If I Can Memorize It or Show It Off, Then I Know It!

Only a bold, liberal tradition like the Vedas would dare to proclaim that we can be unconscious even in the pursuit of knowledge. In the quest to know ever more, our ego can get obsessive. The intellectual thrill we get from studying ancient wisdom is not the experience of the truth; it is like mistaking the menu for the food.

Traditional Vedic teachers say to the disciple, "Don't stop here. Don't become a hoarder of magical words alone—inner peace is your first destination. Go beyond to your truth, which is the source of this peace."

Baba always repeated this Vedic verse to his students, including me: "As one takes rice, discarding the husk, the intelligent seeker must grasp the truth and leave the books behind."[3]

Sadly, under the sway of the obsessive mindset, some students want to hold on to the words and are content with that. The precious words from the Vedas are like a boat on the perilous ocean of suffering that will take you to your joyful destination without fail. It is imprudent to get off the boat too soon, and it is equally unwise to stay on the boat too long once you arrive. At some point, you will have to get off the boat and make the leap by yourself to reach the shore.

The teacher's words will evoke the truth of the seeker, a truth that lies beyond words. Then, one must drop the words and hold on to the truth that the words point to. This is the stage of experiential spirituality, where the seeker transcends the words to enter a mystical dimension.

In some sense, this third type of obsession, that of knowledge, is most tragic of them all. That is because when we are self-ignorant, we may hope that spiritual knowledge will free us from the bondage of our obsessions. But subconscious cravings, or vasanas, are often so sneaky that we may even turn acquiring knowledge into an obsession, never asking when it is enough.

When we suffer from knowledge vasanas, we tend to acquire knowledge at a superficial level, without understanding, internalizing, or living the knowledge. Our sorrow-perpetuating beliefs remain unchanged. Our mind does not rid itself of myth-realties, and our ego continues to spin its delusory realities with its tales of woe, self-pity, blame, and rage.

You may be suffering from knowledge-related obsessions if:

- You already have read a lot of spiritual books, and yet you are still buying new ones. Your bookshelves are filling up, but you still feel lost, sorrowful, and uneasy deep inside.

- You have found a teacher, like myself, who teaches from primary source texts; you may even have studied entire scriptures word-for-word and yet you crave to study more scriptures, without really living the import of even one verse from one scripture.

- You have spent time memorizing (not understanding) verses or lofty phrases that thrill you (and impress others).

- You may be changing your spiritual teacher frequently, unable to satisfy your vasana for better, more, or the perfect knowledge giver!

- Despite having a guru that you publicly proclaim as "your teacher," you may be frequently scanning the internet for additional teaching videos and articles, rather than settling down with your teacher's wisdom and going deeper with it.

- You may be ready to declare yourself as the next "celebrated teacher," "master," or "messiah" without adequate preparation and self-mastery.

All these activities make us happy because they create the illusion that we possess spiritual wisdom or are working hard to acquire it. Yet, it may be all an illusion. True transformative, liberating, paradigm-shifting wisdom remains out of reach. This is tragic because we are so close to the source of wisdom. We may even be exposed to a pure tradition or earnest teacher who has that wisdom, and yet due to knowledge vasana, we are so far from it!

Theoretical knowledge alone cannot liberate us; this, after all, is not hard to attain. If such knowledge were all that was needed, many a scholar would be self-realized by now. No wonder the father of Vedic nonduality Adi Shankaracharya observes, "There is no freedom for a person of mere book knowledge, howsoever well-read in the philosophy of Upanishads, so long as one does not give up false identification with the egoic identity [body, mind, intellect], which are unreal."[4]

What the Vedas mean by "knowing the truth of truths" is much more fundamental than this. It has little to do with an accumulation of facts or the subject-object mode of knowing and everything to do with a profound change of our core identity: a lived realization that we are not what we have always thought ourselves to be—a limited, individual human being subject to continual change, birth, and death—but rather we are an immortal, limitless truth despite our material existence.

Unfortunately, even the study of the very scriptures that are meant to free us from the prison of the suffering mind may fill us with new egoic beliefs of a spiritual nature. An ancient Vedic commentary says, "The labyrinth of words is a thick jungle that causes the mind to wander in its own confusion. Therefore, true seekers of highest truth should earnestly set about to experience the real nature of the Self after acquiring the knowledge from the master."[5] Some students prematurely disconnect at this stage from the path of learning, thinking they have already realized the Ultimate since they now have the words describing it. Sadly, all they are holding onto is a mirage.

How can Self arise merely by repetition of words…
without knowing the truth of Atman?

In today's world, when we all experience information overload, knowledge obsession can also be viewed as a preoccupation with acquiring worldly knowledge of the arts, sciences, and humanities. On the spiritual path, how much worldly knowledge is enough? I would not suggest that anyone underachieve at school or in their profession. You can be a scholar in your field and a recognized one at that. But do ask yourself this question: If I am seeking the truth that is beyond this world, what is essential to know about this world, and how much? Can you separate your identity from what you know and practice or advocate in this world as a profession so you can go deeper in your journey toward your Self?

In a more general sense, knowledge vasana is happening everywhere around us, not simply with spiritual scholars. The one possessing knowledge obsessions may content themselves with reading, memorizing, and quoting wisdom from diverse fields of knowledge or books on health, spirituality, nutrition, exercise, relationships, meditation, and so on, but they do so unconsciously rather than living these teachings.

Can our mind be content with enough knowledge to get by in the world and keep it a bit simple so wisdom can be cultivated within? Can there be space so intuitive revelation of knowledge can happen from within?

Must our mind be crammed with daily news, traffic updates, and the latest videos going viral? A return to intellectual quietude is essential. When we focus solely on becoming "brainy" and gaining knowledge in more and more worldly fields, we build a wall between our mind and our true Self. It does not help us dismantle samsara, nor help in deepening our own study of self-realizing teachings. To assimilate self-knowledge, we need a quiet, centered, and inwardly focused mind, not one swarming with facts, figures, and daily news bulletins.

Even if you are fortunate to learn under a great teacher's personal direction, it is up to you to shake off your intellectual obsessions. We may say wise things, write amazing blogs, engage brilliantly in spiritual discussions, and even give speeches and lectures, but tragically we may still fail to connect with the true transformative opportunity that a teacher who imparts self-knowledge to our sleepwalking ego can provide.

Decrying some seekers' tendency to satisfy themselves by reading accounts of the Self by other saints, Shankaracharya writes: "The true nature of Ultimate Reality is to be known by a firsthand personal experience through the eye of clear understanding, and not through the 'reports' of learned beings. The beauty of the moon is enjoyed through one's own eyes. Can one appreciate it through the word-based description of others?"[6]

The Vedas are clear that the Self is not attainable by mere study or great learning. If we are studying for the thrill of the intellect but not living by the message, then we are not coming any closer to spiritual freedom and liberation. Baba used to say that even if one studies the four Vedas many times over, one cannot know the essence of the Self, just like the ladle cannot know the flavor of the food it is used to serve. You must try to catch a glimpse of the light within you.

THE CASE OF THE MAN OBSESSED WITH SILENCE

Recall the man who wanted silence for his spiritual journey from chapter 4. He was under the spell of knowledge-obsession. He had heard how silence supports our spiritual process. That is true. What he had not understood was the real import of the words. Nor was he trying to go deeper, beyond the words into practice—namely, that silence is not an external condition that one can turn on or off but an internal value that one cultivates, despite outer noises, disturbances, and even chaos.

A true seeker, yogi, or sage is silent inside, even when standing in Manhattan's Times Square on New Year's Eve. A person who has not cultivated internal silence is loud inside himself, even when standing alone on Mount Everest. Silence is not the opposite of speech. Simply keeping our mouth shut can lead to physiological silence but does not lead to spiritual silence. Silence in the context of spirituality is an independent faculty, the choice to be opinion-less and angst-free in the moment and cultivate contentment with whatever shows up in pure existence.

The man in our example was flitting from teacher to teacher, picking up morsels of spiritual information. This is typical vasana-driven behavior. He claimed that he meditated regularly and even offered to teach meditation at my wisdom school, but he displayed none of the benefits of meditation, such as a more inward consciousness, calmer mind, and peaceful demeanor.

When the claimed benefits of a practice don't manifest in noticeably positive behavioral changes, this "all talk, no substance" is another indication of an illusion at work, not reality. His obsession with spirituality simply made him attached to outer silence and averse to outer sounds. Ultimately, his suffering mind got out of control, and he went nowhere. Such is vasana.

The Case of the Man Obsessed with Harmony

The man who wanted harmony in his family at any cost suffered from excessive worldly and bodily obsessions. He had worldly standards of how he wanted his family to look. He had a mental picture of the perfect family, perhaps borrowed from movies, books, and social media. He wanted to translate that "perfection" into real life. Driven inwardly, he was busy controlling what emerged, suffering at every step. Obsessions were shaping his likes, dislikes, and mind in a very specific manner unique to him.

Next, bodily vasanas trapped his consciousness at a surface level. As long as his family members were not in open conflict, but instead watched movies together or happily chatted at the dinner table, all was well for him in his "perfect" world. He was unwilling or unable to look deeper, beyond their physical bodies and superficial interactions!

Did I tell you yet that your Self is ever blissful and devoid of desires?

Another name for Self is *purnam*, which means "radically fulfilled, whole, or complete." In this state, one is totally relaxed, there is no longer any distress or dissatisfaction, and there is a sense of total fulfillment within oneself. In other words, one is satisfied with oneself as they are because this fulfillment is sourced from the Self and not from the outside world. So, wanting, craving, and desiring external gratification are not the natural states of our true Self.

But the mind, ignorant of its real nature, plunges itself into the ocean of unexamined and inexplicable obsessive desires, which go beyond basic need fulfillment to quench a thirst that is not only of this lifetime but accumulated over many lifetimes.

A sincere attempt to live this wisdom is perhaps the key to true spiritual transformation from our identification with our mind, body, and ego alone to our discovery of our true spiritual potential for abundance, peace, and inner fulfillment. The Self is more than and beyond what we know intellectually. Its peaceful inner presence is certainly more important than having an impressive spiritual résumé of books, litany of gurus, pilgrimages, or out-of-body visions! All these things give us a thrill that is, alas, short lived . . . but not the realization of the inner light.

Sleepwalkers high on maya-dope, unaware of their deeper reality as Self, spend all their time diminishing the "roles" of others while covering their own "role" with obsessive fulfillment along with its sorrowful aftermath. But the awakened one appreciates what is already beautiful, perfect, and blissful: the Self. Awakening to spiritual knowledge means awakening from your own unconsciousness and reclaiming your true soul power to withdraw energy and investment from vasanas that no longer deserve your attention. As one enlightened seer put it, these obsessions are like chains that are holding us back from awakening to our own potential: "For those who wish to obtain release from the prison of samsara, the three vasanas are like iron chains binding their legs. Only the one who is freed from vasanas attains liberation from sorrow-causing samsara."[7]

We must sincerely work to diffuse and disempower our suffering minds from the obsessions of worldly acquisitions, bodily pleasures, and intellectual hoarding.

Only then, in quiet contemplation on the Self—such as *I am pure being, who is complete, full, and immortal*—will the eternal joyful divinity reveal itself, the non-hallucinating, not overly intellectual, nonpretentious, restful mind blessed with an inner experience of inexplicable wholeness, power, and bliss.

In the next chapter we will look at some ways to be free of vasanas.

6

⟡⟢⟣⟢⟡

Manoshuddhi: Shining the
Light of Consciousness

*"Sunk in the sea of samsara, one should lift oneself by one's own effort, by
holding onto right knowledge, until one reaches the state of the attainment
of union with the Self."*

VIVEKACHUDAMANI, 9

When it comes to sorrow born of desires, we often ask why we keep coming
back to square one. It is because square one is a point on a revolving circle of
psychologically fixed patterns of suffering—samsara.

It should now be abundantly clear that our delusions and obsessions sculpt
an unconscious samsara for each one of us, so much so that we completely forget
our sovereign nature. In this chapter, I will help you bring a greater light of consciousness to your samsara. We are going to open the curtains and crack a few
blinds open in the mind-attic.

Given that life is ridden with change, transience, death, and loss, how do
we reach a state where we can be truly inwardly conscious in a realistic sense?
Knowing deep inside that no one and no thing can complete us in a worldly
sense and that any semblance of completion or wholeness lies only inside us,
why do we keep chasing unconscious desires, vasanas? What can we do about
these blinding and binding patterns? I encourage self-inquiry, self-reflection,
and self-piloting to make the mind free of unconsciousness.

The Vedic process of mental purification is known as *manoshuddhi*. The word "mano" refers to the mind, and "shuddhi" means "the purified or illumined entirely conscious state of the mind." But usually it is easier to keep repeating unconscious patterns.

When we search for physical, mental, or intellectual satisfaction via our delusional mind, our every endeavor results in even more sorrow, pain, and existential incompleteness. Alas, our obsessive desires don't stop encroaching on our mind just because they cause us emotional pain. Instead, we try fulfilling *other* desires we believe will mask the pain caused by our previous desires.

Often, we simply oscillate back and forth among body, world, and knowledge obsessions, trapped in a delusional cycle. To break such patterns, we must expose our mind to self-knowledge, acquired earnestly from a reliable, stable source (such as this book), and assimilate it patiently, contemplating it long term.

While you may not identify with the real-life stories I have shared in earlier chapters, perhaps you recognize a similar unconscious state that overtakes you when it comes to needing the company of a certain person, a food you must eat regardless of cost to your health, or even a daily glass of wine. Like an addicted smoker who cannot imagine life without two inches of tobacco wrapped in paper, we get used to a desiring, seeking, unconscious way of life. We never question the fundamental assumption that happiness lies outside us and that we must make efforts to attain it. This is the root cause of collective unconsciousness.

Ask yourself this: Do I really need certain people to behave in a specific manner toward me and certain circumstances to transpire in a specific way to be happy? Perhaps to be happy, I need to learn, through Vedic wisdom, how to look for my joyful self, within myself.

Baba said it boldly:

"You need not depend on any external factor. You have got within yourself an eternal source of security, an eternal source of fullness, an eternal source of joy. That source is within you; that is you, yourself."

Beyond Pop Spirituality

In our quest for embodying higher consciousness through mental purification, or manoshuddhi, it is important to evaluate our spiritual tools. This is especially important today, an era of pop spirituality, a trend created by market forces. After all, ours is an age of nearly neurotic self-obsession with spiritual awakening. Our buzzing gadgets assault us with bewildering, clamorous, unsolicited claims of a quick path to spiritual powers, promises of superhuman attainments of bliss, wisdom, and health, without our ever needing to demonstrate our readiness, motivation, or even basic knowledge, let alone preparation of our ego-mind, for receiving these gifts. Can we ever hope to resolve the very real existential illusions eating away at our hearts and blinding us from our own Self? Band-Aid spirituality will not be enough.

Can a positive affirmation or two (without in-depth context), a mystical mantra, a spiritual breathing technique, a series of yoga postures, an online diet protocol, or even a twenty-minute, twice-daily meditation prescription by a great guru with a mass following really offer us salvation from unconsciousness? I call the so-called benefits gained from such gimmicks "drive-through spirituality."

Let us keep what is already whole, whole, shall we?

Frequently today, bits and pieces of a "whole" and often ancient knowledge tradition, like the Vedas, get apportioned into bite-size practices. Meditation, for example, was never a full ticket to nirvana, but today is promoted as such. The quest for true meditation and yearning for real self-knowledge are as old as time itself. We must keep them together and whole.

Even Sage Patanjali, the author of the famous text *Yoga Sutras*, who is given credit for teaching a meditative way to self-realization, stressed the importance of studying Vedic scriptures daily to remove the root of self-ignorance before practicing meditation. But currently, we see that the importance of a foundation of knowledge is given minimal attention, while meditation alone is promoted as a "technique." When meditators (who undoubtedly benefit from meditation) return home after "doing" the meditation, an old set of situations and the same old sticky points of relationships, finances, or what-have-you lead to the same mental patterns reasserting themselves as the same old mental bondages!

Lord Buddha, who stressed the importance of meditation, also provided deep context and philosophy around it. But how many modern meditators live, love, marry, raise babies, age, and die by Buddha's wisdom? Before Buddha became Buddha, he wanted to *understand* samsara and its root suffering and misperceptions, not only for himself, but for all beings. He did not simply want his samsara to quickly go away by just meditating for twenty minutes twice a day. His understanding of the wheel of life and death deepened as his meditation deepened, side by side; this is how a crown prince, husband, father, and truth seeker became an enlightened one, "the Buddha."

The Vedas, which precede both masters by several thousand years and influenced both, always advocate meditation and the cultivation of wisdom together. Each fulfills the other. Seekers should not even start meditating until they have shown they are qualified to begin this inward journey. What is the point of forcing one's body to sit still if one has not yet acquired and internalized the knowledge to value mental tranquility?

This is not only about the vendors of pop spirituality. It is also about the seekers who drive the trend. Most of us, distracted by busy lives, our smartphones, and our online excursions, don't have the time or inclination for going deeper into our spiritual paths. Most of us want quick, feel-good techniques.

But, the best things in life are gained with preparation and patience.

Therefore, the oldest Vedic, Buddhist, and Zen spiritual traditions—from India, China, Tibet, Japan, and other ancient cultures—insist that we spend enough time refining, studying, and purifying our own motives with an authentic master and then acquire knowledge from reliable sources, such as time-tested sacred texts, while taking the necessary time to get it right. They warn to be apprehensive of promises of a spiritual quick fix, as we know this does not work in any sphere of life. Can you master arithmetic by repeating a single equation? Can you attain mastery as an artist after using just one box of crayons? Can you learn music from the first or loudest street musician who catches your attention?

*Why would we settle for such a quick solution for
the most sacred of our journeys?*

We should restrain our overeagerness born from subconscious obsessions. For achieving manoshuddhi, or a pure mind-state, we need to settle down to let the Universal Intelligence reveal our next steps—wisdom steps that have been tread for thousands of years by lofty seers. These seers did not sell their knowledge, nor patent it, nor copyright it—they just gave it away to any sincere heart who genuinely wanted to be free of psychological suffering and shine in the light of the Self.

Ask yourself some hard questions:

- What is coming in the way between me and my true Self, even if I meditate daily?

- Which thoughts do I need to see through and set aside, and which do I need to focus on?

- What can I change in my attitude right now—in my daily activities, while at my job, in my relationships, as a parent, or while relating, communicating, or praying—so I can be free and spontaneous at every level, all the time, not just when I am meditating, sitting at my teacher's feet, or on retreat?

- How do I deal with so many factors, including my own likes and dislikes and things I want and things I have an aversion to (but still must put up with), that bind me in psychological chains?

- What about spiritual practices? Isn't there some daily practice that is not simply an exercise for few minutes a day, but an all-suffusing transformation of my ignorance to illumination?

Some teachers say to meditate more and that eventually you will overcome all the "bad stuff" in your mind. Some say pray and you will receive guidance. Some say get hot and sweaty while doing yoga, and then you will be free! Some say retune your chakras! Others say apply essential oils. Some say go to the Himalayas for emancipation. Other say come join my religious sect or study with my teacher's tribe—they alone grant liberation by touch, sight, or lottery. Some say liberation lies in sacred sex—let's "do" liberation tonight, shall we?

Some teachers, influenced by Hindu ethos, help eager seekers by imparting a "mantra" as the ultimate answer to the problem of samsara being overrun by compulsive vasanas.[1] Chant away, they say, and everything will come to you, including moksha, mukti, nirvana, samadhi, or whatever you wish to call awakening; the mantra will get it for you; your life and attachments will sort themselves out. Chant to activate the superconscious mind and you will gain untold power since it is all about "positive vibration," you know!

But without purifying the mind and seeing through maya, the vibrations can't be activated—anyone who truly knows the Vedas knows that.

Otherwise, millions of happy Hindus would be walking around India, where chanting mantras is a way of life, enlightened. I know people who spend two hours daily chanting to gods, demigods, planets, gurus, and whatnot. But the last time I checked, they are as much tied up in their mind and lives as anyone else. The root ignorance that renders them powerless to their own obsessions and erroneous belief systems does not move an inch.

I teach Vedic chants too and have included one of the most important ones in this book (the Gayatri Mantra, chapter 10), but only within the greater context of how you can consciously think, believe, and act so that wrong thinking is not a by-product of your unconscious obsessions. Only once the mind and heart are purified with right knowledge can chants do wonderful things and introduce us more deeply to our spiritual potential.

"Abiding in the midst of ignorance but thinking themselves wise and learned, fools aimlessly go hither and thither, like blind being led by the blind."

MUNDAKA UPANISHAD, 1.2.8

Thus, until we start shining the light of greater consciousness and stop settling for quick, feel-good spiritual tricks and techniques, we will remain collectively deluded and continue chasing phantoms of Self.

The Law of Attraction: Attracting Consciousness or Unconsciousness?

Ironically, we may need to purify our minds of manifestation teachings. Some clever people have profited greatly by telling humanity, "We can attract what we want"—once we buy the book, course, or workshop that tells us how.

If we could all magically manifest what we want, by now half the world's vasanas should have been fulfilled. Alas, sleepwalking and mass hypnosis continue, feeding the fire of our voracious delusions. Meanwhile, knots of ignorance continue to tighten, binding us to the wheel of existential suffering and taking us far from our beautiful, soaring potential.

Not only do we naturally revolve around the three vasanas, but we are rewarded by society for pursuing them. Our world is like a vasana bar, where everyone is drunk on vasana cocktails. We get high from the experiences of the world, the physical body, and learning. Those who don't display "enough" of these vasanas are scorned for not having them.

The modern teachers of law of attraction and manifestation say, "Keep thinking about what you don't have but want or feel you deserve to have, then use your mind to attract and visualize those things until you get them (or manifest them) because *thoughts become things.*" Modern law of attraction teachers have even made false, sorrow-causing, illusory "universal laws" around our entitled obsessions. And yet the bulk of humanity remains deprived, while the preachers of this law are getting richer by the minute—not because their thoughts miraculously became money without them lifting a finger, but because they are working hard and smart to sell millions of books, audio programs, retreats, and apps.

Such teachings, in my opinion, are only making humans more entitled, yet desperate and delusional. Oops! How did this grand, outstanding, and magnificent universe go so wrong as to serve humanity the sandwich of suffering when we ordered the pasta of pleasure?

It is important to understand why the law of attraction fails all the time and why it is not going to help us achieve sovereignty over our life circumstances. Let me begin by comparing what modern authors are claiming about the law of attraction versus the subtle truths Vedic masters have offered for over five thousand years.

Vedic Law of Attraction vs. the Modern Version

While the modern teachers proclaim thoughts become things, ancient teachers say thoughts can only attract thoughts, not things. Things are not up to human minds to manifest or manipulate at will, at least not with ordinary unawakened minds that are still drowning in delusion. There is a difference between daydreaming versus using the mind to make intelligent effort in a fixed direction.

It is true that better thoughts enable us to create a better life for ourselves and improve communication in an otherwise challenging relationship. However, we won't get any closer to our goals by fantasizing, for example, about a miraculously transformed partner without taking action, such as going to counseling.

All this energy and time spent actively visualizing what we want will take us away from using our brain to turn toward greater wisdom sources, genuine teachers, and tried-and-tested wisdom that helps us internalize, embody, and execute concrete next steps.

The law of attraction presented in the Vedic scriptures declares that "our life and our character becomes what we deeply believe" (*yad bhaavam tad bhawati*). Therefore, we must reexamine our deepest core beliefs, and we must ensure our beliefs are not delusional, for starters. No wonder it is critical, as I pointed out earlier, that your mind remains samsara-free and your ego (jiva) committed to maintaining higher consciousness (manoshuddhi). This alone will aid your mind to support you in leading the life you wish to lead.

Also, caution the Vedas, we must pay attention to our mind's basic quality or core vibration in consciousness. If our mind is generally anxious, agitated, distressed, depressed, dull, or lethargic, then we will simply attract more thoughts and ideas of the same or similar vibration. Our psychological reality will be skewed and our life interrupted. We won't be able to achieve the goals we set out for ourselves. (In chapter 11, we will explore how you too can embody the pure, balanced, and ultra-focused quality of the mind.) Your mind will naturally align with Universal Intelligence to quickly discern between reality and illusion, eternal and transient, right and wrong, and see through delusory thoughts easily.

But modern law of attraction teachers generally do not suggest prequalifying the mind or refining its core propensities and beliefs. They open the gates to a free-for-all buffet to every and any mind, even if filled with unenlightened, confounded, and destructive thoughts.

Furthermore, our mind can be at peace, and even be blissful, despite material lack, say the Vedas—a point of view completely missed by the modern exponents of the law of attraction, who became rich by stoking the desires of humanity. Happiness does not always mean wealth or power, but a sense of satisfaction and a feeling of wholeness and completeness.

Higher than the use of mind to seek out materialistic pleasures and fill material gaps in relationships, the more mature perspective is to cultivate a pure mind and recognize one's own blissful spiritual nature, which can bring permanent happiness from within. And that infinite source of inner fullness, contentment, and peace, and how to access it, is what the Vedas have been presenting and helping humanity attract from within, for decades. Reshape your own mind through the power of your sovereign will.

Law of Attraction, Meet the Law of Karma

Next, the Vedas clarify that when it comes to desiring material wealth and material bodies—be it a house, car, property, inheritance, or relationship—another universal law, the law of karma, starts operating and often supersedes the law of attraction or manifestation.

The law of karma is based on a core belief of the Vedas that death does not end the living entity, the jiva. The jiva (the ego-based self) takes on many bodies until it awakens spiritually to its identity as the Self. In the meantime, actions performed in any one lifetime by the jiva may bear fruit in other lifetimes. *As is sown, so must be reaped*, clarifies the law of karma. Once the jiva acts, be it delusory or reality based, fair or biased, kind or cruel, the seed is sown.

This universe, which is really our jiva's classroom, ensures that we don't get to simply attract what we want using our minds like cosmic shopping carts, but that we get to experience karmic consequences because doing so will serve our spiritual growth. And that is why, despite trying to attract wealth, romance, true love, and health, we may experience financial or job losses, tragic deaths of loved ones, unwanted disease, accidents, and even betrayers in love, all thanks to karma.

The law of gravity impacts you whether you accept it or not. In the same way, the law of karma is a fact of your existence. Accepting its existence helps us cultivate an attitude of greater acceptance of our material life—whether good or bad, rich or poor, happy or unhappy—and experience less envy, jealousy, judgment, and therefore, less desperation as a result.

In that sense, karma is your friend; it is your own unfinished business coming back as lack, limitation, or emotional pain. Law of attraction authors miss this point: that we have not incarnated as human beings simply to have all our wants fulfilled by the ever-willing universe. We are also accountable to the universe for our actions and deeds. It is an intelligent universe, after all. We can't simply act upon it and demand from it and not expect a reaction.

Here is the good news. While predetermination is a reality that we all encounter, you can adopt Vedic beliefs about the Self so you can think empowered thoughts in the face of karmic life challenges and attract more positivity, courage, ingenuity, and inner resources from your higher Self as a result. Then you won't get caught up in self-shaming or other-blaming thoughts. You will be able to think thoughts that support ethical conduct and inner freedom. (I elaborate upon this in chapter 13.)

Whether we experience the inevitable in an emotionally mature way, in a childish way (protesting and screaming), or in a numbed way (medicating or distracting ourselves), we have no true out, except through the self-knowledge that enables emotional strength.

The Serenity Prayer, often associated with Alcoholics Anonymous, is very helpful: "God, grant me the serenity to accept the things [sorrow] I cannot change, the courage to change the things [sorrow] I can, and the wisdom to know the difference."

Deeper knowledge of the law of karma allows us to appreciate the discomforts, difficult relationships, and lack of wealth we encounter along our journey to sovereignty. Karma is our own unconscious actions and behaviors coming back to us, full circle, to be addressed in the *now*, for self-growth. By stepping back, we can see the patterns of the whole gestalt. This insightful "seeing" enabled by the Vedas is, in my opinion, a great gift. It allows us to take appropriate actions to meet our legitimate needs in a realistic manner, without egoic huffing and puffing to get our vasana dope at any cost!

And finally, the Vedas say there is a kind of mind that becomes one with God's own mind, that achieves union (yoga) with Universal Intelligence as represented by the Self within. Such a mind is no longer lost, looking for tidbits of material pleasure and security while sleepwalking in maya. This inwardly anchored mind transcends illusion and its limitations, such as physical laws (like gravity) and spiritual laws (such as karma). In that awakened or super-enlightened cosmic state, the mind can go beyond maya and manifest whatever object it desires. The Vedas identify several latent spiritual powers that spontaneously arise with awakening; the supermind can manifest entire universes with a mere thought if it so desires.

> "*Whatever object the person who truly knows the Self desires, whatever desire their heart fixes upon, they will obtain. Therefore, one who is desirous of prosperity [et cetera], should seek knowing their own amazing Self first.*"
>
> MUNDAKA UPANISHAD, 3.1.10

But as Krishna explains in the Bhagavad Gita, a clod of dirt, a stone, and a piece of gold are the same to self-realized beings anyway. At that time when the lotus of mind has blossomed, one has gone beyond insecurity and the need to accumulate material comforts and pleasures. The being who realizes their true nature as the Self overflows instead with love and compassion for other beings still stuck in the sleepwalking ego's soup of illusions and appearances. Does a self-realized being even want to attract what the rest of us may be trying to attract? I think not.

The greater question is, How many of us possess such minds that can attract what we wish to attract? And does it not point to the value of well-developed spiritual traditions and disciplines that show humanity a slow but sure path to accessing our cosmic mind?

Yes, by achieving union with your own truly miraculous, magical, and godly Self, you will be able to attract and manifest what you want. In the meantime, you must practice recognizing the treasure of Self within. Fortunately, this entire book is about making you familiar with this path and goal.

Due to self-ignorance, we don't really like ourselves as we are. Therefore, we constantly have obsessive inclinations to attract or manifest something more, better, or bigger to somehow embellish our lives and become more pleased with ourselves. This ignorance is the root cause of our gullibility toward law of attraction teachings in modern times. No wonder we blame ourselves when we try to manifest what we think we need to be whole but cannot.

Egged on by false knowledge and enabled by false laws, we chase our insatiable desires, becoming increasingly unhappy and frustrated. Each pact of "ownership," each temporarily fulfilling experience holds a sad discharge, a breakdown, an equal and opposite reaction. Emotional emptiness and a perpetual sense of lack are the fate of all short-lived "fullness experiences." Then we become even more desperate, more determined, and we talk ourselves into believing that we are "almost there." We want more and more. Exhausted, but undefeated, even death does not end this surreal chase. When one body expires, we return, again and again, in more and more suitable bodies, until (we hope) all desires are exhausted.

To get what we want, we undermine ourselves in numerous ways: We undermine who we are and everything we know to be true and noble. We give away our integrity just so our "hooked" mind can have one more vasana-based high on the drug of outer approval, with another body holding us close, or with another degree hanging on our wall.

The Vedic law exposes our wanting-grasping-craving-suffering mind and points the way to inner contentment: *desires grow by quenching them.*

So, we must stop entertaining desires that are obsessive. But how?

What Lies Beyond Desires

The more you chase shadows, the more real the shadows will appear in your mind. Just as a silkworm chokes on threads of its own making, so the ignorant mind binds itself in its own allurements. Therefore, think like this: *O craving, I know where your root lies. You are born of thought. Therefore, I shall not think of you, and you shall cease to exist along with your root, the suffering, discontent, delusional mind.*

Ultimately, vasanas are born out of our forgetting that we are the fulfilled Self and not our grasping, needing, perpetually hungry, and desiring ego. Obsessions are like the ego's wardrobe, and unless we mindfully shed these clothes and accept our Self as we are, awakening to our greater desire-free power remains a distant goal. I urge you to go for the real deal, not its reflection as viewed through the lens of the ego. No matter how beautiful, how learned, and how shiny the reflection in the mirror is, it remains a virtual image of the original Self, which is there all along with you. You are simply looking in the wrong direction.

Here is a suggestion: rather than investing your every waking moment trying to make perfect what is imperfect (your egoic persona, jiva), maybe you can attempt to familiarize yourself with your preexisting inner perfection, the Self.

Compassionately challenge your own limiting or compulsive belief systems to lead a life aligned with your new ideals and give your life your deepest, fullest, craving-free soul expression.

There is a higher purpose to your existence. You are none other than Self, ageless, timeless, limitless, pure consciousness that animates your body and mind, but is never circumscribed, defined, or confined by anything, least of all your vasanas. *Aapnoti sarvam iti Atman* . . . "That which is boundless is who you are, Atman."

I suggest that you read the following verse from the *Mundaka Upanishad* out loud, and then take some time to contemplate its meaning.

"Bright but hidden, the Self dwells in the heart.
Everything that moves, breathes, opens, and closes lives in the Self.
Self is the source of love and may be known through love, but not through
    thought.
Self is the goal of life. Attain this goal!
The sovereign Self dwells hidden in the heart.
Everything in the cosmos, great and small, lives in the Self.
Self is the source of life. Self is truth beyond the transience of this world.
Self is the goal of life. Attain this goal!"[2]

The Power of a Well-Instructed Mind

You cannot physically destroy the fixations entrenched in your personality, but you, the Self, can disempower vasanas by recognizing them as no more than a cluster of grasping thoughts and then no longer giving them the attention you used to give them. You don't push them away, but you don't act on them either. You simply change your relationship with those unconscious desires that had previously ordered you about and left you so needy.

When grasping, unfulfilled, and discontentment-arousing thoughts arise, you can simply let them arise and then see them fade away as if from a distance. Or, you can think and hold a new thought. This new thought must match your emerging higher consciousness, like *I am Self, I am enough unto myself*. (See chapter 13 on thought management.)

When you reacquaint yourself with your true Self, which is already inherently fulfilled, then the nightmare of your estranged ego seeking joy, esteem, and even identity through the illusion of externalized fulfillment will fade away. As your existing unconscious thoughts are exposed one by one, you will regain the power to begin laying them to rest. Then, increasingly, your own true abundance, bliss, and wisdom flourish: what has been within you all along is revealed. You will experience a deeper fulfillment, irrespective of who or what comes into or goes out of your life.

To do this, you must vigilantly observe your thoughts and impulses while asking yourself, "Is this desire coming from consciousness or unconscious obsession?" When you find that a simple desire is becoming urgent and compulsive such as, "I must have sex tonight," "I must eat dessert right now!" or "I must make more money at any cost," rather than blindly obeying that compulsion, choose to turn the tide of suffering by replacing that thought with a new thought transformed by knowledge of eternal principles.

Ignorant vs. Instructed Ego

It's important that we continuously discern between uninstructed, ego-based motivations versus the motivations of our ego when it is exposed to enlightening wisdom. I developed this ignorant-versus-instructed ego matrix in the process of counseling my students. I am confident it will help you too.

Desire Matrix

Ignorant ego is never satisfied; driven almost 100 percent by unconscious compulsions (vasanas); experiences quick discontent, massive frustration, even jealousy. No thing, person, wealth, or even fame can ever fulfill the ego's virtual black hole of desires (glass is always half empty).

Instructed ego learns to recognize unconscious compulsions and chases them less and less, or within limits. It is satisfied, peaceful, and content after essential needs and valid desires are met, and experiences gratefulness and appreciation (glass is also half full).

Validation Matrix

Ignorant ego is heavily dependent upon the world and outer sources for validation; craves constant attention, credit, and recognition; feels resentful or self-pitying without external approval (and it is never enough).

Instructed ego works from inner approval—outer approval is welcome, but not critical for well-being and survival; prefers being validated from conscious role models, ethical traditions, and universal spiritual ideals over approval of random people or society; works toward what is right, versus what is popular.

Esteem Matrix

Ignorant ego has perennial low or fragile self-esteem; often feels undeserving, broken, limited; needs to fulfill unexamined cravings to have more esteem. When desires are thwarted, ignorant ego feels less esteemed and when fulfilled, experiences more esteem.

Instructed ego enables healthy and stable self-esteem that is independent of all and any kind of desire fulfillment, least of all the unconscious ones (vasanas); feels reasonably whole and inherently worthy—despite not fulfilling all desires; feels no need to prove oneself.

Love Matrix

Ignorant ego cannot understand love beyond the body; also converts love into a worldly accomplishment (love haves and have-nots); can never have enough; feels devasted when love is withdrawn or thwarted.

Instructed ego understands love as a state of consciousness that is generous, understanding, compassionate, and at times even sacrificing for the one who is loved. Only this love dares to explore a commitment beyond body and worldly standards of a given society.

Focus Matrix

Ignorant ego wastes energy, time, and money, and above all remains focused chasing its unconscious compulsions in obsessive pursuits of more money, romance, physical beauty, sex, approval, recognition, and so forth. Even time spent with a teacher is wasted since ego is besotted with knowledge (but more important than knowledge is freedom from knowledge that lies within). It thinks and talks excessively about one's challenges in accomplishing these so-called important pursuits.

Instructed ego has right focus on healthy goals after due consideration; picks and chooses pursuits; believes that *I am emerging infinite and will be at peace with any situation, job, parents, country, and so on.*

True self-acceptance comes from knowledge of our true Self. With wisdom, your ego gradually centers in a spiritual awareness and no longer desperately seeks external fulfillment at any cost. You are always sovereign, and the moment you recognize this and begin acting that way, the mind's chains of ignorance come unshackled that very instant. Self is never attached. It is eternally unfettered!

No wonder an ancient text comments: "As oil is to be found on pressing sesame seeds, butter by churning yoghurt, water by digging a river bed, fire by rubbing dry sticks, even so this Self is perceived in the small self, by practicing truthfulness, self-restraint, and meditation."[3]

Prune the Plants of Unconsciousness When Young

Seeing through unconsciousness is easier when it is expressing itself as baby cravings than when it is fully entrenched in your mind, making your life miserable from the inside out. Subconscious cravings, or vasanas, initially arise in the mind as tiny, weak urges and, in the beginning, have much less power! Now that you have been alerted to the three types of obsessions, you will be able to catch them when they have just sprouted and squash them forever.

Teaching this point, Baba said to me:

"Shunya, whenever a grasping tendency arises, see suffering built into it. Step back by establishing yourself in firm dispassion, be free of it. The essential nature of bondage is nothing other than this need to grasp, and its elimination is known as liberation. It is simply by not being attached to grasping for things at any cost and accepting what is, with inner contentment, that the everlasting bliss of Self is attained, from within."

Sometimes our mind can convince us that we must meet our every desire, whether it is legitimate or not. It even offers us sneaky justifications as to why it must be met. But as Baba advised, step back and watch it dispassionately. The urge will fade away . . .

Even if a desire is healthy, we still need to ask when and to what extent it should it be met. This is taking stock within and discerning reality from any myth-reality that our delusional mind is so good at painting.

Learn to Take Only Conscious Actions

To be free from unconscious seeds, you first need to recognize you have them. Once you know they are playing a role in your mind and you know their nature, then the next time they start dictating your behavior, you have the power and freedom to choose "no." In the end, you decide if unconscious desires rule you or if you rule over your unconsciousness.

Baba taught me to differentiate between three types of actions I can take. Use the list below to determine whether you are taking obsession-free actions or actions tainted by obsessions.

- *Unconscious action*: Most of us think we are intelligently following our desires and goals, but alas, we are simply following our senses, quite unconscious while we're hot on the trail of whatever fascinates us next. We jump in headfirst and then find our entire being is stuck in a sticky jam of vasanas! We do almost no examination prior to making our move. This passionate trajectory often lands us in a compromised position.

- *Unconscious inaction*: This is marked by giving up, such as not acknowledging our legitimate desires or not bothering to know the difference between what is okay to pursue and what is not. This response also creates a prison, the prison of victimhood, depression, and escapism. Inaction toward changing our life situation by not following through on our valid desires is simply another kind of prison.

- *Conscious action*: This is when we use our senses, mind, or intellect in such a way that we respond from a detached and well-considered position, thoughtfully, after due discernment between true and false, truth and illusion. (I teach these practices in part II.)

The Conscious-Mind Checklist

If you are exhausted from being overrun by unconscious desires and cravings that leave you feeling unfulfilled and passed over by destiny and are now ready to cultivate only conscious desires, this checklist I developed will be an aid to you.

You will know you're not unconsciously obsessive when:

- You don't feel inner pressures or mental stress in your daily actions. Even the goals you set, whether personal-, professional-, or lifestyle-related, will be met with ease. Absent will be a sense of comparison with others or with an imagined ideal scenario. You will not have the need to prove something to yourself or someone else from a chronic, unexamined sense of lack, compulsion, or sheer habit.

- You experience inner freedom to review and change your goals as required and communicate the goals and any changes with ease to people who must be kept informed.

- You don't shame yourself for changing your mind or blame others.

- You are not thinking about your goals, desires, or ambitions all the time. (If you do and you can't let go, relax, or find joy in something unrelated to a goal, then there's a good chance you are in bondage to a vasana.)

- Conducive situations seem to arise naturally; you receive signs from Universal Intelligence (spiritual signposts, increased synchronicity, intuition, or appearance of a timely teacher in your life) to proceed forward, pause, or change course. In doing so, you may experience some outer inconvenience or even challenge, but with minimal or no inner angst.

- You feel something greater is guiding you, even in so-called hard times. If desires are thwarted, you are okay accepting that too with ease, without getting into attachments and aversions or even feeling bitter.

- With self-knowledge, you feel pleased thinking, *In the denial of my desire by Universal Intelligence, something beautiful and more real is awaiting me since I am that Universal Intelligence. There is no conspiracy against me—this whole universe is flowing from my own true center, the Self.*

- You start cultivating your mind as a garden of ease and start planting seeds of well-considered, vasana-free desires that shall bear fruit in due course for you and for all beings to enjoy. You put having a peaceful mind over and above all goals and pursuits. You have new, expanded goals like spiritual self-approval, spiritual self-esteem, spiritual self-contentment, and spiritual self-love.

- You enjoy creating a less outwardly busy life without compulsory, unexamined activity and make time for meditation, a quiet walk by yourself, perhaps reading this book again and making notes to yourself or journaling, finding your teacher, and showing up for classes.

* You no longer experience urgency to do things or the need to respond to people instantaneously. There's a feeling of "no worry, no hurry"—a real patience and trust in the process of life unfolding versus obsession over outcomes.

* The Self takes center stage, and your ego starts taking backstage. You find that new values have emerged, like nonviolence, compassion, altruism, and generosity, which make you frame your goals differently. With the application of self-knowledge, your obsessions quiet down, and the samsara-causing fuel is emptied out. The mind becomes your friend and helps you in the discovery of your own joyful, truly expansive, sovereign inner nature.

Every true leader, such as Gandhi, Nelson Mandela, and Martin Luther King Jr., connected with something original and forever free inside of them, beyond their unconscious chains and limitations, and then shared with all of us the gifts that they were meant to share. Similarly, by freeing your mind from unconscious pulls and desires, you too can connect with the most creative, original expressions of your inner radiant Self and thereby produce your best work. This freedom, born from a conscious mind, supports your true creativity to shine forth, not for attention or approval, but simply because the nature of the Self is to shine.

The Craving to End All Craving

Vedic tradition does not require physical separation from all desires, worldly objects, or activities, but simply aims for a pure state of awareness without any impure desires pushing and pulling at you; this leads to the natural dismantling of the unconscious suffering mind. As your mind becomes less and less hospitable to the three unconscious vasanas, it increasingly can give wings to a superconscious desire known as *Atman vasana*, the "longing for the Self."

This is the only craving permitted by the Vedas. It pertains to discovering your Self. When you make your spiritual quest important over and above other quests, and make your spiritual lifestyle, peers, and teacher your priorities, you are fulfilling the only positive obsession you can afford to indulge on this planet: *the obsession to awaken to your own truth!*

Nowadays, when we modern folks discover the existence of Atman vasana in our mind, we start searching for our life's meaning. Our previous relationships, even beloved ones, begin to feel a bit empty and lacking energy. We start searching for not just any spiritual teacher, but our guru. We keep hoping for someone pure, with no ulterior motive, to come and enlighten us. As a last resort, we at least sign up for long-term psychotherapy to figure out the existential muddle! We become students of life, take spiritual workshops and wellness courses, read books like this one, take long walks in nature, and rediscover the joy of solitude. Some of us even make that long-planned trip to India or other holy sites in the world.

When this desire is gaining strength, we may prefer meditating over shopping with our best friend, contemplating our teacher's words over lovemaking, choosing solitude over socializing, or selflessly serving or sharing generously over accumulating wealth just for personal pleasure.

It is my belief that inside each of us this vasana lies concealed, waiting for its turn. Sooner or later, it must appear. Otherwise, the crowds and deluges of body, world, and knowledge vasanas, with their accompanying noise and pomp, will keep us forever distracted and occupied in the chase. If you are already in touch with your Atman vasana, you will value every word of this book (and other books that deal with such topics) and nod in agreement at every page you turn. You will not simply talk about this ancient wisdom, but you will try to live it, quietly, earnestly, and often privately.

To satisfy Atman vasana, the desire for your Self, you must guard your mind fiercely from sleepwalking, mind-polluting, gossiping, negativity-spinning, mocking, or shaming others. If you are in a committed relationship, you will need to nourish that relationship with higher consciousness (not mere vasanas guiding your behavior) alongside your spiritual quest of Self. In no way can you put your quest last on the list. You may enjoy the new way of being conscious in relationships—as a conscious and conscientious mom, dad, sibling, partner, or grandparent. (My teachings on empowered relationships in part III will be a help.)

Make time for a few serious conversations with your partner, significant other, or parents. If you have children, you may cherish the times you can engage in your spiritual disciplines, like meditation and practices, when they are happily asleep. You may tell them spiritual bedtime stories and sing spiritually uplifting songs on the way to school. You may start your day earlier to meditate or journal, study, or pray. Your family will become your spiritual laboratory, and your growing sense of ease within will radiate outwards and help everyone relax as you evolve in your own understanding of your true limitless nature.

If your parents, friends, or significant other do not support you, or even challenge you, I suggest retreating inside to discern between what is permanent (Self) and what is ephemeral (people who come and go). What should be important to you: truth or myth, reality or appearances, bondage or your right to choose your next steps? Your path to your own truth or friends and relations who mock your choices?

Watch out, however, if you leave your family behind in your spiritual quest or dump all your friends because they obstruct you from "your true Self." You may want to throw out your lover, your job, and your nice things to prove your spiritual progress. Don't be in a hurry to do that. As a householder, your conflicts will increase rather than decrease when ego is active in this stage. Educate your ego with inner discernment and commitment, not outer egoic display. Instead, gently include your loved ones in your growing light and being there for them, not abandoning them because you are on a spiritual train. This stage of Atman vasana, when it is real, is inclusive, not exclusive. It makes us more patient, more giving, more understanding of others who are not yet bitten by the spiritual bug.

Let your partner and friends gently know that you are in a new stage of life, a path of inner quest, and that this is a priority. Avoid giving long explanations to people who don't understand these impulses and language. You can also keep silent in cases where it would not be considered rude. You may choose to be in a relationship with a person who is on a similar journey or who at least respects yours.

Sometimes, Atman vasana can show up unexpectedly and even surprise you. We hear accounts of people from all over the world who make a complete 180 in their life. They begin to read spiritual books, sign up to serve in genuine spiritual and socially altruistic causes, meditate on the steps of temples, wander away into forests and the mountains, and write ethereal odes or blogs to free birds, soul, god, and glorious sunrises. Others may comment upon this "odd" behavior and counsel them to return to sanity and regular life. However, the inner urge to know your own truth, as embodied by the wonderful Atman vasana, will not rest until you do.

Indeed, if you are in the grip of this spiritual desire *to know thy Self,* you are on another life mission altogether. Galvanized by a deeply embedded inclination for seeking spiritual wholeness, you are resolute to realize your divine truth despite all odds against you. If this feels familiar, then acknowledge that, openly, first to yourself and then to society. Only when you embrace your inner quest will you manifest support for it in your relationships.

Not everyone can change as you change when you embrace Atman vasana. Your efforts to gain your true Self will only make you a better person, a beautifully conscious person across your relationship spectrum. My students begin succeeding at home and in work relationships since they have tools to have a better relationship with their own Self in this stage. Atman vasana is only a start, not the end of the journey. But it is a splendid start to a whole new journey of a conscious mind that ends its bondage to cancerous desires and heralds the freedom implicit in Self.

There is no greater mission than your own self-discovery. Those who are fulfilled from within, having drunk from the cup of inner freedom that overflows in divine consciousness, come back as gifts for the rest of the universe. Such embodied spirits slay the three-eyed dragon of vasanas, light the path to self-ascension, and become role models of the way to live, love, and let go in sovereign inner fullness.

7

⟨⟩⟩⟩⟩⟩⟩⟩⟩⟩⟩╼━━╾⟨⟨⟨⟨⟨⟨⟨⟨⟨⟨⟨⟨⟨⟨⟩

Viyoga: Cultivating Detachment from Possessions and People

"When the perfectly disciplined mind rests in the Self alone,

free from longing of all objects of desires, then,

it is said, the mind is united with Self.

One reaches the state of yoga with Self."

BHAGAVAD GITA, 6.18

We now understand that we humans universally feel unfulfilled because our sense of "I" is derived from our sense of "mine."

We all think we know who we are, but do we really? To an extent, we're all defined by our things and relationships. But to become abidingly joyful, whole, and abundant, it's imperative that we try to detach our identity from what we possess and discover who we are, without our stuff.

When we fail to do this, our attachment to objects activates a sorrowful samsara, clouding joy and holding our happiness and well-being hostage to emotional bondages. We need to break free from all forms of bondage to truly enjoy all our relationships, with deliberate consciousness and knowledge of our Self.

Separate from All That
You Are Not with Viyoga

The word "yoga" means "union." It aims to connect us with something higher, like Self and God. We are fascinated with the concept of union. Every religion promotes union in marriage, and we all dream of that perfect union.

But before you can have union in your relationships (that is yoga), it is important to learn about *viyoga*—an emotional, although not physical, detachment within relationships.

Viyoga is less well known than yoga. It is its opposite. Viyoga means to consciously step away from things we relate to so we can first be in yoga with our own Self. Instead of an instant desire for yoga in relationships, we should have the goal of viyoga: intelligent inner separation to discern and detach, to connect with what is true versus false.

Viyoga means you consciously separate to first have a comfortable relationship with your own Self. *Who am I? What are my values? What are my goals? What is negotiable, and what are the nonnegotiable issues in my life?* With viyoga, any necessary actions we take in the future proceed from a relatively neutral, less attached space. Only then can we know our gifts, visions, needs, and priorities and relate with our spiritual wholeness. Only then can we know our true power, which all too often we give away in the chase, seduction, or manipulation of a relationship embarked upon without prior self-reflection.

While heading toward yoga, a beautiful union, we must all first actively practice viyoga. You can initiate viyoga in all your current relationships. Do you have clingy and needy friends? Parents who still undermine your decision-making capability? Or a spouse who doesn't give you attention? All these relationships need viyoga, not yoga. And check out your positive relationships. Somewhere, you must be acting from viyoga. That is why they are thriving. The moment either of you turns needy or desperate, the relationship won't remain so positive.

You need to know where your value, wholeness, joy, and power lie—with them or with you. Without that contemplation, sorrow-engendering patterns simply repeat.

We need viyoga for ultimate emotional health.

With viyoga, you can cultivate a healthier, more empowered, less codependent mental state. You will not need the other person to approve, endorse, or confirm your reality. You'll be in your joy because you will recognize that your truth, power, and wholeness were never dependent on that person.

From this perspective, then, you will be able to influence a change in the person, leave the person, or attract another person.

I love my husband of two-plus decades. I am grateful to have him in my life (he makes me laugh, feel comfortable, and cared for). But thanks to Vedic knowledge, I embody my wholeness and my own light; I do not outsource it to him. I practice viyoga for a beautiful state of union (yoga) with him.

The only way we can really influence another is by walking the path, not just talking the talk. I obsess less over what my husband is doing or thinking and focus on myself. Everyone is a free operator. Everyone is Self, ultimately responsible for their own samsaras and degree of sovereignty or bondage.

My wholeness, power, and joy are, indeed, mine alone to acknowledge. They are not coming to me from my external relationships that at best give me occasional pleasure, strokes, or recognition, and many times displeasure. But there must be a specific reason for me to choose my husband as my life partner. Whatever he's doing or not doing may be a gift for me, to see through my own mind and the degree of consciousness or unconsciousness I am embodying. Once I realized this, I stopped my experiments with unexamined yoga in relationships (union at any cost) and instead started exploring my own truth and designing my own spiritual lifestyle and goals with mindful viyoga.

Now, we have weekends when I'm meditating and he's experimenting with cooking a new recipe (he is an Ayurvedic chef). The kitchen does not call me much, and meditation is not his thing. Some days, I walk into our backyard, and he is cheerfully tending to the plants, vegetables, and Ayurvedic herbs we both grow with so much love. Then I join him, and we have fun together, tending to our plant babies. It feels no less meditative, that time spent together in our vegetable and herb garden together (our moment of yoga)!

In our relationship, there were some things that were nonnegotiable. Some things were entirely negotiable. And I know the difference now, thanks to exercising viyoga before striking yoga.

Somehow, I've noticed that the brighter your light, the more convinced you become of your own Self, its gifts, power, wholeness, and joy. You learn that by saying nothing, simply being who you are, and living your truth, you positively influence the world.

"Let it be known that the mindful separation [viyoga] from union with what causes suffering is yoga."

BHAGAVAD GITA, 6.23

My Personal Journey
with Viyoga in Parenting

Questions I constantly faced as a parent while raising my son were, *Should I relate with him as one bound inside a body made of matter of a certain age and bound by a mind of certain beliefs (ripe and unripe)? Or shall I continue trusting his inner-most nature, which is unbounded, free to express itself?*

When I regarded him as body alone, a body I own, possess, and claim as my child, I became bound mentally to his body in dense emotional attachment. Clouds seemed to cover my inner sun of clarity. I was fearful and agitated at the same time, wanting to protect and enjoy what I own . . . forever, yet, deep down knowing that all control is mere self-delusion. As I clip his wings, I sabotage my own sovereign flight in a free sky, psychologically speaking.

Control and love can never coexist. They never have. They never will.

The mental vines that bound me to him were thick with the glue of attachments, and the control, compulsions, scripted roles, and self-defeating expectations arose from unexamined attachments in the mind. I suffered as a result and made him suffer, pulling at his strings, making him an object to please my delusory "mom" unconsciousness parading as love, care, and concern (while really being control, panic, and sheer ignorance).

But when I see him as the unbounded one, the Self, I give myself the gift of inner freedom to relate to my son in all new ways. The clouds seem to float away spontaneously, and my inner sun of happiness, poise, and freedom begins to shine again (or rather, it shone all along, it's just that clouds of self-ignorance had seemingly covered it).

Then, in the right light of my own mind, I see that we are not just another worldly mom and son defined and divided by conventional power struggles. We are no less than untethered spirit, mutually coexisting, supporting, understanding, and celebrating both of our flights in pure potential.

Bounded and Unbounded
Relationships with Viyoga

Bound humans are psychologically dependent humans. They hold each other back. Unbound humans fly and help others fly too. Unbound humans give each other much-needed strength and support to be and become what their heart desires, but to always, first and foremost, be free inside. Emotional sovereignty, or what is called *mukta*, is, after all, our inherent nature. Any relationships (even our most valuable ones) that bind us in a web of expectations and obligations will eventually cause us suffering. We must neither depend emotionally on others for our fulfillment, nor encourage others to make us their crutch.

The Vedas say that the universal Self, Atman, is always one. Bodies and minds are countless, but share a splendid, united Self—One Consciousness manifesting in diverse matter-suits—unconditionally supportive, accepting, and equal.

The man who wanted harmony in his family at any cost had no inner sense of Self. When his family members bickered, he could not keep inner and outer realities separate. If he only had chosen viyoga, to be a detached "observer," separate from other people's life scripts and questionable choices, he would have found creative ways to deal with outer disharmony. His soul would have sung the song of inner harmony. Through viyoga—detachment from others and attachment to self-knowledge—he could have stepped away from the attachment merry-go-round and found the inner wholeness that he craved.

Because we're keeping up with two demanding relationships that we believe will fulfill us, the first with inert, pleasure-giving objects (house, car, gadgets, clothes, jewels) and the second with human relationships, we don't know when we sell ourselves short. We don't notice when, despite our best intentions, we begin sleepwalking again, blindly chasing elusive fulfillment criteria, trying to feel secure.

Except for our Self, which is changeless (*nityam*), everything and everyone is under the law of perennial change (*anityam*), say the Vedas. This third relationship with the Self is therefore the one that offers true security.

We cannot expect sand in a desert to not swirl and change the landscape's contours; it will because that is its nature. We must not expect a river to stop flowing and for the water to stand still. The river will continue flowing because that is its nature. Can we censure the unstoppable river and the changing sand? Or should we instead rewire our expectations and look within for stability?

Perhaps as you let go of demanding, controlling, and fiercely expecting from others to the point of exasperation, indignation, and rage, you can deepen and cultivate a relationship with a deeper awareness and self-worth inside you. This is a thought worth exploring.

You have the power to fulfill you—only you, and you alone!

Things begin changing when we care to remember who we truly are, beyond the roles we play in our relationships. Remember you are a divine light, not merely the role in your relationship. Enjoy your relationships, but don't forget to nurture the relationship with yourself in the process! Your true Self is forever beyond all worldly roles.

Remind yourself often: *I am a soul. None of these roles define me in any ultimate sense. Rather, I give power and lend reality to all my roles and relationships.*

It is never too late. Your Self will always give you gifts anytime you turn inward. You can still choose you first, and then enjoy everything else from this *Self-first* perspective!

Projected Value vs. Intrinsic Value

Everyone knows that the happiness we feel from the first bite of a juicy apple is not the same several bites later. We may even toss the apple, half eaten. We all know about the fading pleasure of sex with a body that is no longer a novelty. The lover is the same, the body that we once craved to touch and even obsessed about is the same, yet the enjoyment we draw from the sexual encounter is no longer the same. It may even be completely missing. One too many bites or one too many sexual encounters, and the object we once sought enthusiastically may even evoke disgust in us. When we walk down the aisle in marriage, we are doing so often for all kinds of security. We can't hold back our glee. But so many times, the person we married becomes the cause of sleepless nights and threatens our sense of security, financially, physically, or emotionally, in unprecedented ways.

No finite object of the world possesses intrinsic value; it has only borrowed value, the value we ourselves have transposed onto it, by our likes and dislikes in the moment. It is our own state of mind after all that makes us pleased or displeased, secure or insecure. That is why, if you contemplate the true source of happiness—which is not the objects you seek, nor the confused mind—you will know it is your own Self.

From this point forward, I invite you to assign value to any external object of desire from a spiritual perspective, understanding that your Self is the absolute value and all other values that the mind projects, assigns, or withdraws are relative. Searching for values in objects outside the Self is a futile wild goose chase, as is expressed in this ancient text in which the teacher instructs his student (who happens to be his wife): "Everything is dear or valuable in its relation to the supreme Self. The partner is dear not for their own sake, but for the sake of the Self, which is loved above all else. Riches are valued not for the sake of riches but for the sake of the (common) Self that is valued above all else."[1]

This distinction allows us to stop being desperate in our seeking and, at last, through systematic internalization of self-knowledge, turn to the original source of all happiness and fulfillment: the Self.

Two Types of Emotional Bondage

Bondages can be of two types. When an object is present, its presence can cause bondage. For example, when a relationship is present, it demands a lot of time, emotions, and sometimes even wealth to "maintain." But, when an object, such as a relationship, is not present, it creates another type of bondage, that of chronic inner stress from perceived lack or loneliness. Either way, objects can bind us—through their presence and through their absence.

Either way, you are dependent. You have forgotten your truly sovereign (mukta), inherently full (purna), and eternally blissful (ananda) inner nature.

The Difference Between
Possessing and Needing Objects

It can be a source of frustration when we rely excessively on our romantic partners or significant others. The illusion that someone out there will fulfill us exactly as we would want to be fulfilled gives birth to a host of illegitimate desires and expectations; each, when dashed, leads to disappointment, rage, resentment, and ultimately, emotional bondage.

While emotional interdependence is what mature people offer each other, emotional dependency—leaning on others for our emotional fulfillment—is spiritually damaging. It can become a slippery slope to bondage, especially when we are unconscious and enslaved by our expectations, attachments, and aversions.

Additionally, when we believe another person will meet our inner needs, we stop meeting our own emotional needs. We stop cultivating a relationship with our self. We could have been our own consoler, guide, cheerleader, parent, caretaker, celebrator . . . but alas, we outsource our emotional well-being to our relationships. Relationships are invariably afflicted by transience. Sooner or later, someone is bound to disappoint you, betray you, or die on you.

Emotional leaning on others, instead of consciously staying emotionally autonomous or self-sufficient in relationships, gives birth to samsara sooner or later in one or both partners. It leads to yet more clutching, grabbing, controlling, and manipulative behavior. And again, sooner or later, it spells loss of emotional freedom, powerlessness, and helplessness.

Understand this: you may possess things and relationships, but you do not need them. When you possess something, you need not be bound by it—you can remain aligned with your inner sovereignty. But when you *need* a thing or you feel emotional dependence or attachment, then you are possessed by it. This is where you lose your sense of Self to your unexamined needs. Therefore, go ahead and have things, use things, but don't *need* them to the point of dependence.

Remember, your relationship with your Self is primary. Your relationships to objects and people are secondary. Only Self leads to inner fullness and abiding contentment. One can possess and pursue potentially everything (house, car, lovers, awards of nobility, and ribbons of dharmic honor) but never as a sleep-walking mental slave to anything.

When you find this transcendental, infinite source of "receiving" unconditional love and security from within, you become highly self-sustaining emotionally. Have you heard of Indian yogis and mystics, living without relationships, fancy clothes, or even a bed in the stark and frozen Himalayas, yet resplendent with health, charm, beauty, and joy?

That's perhaps an extreme case to cite, so let's look at something a little closer to home. Any one of us who starts meditating, contemplating, letting go, surrendering, and just taking a moment to check in, starts becoming more emotionally self-sufficient. We radiate another level of peacefulness and joy, which communicates, "There may be overwhelming turmoil around me, but my Self and I are just fine." Both the yogi and the contemporary seeker are connecting with the inner center, the Self, an internal reservoir of invisible but indivisible security, pleasure, and peace.

Meditate on the reflection, *I am Self, the Ultimate Reality. I am enough unto myself. My freedom, power, joy, and fulfillment lie within me. It is up to me.* As you meditate, you will become what you believe—the Vedas say—the knower of Self as Self.

Happiness Is a State of Mind

We are happy with our new phone or relationship when it functions to our liking. If it does not, we become unhappy and want to be free of the offending object, be it a phone or a person.

Your happiness and unhappiness are only mental states. Happiness does not lie in the object itself. If it did, we would never want to get rid of any object. Joy, therefore, comes from recognition that *I, the Self, am an independent happiness-engendering entity and not dependent on any objects I interact with, living or nonliving, for my security or pleasure.*

Maybe you wrongly entrusted your happiness to external objects or assigned them greater value than they ever deserved. Happiness is something you must claim inside you, as your own.

And here is the best part. When there is no emotional dependence, there is no fear of losing the object. People, for example, can no longer manipulate you to put up with disrespect, just because you fear losing them. The more you operate from your inherent wholeness, the more fearless you will become. Yes, being prepared to lose anything (but not your Self) is the ultimate inner strength and best preparation for human relationships.

Trikanataka: The Three Thorns of Material Fulfillment

Baba explained to me that a beautiful rose blossom is very beguiling in its fragrance and beauty. But when we grab it to make it our own, we must contend with its three thorns—*trikanataka* ("kanataka" means thorn, and "tri" means three): mental dependence, chronic dissatisfaction, and unavoidable sorrow.

The Thorn of Mental Dependence

Once we've enjoyed an object, or soon after, it makes us dependent. It takes away our sovereign power when we are unconscious. Have you noticed that if you've had one slice of cheesecake, you wouldn't mind a second one? If you have one scoop of ice cream, you don't mind a second scoop? By then you are hooked and don't mind a third scoop!

This doesn't happen only with ice cream but can happen with anything! Object gratification doesn't end with gratification. It leads to subtle or gross addiction.

Initially, we think we're enjoying our objects. But soon enough, we get trapped by them. Be it coffee, the morning newspaper, or our lover, we *depend* upon these things for our well-being. Therefore, any object that promises us security or pleasure is addictive, just like alcohol is addictive.

The Vedas are not saying that to be spiritual, we must walk away from objects. In fact, it says, do gratify yourself; you deserve all worldly pleasures. But if you are aware of this thorn, you will have a more balanced relationship. You will know how to enjoy your objects without becoming addicted to them.

Most of us have not received this kind of teaching. We've grown up understanding that we need to try to make more money so we can have more. And, more. And yet more.

When we are children, our needs are simple. We need Mom and our favorite toy at bedtime to be happy! As we grow, our dependency also grows, from a plush sofa under our bottom to the fastest possible internet connection. We panic if we are without our smartphone for even an hour.

As children, we needed perhaps ten conditions fulfilled to feel secure and happy. Now we may have hundreds marked as mandatory on an ever-growing list! Can we moderate our desires for object-based happiness, whether for material objects, like food or jewels, or living ones, like lovers, children, and pets? Yes, we can.

Objects give comfort. But we will find that as our relationship with the Self improves, our need for objects (inert or alive) will naturally diminish. It happens. Our needs reduce dramatically.

When I was in my twenties, I thought I could not live without my family. I was devastated when my sister passed away suddenly. I missed her so much I hurt everywhere in my body. My heart felt numb. But slowly, as my self-awareness grew, I was less and less susceptible to any pangs of "missing" someone. Now, nobody's absence has the power to make me distressed, and nobody's presence has the power to excite me. I feel self-pleased and cheerful most of the time, whether alone or in a crowd, with whatever is flowing in existence.

The Thorn of Chronic Dissatisfaction

If we do get the object we want, it only pleases us temporarily. Sooner or later, it gives birth to dissatisfaction.

Acquaintances of ours owned a house in the Bay Area of California, but they lost it when the husband got laid off. Then, the wife began to complain. She wanted a new house, not just a rental. She made their lives hell, complaining nonstop.

Finally, the husband gave in. He bought her a beautiful new house in a small town on the East Coast, where it was more affordable, given he still did not have a job.

In a phone conversation after their move, I congratulated them for the new home. The woman said, "Thanks, but I miss you." I thought, *That's nice.* But that was just the beginning. She went on, "I miss you and the weather in California; I miss you and the circle of people you knew, the classes you offered, the retreats and festivals you and your husband celebrated where I had so much enjoyment meeting your spiritual colleagues and students. I miss you and the walks I could take in California under the sun, unhampered by snow."

No matter how much effort you make to secure or please yourself by means outside yourself, you will never feel fulfilled. Material things rarely fulfill a spiritual gap.

Our lack of connection with our inner wholeness will not be completed by one more red dress, new car, or candy. You can have them if you want, but you should know that your wholeness has nothing to do with these objects. Whether you have a red dress or not, you should flow your inherently attractive and amazingly potent wholeness like you're a diva all the time. Objects come and go. In a fire or a flood, often people lose everything they once owned. Anything can happen to our objects, so you can't put your heart into them.

All finite objects—including vacations, relationships, and life partners—can give us finite, time-bound, transitory pleasure. It is the law. Each fulfilled desire leads to yet more unfulfilled desires. They all lead to chronic dissatisfactions that eat away our happiness and peace of mind, like tiny critters can destroy an entire healthy plant within days. No wonder the Bhagavad Gita observes: "Desire for pleasures is difficult to appease like a fire."[2]

I've met people who spend their entire lives amassing wealth, assets, or pleasures, yet they feel empty and chronically dissatisfied. The wisdom that all finite pleasures are illusory and that desires for more grow with each fulfilled desire helps me cultivate a healthy detachment from everything I own.

As for my acquaintance, she had outsourced her wholeness to objects outside of herself. She felt powerless and unhappy. Not even the home that she'd wanted fulfilled her. To be free of discontentment, we must separate our wholeness from objects, which come and go. We must recognize our Self within and look there for our fulfillment.

The Thorn of Unavoidable Sorrow

The task of acquiring objects to fulfill our inner lack is not necessarily stress free. Whether we are earning money to fill our life with pleasure and security-giving objects or are pursuing a relationship, it all takes work and generates at least some inner stress! Maintaining the relationships or objects can also be stress inducing. Finally, the worst pain is the pain of loss—as all finite things or relationships come to an end, sooner or later. The emotional pain or loss you experience will be directly proportional to how much security or happiness that object had once given you.

As human beings, we arrive naked and leave this planet naked. In between, we try to accumulate what we can, but nothing lasts eternally. There are gradations to this reality. Nothing lives eternally, not even planets and stars. People, pets, pleasure, security, name, and fame are all ephemeral. Therefore, pursue your worldly goals happily, but consciously; keep your head on your shoulders and constantly question: When is enough, enough?

Predetermined by Unseen Forces: Karma

Your relationship with objects is predetermined by the unseen forces of karma. People born into wealthier families by default have more material objects surrounding them. Some people may get lucky with sudden inheritance or unexpectedly winning lotteries. Some may lose everything, when they least expect it! Life doesn't always give us what we want. It's not set up that way. But karmic lack may be exactly what you need to progress spiritually and open a very special door! If you don't lose heart but keep sowing seeds using discernment and willpower, you will surely reap what you have sown, tomorrow or soon after.

The Third Relationship Is Your Lost Treasure

The unique goal of the Vedas is to positively empower us humans in our search for our lost treasure, the Self.

Not knowing that a golden treasure lies buried beneath our feet, we may walk over it again and again without ever realizing that a hidden treasure is buried there. Sadly, we have all forgotten to claim our treasure because we are so caught up with our other two relationships—with our things (boat, house, jewels) and the people who purportedly "belong to us"! Because it is not material, our true Self remains invisible, unknown, and hidden to our senses. Because the true Self is beyond our perception, we conclude that it cannot possibly exist. Most of us happily (or unhappily) spend our lives unacquainted with anything beyond what we own or call our own. That is why, unless they are spiritually instructed, most humans never cultivate the third, and I would say, the most important relationship, with their own invisible but true Self!

The Self is truly a treasure.

If we put our worldly possessions and human relationships into their proper perspective, the Self will find us.

The quest of the Self is perhaps the worthiest of our quests. A particle of its bliss supplies the bliss of the whole universe. Everything becomes enlightened in its light. The knower of Self revels in the light of their heart, an ecstasy that is indescribable—pure bliss, transcending time, ever free, beyond desire.

8

Guru: Recognizing a True Teacher

"The truth of Self cannot come through one who has not realized that he or she is the Self. Awakening comes not through logic and scholarship but from close association with an awakened master."

KATHA UPANISHAD, 1.2.9, TRANSLATED BY EKNATH EASWARAN

I believe that every single human being on this planet who possesses Atman vasana, or the sincere desire to irrevocably awaken to the truth of Self, also possesses a private desire to be helped along this inner journey. We all secretly hope we will encounter a sincere mentor, a way-shower. This desire is natural. An important Vedic text even dictates: "One who is searching for the Self must seek and submit one's ignorance unto a realized master, a guru."[1] A guru is one who knows the inner meaning of the sacred words, is fixed in the Self, and is expert in the revealed knowledge (awakening wisdom).

Yes, when your soul is ready to make that leap from unconsciousness to consciousness and, finally, to experiencing your own superconscious divine nature as Atman, the universe will match you up with that special soul who will help you along and lead you to the home inside you. Consider that teacher as a representative of that divine universe.

If you are looking for wisdom that does not ask you to become something more (and somehow prove your worthiness) or become less (and demonstrate your submissiveness), but simply to turn within and quietly rest in who you already are, a proud and beautiful sovereign being, then you may be seeking a Vedic guru.

Katha Upanishad summons all of humanity to undertake the great commitment of raising our collective consciousness from bondage to freedom so our default sleepwalking and darkness-filled minds shine with purity, luminosity, and universality. The seers of this Upanishad exclaim, "Arise! Awake! Enlighten yourself by resorting to the great teachings and teachers."[2] The dialogue between master and disciple is a fundamental component of the Vedas. The term "Upanishad" itself is derived from the Sanskrit words "upa" (near), "ni" (down), and "shad" (to sit)—"sitting down near" a spiritual teacher to receive instruction.

Gautama Buddha shared some beautiful words on this topic: "Like one pointing out hidden treasure, if one finds a person of intelligence who can recognize one's faults and take one to task for them, one should cultivate the company of such a wise one. He who cultivates a person like that is the better for it, not worse."[3]

Searching for a genuine guru nowadays, however, is like looking for a needle in a haystack. Even if one is a genuine teacher, the word "guru" has earned a bad reputation, thanks to the scandals surrounding lamas, swamis, rinpoches, and self-declared enlightened masters and avatars not yet ready to be a guru figure! They have not yet slain their own samsara snakes.

But you should not let false gurus keep you from finding your true guru. In this chapter I will shine the light on the Vedic concept of guru and the criteria to keep in mind in following or "unfollowing" of a teacher.

The Gift of a True Guru

My own life has been a journey from darkness to light. And the light is very much a gift of my guru. Fifty-four springs ago, I was born as the grandchild of a legendary, progressive-minded, householder Vedic guru—a remarkable yogi, renowned Ayurveda healer, and scholarly master of the nondual wisdom of the Vedas all rolled into one towering personality known by the name Baba Ayodhya Nath—in northern India, on the banks of the Himalayan River Sarayu, in the holy city of Ayodhya. This was where I grew up with my parents and extended family, in our ancestral home, under the spiritual guidance of my grandfather, whom I lovingly called "Baba."

Baba was my benevolent paternal grandfather, with kind eyes, a deep voice, and a flowing white beard. But he was an imposing, awe-inspiring guru to thousands, and son of Param Atman Shanti Prakash, who was himself a legendary spiritual teacher, Hindu saint, and Vedic scholar. Ours was a traditional family, renowned for countless generations in the Gangetic plains of India because we had shown people who had lost their way in life due to estrangement with their own true nature the way back to re-owning their spiritual truth as powerful sovereign beings, liberated from emotional, mental, social, and religious bondages. We showed them that they could touch something deeper that could be accessed from within their purified minds: their divine Self!

Thanks to tremendous good fortune, the sacred knowledge collectively known as "Vedic wisdom" came to me without my having to go search for it outside my home. For fourteen long years, I was steeped in formal learning of the Vedas under my guru, my grandfather, Baba, alongside regular schooling in arithmetic, biology, physics, and so forth.

I left my home to settle down after marriage in a new home (and as destiny would have it, in a new country), grateful to take with me the wisdom of the Vedic teachings on how to receive and give respect to the cosmos and all its creatures and how to be spiritually liberated from the delusions of my own mind.

Yet, shortly after I got married the first time, all hell broke loose as old, buried patterns of inability to be powerful and self-assured in intimate relationships surfaced as if out of nowhere. When we lose touch with our inner truth, we become shadow versions of ourselves, enslaved and imprisoned by our own self-betraying, self-belittling, self-abandoning minds. We give and receive unimaginable sorrow. This is what happened to me.

I was suffering due to my ego's lostness in maya. In this period, I almost forgot my way and was filled with losses — of important relationships, self-confidence, and physical health. A disconnect occurred between what I knew to be inherently true and how I thought and acted. Apparently, time with Baba studying the scriptures and purifying my ego was my undergraduate classroom, but *applying his teachings* was my advanced course of study.

My guru's wisdom did not let me down.

Cosmic intelligence ensured that the knowledge I had received, which told me I am powerful, blissful, and eternally pure without blemish, could be applied in my relationship classroom, too, to release me from my emotional bondages and claim my inherent soul-freedom. The wisdom resurfaced in my mind and became the boat in which I sailed back to solid ground, back to my worth and esteem. I came out of it feeling not like a victim or a perpetrator, but an "awakened, sovereign, joyous one" in the "now," ready to take responsibility for what I can do to be even more empathetic, and yet have even more clear boundaries.

This was accomplished with the insights I received from intense contemplations on teachings my Baba had imparted to me on the nature of Self.

"Shunya, you are not a physical body. You are a nonmaterial, entirely spiritual entity that dwells inside a body-suit, a soul made up of pure divine consciousness, and this life you are leading is a test for your soul to remember your hidden spiritual essence, celebrate your inherent connection to your creator, shine the divine light inside you, and be the best you can be. Indeed, this entire universe is a soul-schooling ground and evolution of consciousness opportunity. The super-sophisticated and ultra-intelligent yet subtle equipment all souls possess to navigate the universe and pass tests with divine ease and joy, is none other but the humble 'mind.' With spiritual reeducation and purifying self-awareness from the Vedas, the same mind, which is typically the domain of unconsciousness, greed, lust, self-sabotage, addictions, bondage, terror, pain, and confusion, and reduces us often to mere grasping, chasing, lamenting, fearful creatures (estranging us from our higher soul nature), can become our best friend, an illumined torch, guiding us through this mystical and mysterious universe. It will reintroduce you to your own inner freedom and power. It will make you a winner, every single time, in material and spiritual sense."

Thus, I was blessed with a genuine guru, my Baba. A true guru shows the way out of samsara, rather than leading you deeper into it.

Who May Not Be a Guru

Today, when almost anyone can call themselves a guru, it is important to briefly explore first who is *not* a guru.

There always have been and always will be true and ultra-sincere gurus. It's not worth discarding the chance to benefit from the knowledge of a genuine guru just because of a few false gurus in modern times.

Looking around, one could believe that anyone expert in anything is a guru. Today the world is full of "gurus"—tech guru, money guru, food guru. Due to this trivialization of an ancient tradition, we might fail to recognize our guru, even though we are waiting to find one. We may see "the one" as just one among many and allow our guru to wait while we connect with yet another (this time, perhaps a pastry-making?) guru.

There also is a prevalent trend of "seeking the inner guru," so the need for any human guru may be utterly dismissed. Sadly, we may then become disciples of our shadow self. If this means were effective, we would all be self-realized by now.

Some say that this "world" or "life" is a guru. But we can only learn from what we bring to it, in terms of our own state of mind. We deduce life lessons based upon the status of maya in our mind. Are we sleepwalking, semi-awake, or awakened in the world projected by maya? Different people will learn different lessons from the same experience. So, can it be a guru then for all of us?

Due to the publishing revolution—and we are all the better for it—the sacred Vedas and Upanishads are now available online, downloadable at a click. This gives rise to yet another illusion: that a specific book is my guru. While books impart paradigm-shifting new ideas, a book will not talk back to us; it cannot engage us in a dialogue to weed out false assumptions.

For some, their guru is a photo. This is especially of concern if the relationship is exclusively with a photo and not in addition to a full, living relationship with the guru. This is a sincere, but one-way, relationship. The shadow-self talks to its own self while the image simply sits there. Perhaps we should try to find a living representative of that beloved guru and seek living guidance. Or, keep this image intact and, with all due respect, seek out a new, living guru.

According to Vedic tradition, you need a living guru until your metaphysical self-ignorance is fully shed. Your goal is to awaken from the spell of illusions and appearances common to existence (maya) and embrace your own inner guru: the Self. The recent development of revering gurus in absentia is not traditional since it leads to subtle self-deception. The guru who has now moved on, is distant from us, or is inaccessible can be an inspiration—an ideal, worthy, and even reverential role model, but not a guru in a traditional Vedic sense.

A Vedic guru is always a living guru who can communicate with you in real time, and to whom you can pose questions and receive answers, or who can correct your train of thought and respond to your spiritual query. The awakening knowledge is not easy to grasp, and ego presents doubt after doubt. A teacher must be capable and willing to address the doubts.

And finally, let us address the "the internet is my guru" delusion. Nowadays, it is the norm to spend hours on the internet, watching videos of myriad spiritual teachers explaining diverse and sometimes even contradictory spiritual paths, techniques, and practices. There is nothing inherently wrong with looking up teachers online or even taking courses. Some of my best students have found me through my videos and online teachings.

However, if we are already delusional from vasana overload, we can misuse the free information out there and further delude ourselves into thinking we are already self-realized or awake, all the while fast asleep in maya and bypassing the issues we must face in our lives. From such a virtual-knowledge shopping spree, the mind is often seduced into hoarding bits and pieces of information selectively, from various spiritual sources into a grand samsara cart. Vasana-deluded minds cannot discriminate between wise and unwise, reality and myth, truth and falsehood, right and wrong, ethical and unethical to begin with. Despite the best teachers out there sharing what they know, such minds more often than not get even more confused between reality and appearances, fantasy and real awakening!

Even though we can find all kinds of spiritual teachings and teachers on the internet (including me), the personalized and long-term, systematic connection with a living guru is irreplaceable. Technology can be helpful, provided we at some point stop window-shopping, choose a teacher or tradition, and stick with it.

Even if you are studying remotely, you may be able to have a dialogue in which you can expect to have your questions answered, even if not immediately. If you learn from an online spiritual teacher who simply teaches without taking questions and may not even know that you are there, then appreciate them for being powerful beings shining inner light. You may even incorporate some of their wisdom. But they are not *your guru* yet. Why not take the next steps? Approach them. Ask to be a disciple. Manifest your guru through your own efforts, and go beyond the virtual screen into the deeper association that you deserve.

But then again, why rush to give a virtual guru the precious garland you threaded with flowers from your own inner garden, especially a guru who does not even know you or about you? What are you telling the universe? That you are so quick to be satisfied with spiritual guidance that you will settle for what you can get. I suspect that the internet-guru experience is leading even more people to believe that the master-student relationship is insignificant, when what we really need is to grasp maya by the horns and roar like a tigress or tiger, announcing from our inner being, *I am ready for my outer guru—I am here, ready. I am not leaving until I pierce this veil of self-ignorance and awaken to my inner guru.*

If you do settle for less—the world, a book, a photo, a video—then even if the Ultimate Reality were coming your way in the form of an outer guru in a guru body, with a guru mind, guru knowledge, and guru compassion to awaken your inner guru, they would turn back because you had already settled for a shadow. Maya strikes again!

As you can see, even in the matter of finding a teacher, illusion can take many forms in our mind and cloud our ability to judge! Maya is slippery and tricks us, and spiritual delusions can be concealed by the pious ego under glamorous highbrow spiritual outfits and unwarranted miraculous promises. So how do we know when we are in the presence of a true guru?

The Guru: A Classical Understanding

The Sanskrit word "guru" is derived from the root "ghri," which means "to enlighten the mind."

The sound "gu" refers to darkness, the great internal darkness of the mind's self-ignorance. The sound "ru" refers to the light of knowledge that drives away the darkness. This is an internal light, the light of Self. The guru is the one who dispels the darkness of ignorance of our blinding, suffering mind by igniting a steady lamp of knowledge.

According to the Vedas, a true guru's words remind us of our sovereign potential. A true guru won't ask us to worship them, for example, but rather to look for what is worth worshipping within ourselves.

The guru says look within (not toward me) to find the truth, your destination, where you can rest at last, inside you. The only trip that you must now accomplish is to turn toward your own Self. I am a consultant, a guide, a mentor, a professor of the Vedas, not God. The outer guru assists the emergence of your inner guru.

That is why the *Katha Upanishad* observes: "The extraordinary knowledge of Self cannot come through one who has not realized that he or she is the Self. Awakening comes not through logic, arguments, and scholarship (alone), but from close association with a living awakened master."[4]

All spiritual seekers, according to the Vedic tradition, are initially suffering from overexpressed samsaras. This includes the guru, when they were a student. Yet now, the guru should be free of samsara. They can see things for what they are and show us, at last, our own true potential. The "awakening scriptures" are said to act like mirrors. We see our "true spirit face" when we simply hear the description of our true Self.

As the venerable guru shares the knowledge of Self from the scriptures, deep-down concealed memories in the subconscious mind awaken in us, breaking through the spell of maya-dope. At this stage, to receive the knowledge, it helps to have a calm, meditating mind.

As we hear the expert expound on a greater truth, maya-dope relaxes its drugging grip on our mind. When we contemplate upon the truth, the delusions weaken even more. When we begin living contrary to the dictates of our obsessions, when we stop sleepwalking a scripted existence, then obsession-vasanas, which were virtual all along, completely fall away. We had given them way more power than they deserved!

Awakening in the Vedic tradition is like the treatment for someone suffering from amnesia. Various cues of the old personality are presented to the person, systematically and persistently, until full memory returns. Slowly but surely, from remembrance, the intellectual description becomes our living reality. Our body, family life, and eternal situations remain the same, but our consciousness is totally different. Our identity shifts from the small shadowy "i" to the real "I."

A respected Vedic text says this about the one seeking a guru: "To him who, thirsting for liberation from samsara, has sought the protection of the teacher, who abides by the knowledge, has a calm mind, and a serene heart. May the master give the knowledge of the truth with utmost kindness."

To this the guru responds: "Fear not, O learned one! There is no danger for you. There is a way to go beyond your own delusional suffering mind. I shall instruct you in the very path by which the ancient seers have reached that state. Whoever pursues this path is liberated from the bondage of samsara, mysteriously forged by spiritual ignorance, maya.

"You are indeed the supreme Self, but due to your association with ignorance, you find yourself under the bondage of the delusional mind, which is the sole cause of bondage. All the effects of ignorance, root and branch, are burnt down by the fire of self-knowledge, which arises from discrimination between these two—the Self and the ego."[5]

The tradition says that if you are ever matched with such a mentor, you are simply benefitting from the accumulated spiritual merit of countless prior births, and it is divine grace upon you that you are encountering such a teacher.

Therefore, a true guru does not bind us in more ropes but shows us how to cut the ropes and reclaim our inner freedom. You will find the guru is flying in free skies, and they will tell you that you can fly too. They show you where your wings are, metaphorically speaking, that you had forgotten all about after landing on this planet and in this body, thinking you are just a body!

A true guru in the Vedic sense is first and foremost a teacher of what I call the "awakening scriptures." Traditionally, a Vedic guru always belongs to a scripture-based lineage, since having received awakening wisdom of the Vedas from a qualified guru is an essential prequalification to be a guru themselves. This indicates that they have systematically received, know, and uphold the scriptural tradition and will transmit accurate teachings.

These teachings, received from the expert, the guru, impart not only fullness and inner power at every encounter, but a gradual and permanent lessening of maya-dope's grip on the seeker's mind and self-revelation of a higher paradigm of suffering-free existence within. The students become noticeably more emotionally mature and better human beings, and over time they suffer less from self-ignorance. Remember, awakening is gradual but permanent, not a fleeting, one-time event.

The Bhagavad Gita describes who can be a guru to the rest of humanity: "One who is not agitated despite the threefold miseries [physical, psychological, and existential], who is not excessively elated when experiencing pleasantness, and who is not depressed and remains free from attachment, fear, and anger possesses a steady mind in daily life."[6]

In due course, such an emotionally mature guru can grant awakening to ready disciples, not with a secret mantra, magical touch, special glance, or sacred sexual interaction, but through an accurate transmission of sacred knowledge of Self, taking the time it takes to teach, until self-ignorance is pierced and the beautiful Self is revealed in the student's now vasana-free, pure, and self-content mind.

The true guru does not simply teach feel-good tools for mere transient happiness but helps us pierce our delusions and put an end to the delusional mind. They help us discern between what is important versus trivial, eternal versus noneternal, and what we can ignore and what needs our attention to turn inward to our own higher truth. The true guru provides the critical knowledge of Self that leads to awakening as well as how to conduct ourselves in the world until we do awaken from this self-imposed, powerless, and often frightening existence.

In the classical, time-tested, nondual Vedic path, the path to awakening is structured and held within a system of checks and balances, with emphasis upon developing an inner ability to clear the cobwebs of our own false beliefs and discern between the eternal and the transient, truth and appearance, Self and ego. Then we enhance our understanding of Self versus non-Self and finally choose the Self alone. It is a slow but sure process.

Therefore, the Vedas arose from not one lone messiah-type leading masses of sleepwalkers, but from multitudes of awake figures at various degrees of self-realization, who are in alignment with greater truth. Vedic spirituality is not a one-time revelation through the eyes of one messenger or one god alone; it is a divine revelation that is continuous, ongoing, eternal, and ever available to any human of any age, color, or race in any moment.

However, the ultimate guru in the Vedic tradition is the scripture (the Upanishads) since the knowledge contained within them awakens the Self when it is heard or contemplated. I personally like this. It keeps the human ego in check, while knowledge remains paramount in a self-knowledge-based, not personality-based, tradition.

How to Spot a Genuine Vedic Master

It can be useful to have something of a checklist when looking for a true guru.

+ A Vedic master can be a monk or a householder. Either way, they are not confused about their lifestyle or their relationship with sex, and they don't mix up their paths. They never sleep with their students. Period.

- True masters feel secure and whole inside themselves and good about their life. A true master models inner fullness, remains humble and non-pretentious, and always reminds you of your sovereign truth. They don't depend on you to make them feel better or important. They are not narcissistic. They won't ask you to bow to them because they are God or God's messenger. They thrive in solitude and society alike. They don't do desperate things to attract attention.

- Following the Vedic tradition, a guru always has a teacher who taught them step-by-step, not for a few weeks or a few months, but for several uninterrupted years. They are not self-taught, and ideally, they belong to a lineage of teachers that provides cultural immersion so that the teachings are understood in their intended context. Because it is an oral lineage, a genuine process of succession is the only route to access the Vedic knowledge.

- A true master will exhibit emotional maturity and command of their senses. They may have had a personal learning curve and suffered from self-ignorance when they were themselves students, but now that they are a guru, they are aware of their role, duty, and responsibility to seekers and the path they uphold. Therefore, they are in control of their minds, not just pretending to be in control. They don't have "oops" moments or hidden character flaws that may emerge suddenly due to spiritual bypassing. They are truly enlightened; they teach what they know to be true, and they live an internally expanded life.

- At the same time, they are transparent about their humanity; they don't pretend to be superhuman despite possessing an elevated consciousness. They can admit minor shortcomings as human beings and withstand constructive criticism gladly.

- They are friendly and loving toward all beings, but they have healthy boundaries.

- They cite the benefits of ethical living, discernment, and self-inquiry, versus promises of miracles, dreams, blessings, gems, gizmos, mantras, chakras, extraordinary visions, or dependency on them in any form whatsoever.

- They hold the scriptures higher than themselves as the ultimate source of awakening knowledge and do not dismiss or negate them while teaching or giving discourses. In fact, their lifestyle demonstrates how much they have internalized the wisdom of the Vedas. They walk the talk.

- They are always approachable and real. Any association with them will leave you clearer and calmer inside. You will feel more empowered, freer, and more sovereign in their presence because they transmit the self-knowledge that ends the hold of self-ignorance on your mind.

In the Vedic tradition, true gurus never declare themselves as God. They remain awakened humans, albeit ones who know deep inside themselves their divine Self. They do not ask to be worshipped or pampered like gods. They serve others with their divine compassion and wisdom.

A True Guru Is Always Transparent

Transparency bears further discussion, as the lack of it has caused modern seekers no end of trouble. Since maya strikes universally, the Vedic tradition holds that there is no reason for a guru to feel shame or hide their less-than-perfect past or make up stories of divine intervention. Ultimately it is our inner light that we embody today that matters, regardless of what trail of darkness we leave behind.

The tradition acknowledges that a future guru may start out as a regular individual, identified with maya, emotionally suffering to a greater or lesser degree, along with a sincere desire to transcend ignorance. Teachers from the rather realistic Advaita tradition almost never lay claims to a perfect outer personality; they always share how they, too, were once vulnerable, since maya strikes every mind. They will share how they applied self-knowledge from the Vedas to go beyond their shadow, with all its strengths and weaknesses, to claim their true Self. Their own past vulnerabilities, challenges, and inspirations are used to inspire their disciples.

Baba candidly shared with me how his rage colored his samsara when he started out and how he saw through it at last. Then he said to me:

"Let a guru share his or her own past fragility through poem, story, and play, so that the student can know: 'I, too, will overcome. So what if I started as

a meager stream—I am always as pure as the River Ganges herself. I am the Self. I am the splendid Atman.'"

The Vedas tell the story of Vishwamitra, a seer of the *Rig-Veda*. Prior to his own awakening, his samsara was colored with lust, rage, pride, and jealousy, so much so that he even tried to murder a sage he was envious of. But at the same time, he was a true yogi. Despite the attachments and aversions in his mind, he did not give up on himself, and he continued to effort, to purify his mind. Vishwamitra ultimately did break free from his own shadow. He did discover who he was after all. And when that happened, there was no looking back for him. In fact, he became a celebrated seer of the Vedas, renowned as a Brahmarishi, the "knower of the ultimate truth." He gave us the great Gayatri Mantra, which I will share with you in a later chapter.

A Conceptual Difficulty with Submission to a Guru

In contemporary times, the requirement to find and submit to a guru sets this challenge: Isn't submission to a human guru contrary to the goal of sovereignty?

I respond to this important question in this way: To a teacher whom you have accepted after due examination and discernment, submit your self-ignorance, not your self-esteem or your right to self-determine your life!

Nowhere does the classical Vedic tradition ask for the student to become a subservient slave. This exists in certain cults, but it is a pathology emanating from the corrupted minds of false gurus and deluded, sleepwalking disciples. It is not the pure and pristine tradition of the Vedas.

The Vedic tradition is built not on blind trust, but rather trust supported by reason. It supports regular dialogue between seeker and master. The seeker must not accept everything the master says until the seeker has full clarity.

Submission is something we do all the time. We submit our health to the hands of a doctor; we submit our child to the hands of a trusted babysitter. We even surrender our entire body and life into the hands of our trusted surgeon before going under anesthesia. If we want to master algebra, we must surrender our ignorance to an esteemed math professor who has the right credentials. To learn, we must let go of what we "know" and acknowledge openly that the professor is the expert and we are the novice. We must submit our ego's tendency to control or be dominant during the learning process if we truly want to learn anything.

The word "submission" is a poor translation for the Sanskrit word *vinay*. Vinay refers to all aspects of the way in which we engage with an awakened being. Vinay reflects our own respect for this path and our internal commitment to self-knowledge.

Before submitting our ignorance to a guru, what we must ascertain is the guru's worthiness. The Vedas talk about teachers examining seekers before taking them on as students. Teachers are frequently asked to test students' intentions, morals, and commitment to the path. But the Vedas don't give this privilege exclusively to the guru. They ask seekers to examine the guru before taking them on as mentor and teacher. This keeps everyone on their toes.

In its purest form, the tradition focuses on a formal spiritual reeducation process, a systematic study of awakening scriptures, and a highly intentional and sacred journey of ego sublimation under a guru's guidance to awaken our own inner guru (the Self). A self-declared enlightened master who went up a mountain as a normal person and then came down the mountain announcing themselves as an awakened being is an exception in the nondual Vedic tradition. Our scriptures mostly stay silent on such one-off experiences of solo spiritual liberation and suggest that perhaps this person received wisdom from a qualified guru too, but in a previous lifetime.

In every case, a guru is indispensable. When a person is truly ready to experience the truth of Self, a knower of Self manifests miraculously and leads the way.

Avoid Sleepwalking Gurus and Disciples

There are, unfortunately, both sleepwalking gurus and sleepwalking disciples. It is critical you stay clear of their influence. Never surrender your mind to such minds, no matter what you are promised in return, be it heaven, nirvana, mukti, enlightenment, sacred sex, or miraculous healing.

From the womb of sleepwalking samsaras often emerge sleepwalking spiritual teachers, ready to save the world, throwing around Sanskrit jargon without understanding the true meaning of the words in their venerable Hindu and Buddhist contexts. Such teachers rarely comprehend the sacrifices the seers had to make to attain such wisdom. And often equally unconscious disciples emerge out of nowhere for such teachers. These disciples are mostly disempowered individuals, estranged from reality, needy, emotionally delusional, with egos operating overtime under the influence of obsessive cravings.

There is a reason why through the ages the greatest spiritual truths have been transmitted with the greatest care by the master, only to a steady and deserving seeker with a pure and stable mind. Otherwise, when sleepwalking disciples become sleepwalking teachers in the future, who will awaken humanity? Sometimes sleepwalking followers feel taken advantage of and yet are willing to be abused if it will lead to their "awakening." The sleepwalking teacher believes themselves enlightened and takes what they will from their students as their just due. Who should we blame when self-ignorance is a universal phenomenon? All characters in such unconscious situations require correct knowledge to set themselves free from the grips of vasana-obsessions and help them make empowered choices based on correct discernment.

A sincere seeker may reflect on this Vedic passage as a caution: "True wisdom never arises to a person who acts in accordance with what the people of the world will say or to a person who is concerned about pedagogic knowledge from the scriptures and who is subject to delusions such as 'I am the body.'"[7]

Many seekers, consumed with worldly vasanas, take on a guru simply through herd mentality. They may not wait for the teacher who speaks to their heart. In the grip of obsessive tendencies, they may quickly take initiation into a spiritual tradition and devote their entire life to a spiritual path they were never really meant to walk. I know many sincere individuals who lost decades worshipping a false guru or studying a tradition without ever pausing to ask themselves, "Why am I studying this tradition?" When they emerge from such automatic behavior, it is as if they had been asleep the whole time, mindlessly engaged in beliefs and practices that never took them far. When they felt conflicted, they were told that they did not have enough faith, that their qualms were their own fault.

Running on the hamster wheel of worldly vasana-obsessions, you will experience only bondage, never freedom, constantly feeling anxious as you compare your spiritual life to standards set by others.

In spirituality, it is so important to be vigilant
of appearances that make us fall asleep.

When unconsciousness rules, the gender of the body continues to matter, even in the spiritual arena. It makes us seek our teacher in a specific male or female body, with a very specific gender preference, never realizing that it is rare enough to find a true teacher. We must accept the teacher's body, as it comes, regardless of gender, if our teacher's Self is to lead us to our Self.

Body-obsessed people are also quite fashion-conscious too. Even if they encounter a true teacher or a genuine spiritual path, they nevertheless think less about the wisdom coming their way. They remain ultra-conscious of how to dress "spiritually" versus how to think and behave spiritually. Their previous biases, judgments, and worldly assumptions remain fundamentally unchanged, except now they are wearing all-new—even designer—holy garb (shawls, malas, amulets).

Sometimes body vasana compels us to choose the teacher with the largest number of "bodies" following them. The tally of followers and symbols of bodily transcendence, such as a shaved head, dreadlocks, spiritual tattoos, scars or marks of penance and holiness, or other signs, count much more than the purity of the teaching itself. The ultimate question *Who am I?* gets lost in bodily experiences that give us a temporary thrill. Spirituality is reduced to risky sex, extreme sports, drug-induced highs, and body-based yoga fads such as naked yoga, beer yoga, or paddleboard yoga.

It is unfortunate, but in an unconscious, obsession-driven society, the so-called teacher figure is sometimes smitten with body vasana as well. In this case, the so-called guru may claim they can shorten the student's arduous spiritual journey of many years to five or ten minutes simply by having sex with them, couching it as the ultimate transmission of "potency." Or, vasana-smitten disciples may copulate with each other in the search of a beyond-body truth, while still locked inside a body-based mental consciousness.

Therefore, even in spiritual matters, the three obsessions called vasanas (which I discussed more fully in chapter 5) can get in the way of true, lasting transformation. Maya-dope and its hallucinations work overtime on our ego, warping our perceptions and leading us astray from our potential to know our truth of Self.

Unexamined vasanas can bind us to this world, our bodies, and even confuse us in the realm of spiritual knowledge. Vedic words like "guru," "karma," "dharma," "tantra," "chakras," and "yoga" are often abused, and the great tradition of a sincere guru leading a true seeker back to the Self within is sometimes sadly mocked or tainted. In the grip of vasanas, even our spiritual journey can land us back into our delusional samsara as fuel for more suffering.

Three Stages of Gradual Awakening

If we take the time to internalize a true teacher's guidance and take baby steps to live the wisdom authentically in daily life, we begin acting from a greater knowingness. The Vedas do not recognize instant awakening, but rather a gradual remembering of our truth. Traditionally, it is recommended that nondual wisdom from the Bhagavad Gita and Upanishads be imbided in three stages to prevent spiritual bypassing—that insidious trap of imagining ourselves spiritual, beyond our sorrows, awake, or enlightened when we have simply covered up our wounds with spiritual jargon, attitudes, and beliefs.

The first stage is called *sharvanam* and involves the senses. The guru's speech is received in the ear. The guru's writings (and writings of former gurus contained in scriptures) are read by the eyes, repeatedly. Typically, this is a twelve-year-long process, and that alone prevents hasty illusory awakenings! The guru's behavior is watched by the eyes (thus this is a good time to walk away if it is not of the highest standard). I was fortunate to spend fourteen uninterrupted years in this stage with my guru. I listened attentively when he gave discourses. I read his writings repeatedly, and I watched him conduct his life with inner freedom as a bold Self, not a frightened or manipulative ego, despite constraining outer circumstances. It was very inspiring and reassuring that, yes, one can lead a life that looks ordinary outside but is extraordinary within!

The second stage is called *mananam* and involves the mind. This can accompany the first stage or be its own stage. A new problem arises: How do I take this feeling of spiritual sovereignty—this clarion call of a higher truth that makes so much sense in the presence of my teacher—and bring it into all the moments that I am not sitting with my teacher? What do I need to do to keep remembering the Self all the time? The Vedas say it is simple. Contemplate the wisdom you have received in the privacy of your own mind, steadily, repeatedly, until all doubts are resolved, such as doubts pertaining to the technical terms ("samsara," "maya," "vasana," and so on), the goal of the philosophy, and dos and don'ts of the path. Questions must arise in this stage. A true guru provides answers gladly. Mananam brings about intellectual conviction. Because of mananam, after I married and left my Baba's home, my domestic and social life became my school. I got to contemplate my guru's wisdom in the laboratory of my householder life.

The final stage, *nidhidhyasanam,* involves the heart. This stage is one of steadfast conviction. It literally means beginning to heartfully live inside our daily lives with new Veda-empowered emotional convictions, beliefs, and attitudes behind all our thoughts, actions, and engagements in the world. This stage confirms that what we have heard, read, and believed to be true from our teacher and the scriptures is indeed true and that sovereignty is not only possible, but in fact our birthright. Seekers find themselves in this final stage flowering into a new paradigm, making new choices that are more inwardly sovereign right *now,* even amid a million opposing options, obligations, and circumstances. In the middle of our relationship challenges, losses, and adversities, when we begin living and responding as the Self, the sovereign one, we begin remembering our original whole, blissful, beautiful soul nature, soul gifts, soul power, and fearless, boundless soul essence. Our personal experience and validation alone, not hearsay, completes our learning. This brings about the deepest emotional conviction, personality transformation, and spiritual elevation from darkness to light! No wonder an ancient text joyfully exclaims: "In inner union with the great reality, self-luminous like the sun, one goes beyond bondage and mortality to discover sovereignty and immortality, for one possesses ALL; for then you are one with this Great Reality."[8]

Thanks to Baba and this immersive three-step learning process, even though he has transitioned from his body, I am able to irrevocably remember that I am beautiful, whole, and perfect right now, despite any ugliness, brokenness, or imperfections in my relationships. The gifts of remembering my true nature are nonstop. Now I find I am no longer so attached to my individuality because I have reclaimed my connection with something bigger—my universality.

The sovereignty I experience is so enormous, and beyond the mind, that all I can do is release a few inadequate words to describe the truth that lies beyond words, like eager birds, set out to map an infinite open sky. The birds come back, humbled, as their wings must fold in prayer to that one Self, in which we take our flights, seek ourselves with all our tiny might, and return home, at last, to rest in THAT, who always was, is, and will be, here, always. As my guru had hoped and prepared me for, after years of study the bud of his lineage's wisdom blossomed in his disciple's heart. I did become worthy of the gifts of wisdom he bequeathed me with such searing honesty and loving generosity. The fragrance of my Self is unmistakable. It is spreading and awakening the Self in many heart lotuses.

> *Thank you, my guru Baba, thank you for rescuing me from drowning in the ocean of samsara that froths and fumes in my own mind. The knowledge you imparted me, of my true Self, saved me from my own lethal ignorance.*

Do not panic if you long for a guru and have not found one yet. When your thirst for spiritual knowledge becomes intense, it is the responsibility of the universe to match you with one, promises the Vedas.

My student writes:

"Your beloved guru will come forth at the moment you think all may be lost. The guru will reveal the seed that has been lying dormant within your heart all along. Your Self will be unearthed. Your intuition will spread her wings. Your mind, now tranquil, will connect to the teachings. You have given up egoic control for your inner light to emerge. Stability, clarity, and unbounded consciousness will be the fruits you reap."

When you are ready, a living teacher or their teachings will manifest and remind you of your spiritual bigness and blissful wholeness. You may not even be consciously looking for a teacher or teachings, but somehow a great awakened soul's teachings will reach you, awaken you, empower you. Deep-down concealed memories in the subconscious mind will awaken in you, breaking through the spell of forgetfulness. You will recognize your outer guru when you are ready for the final journey toward your inner guru, the Self.

In meantime, let my words guide you forward.

PART II

Tools to Unmask
Your Sovereignty

9

Sakshi: Cultivating Your Inner Witness

"Self is the internal ruler.

Self is never seen, but is the witness;

Self is never heard, but is the hearer;

Self is never thought, but is the thinker;

Self is never known, but is the knower.

There is no other witness but Self, no other hearer but Self, no other thinker but Self, no other knower but Self."

BRIHADARANYAKA UPANISHAD, 3.7.23

Witness consciousness has become a universally popular spiritual practice, but it originated in the ancient Vedic Upanishads, specifically the *Mandukya Upanishad*. Cultivating witness consciousness is essential for the cognitive tools offered in this section of the book, practices such as meditation, discernment, nonattachment, and the management of our thoughts and emotions.

To be a witness of something implies that one is watching and observing it objectively, as if standing apart from the situation and not identifying with it. The practice of witness consciousness teaches us that our emotions are passing phenomena and not our true nature. By developing this watchfulness along with an ability to observe ourselves even in difficult circumstances, we can gradually weaken the roots of self-ignorance and transform our mind.

With constant practice, the *sakshi bhava*, or witness awareness, can be invoked at will and remains constantly with us, through day and night. It becomes a way of life. We become aware of a part of ourselves that is the observer and a part that is the actor; the observer watches without judging. By virtue of a greater awareness, the actor in the mind starts making better choices. Being in this observer mode means that you are constantly alert, examining every action and thought, even if subconsciously. It helps the mind see the motives behind an ill-advised action or thought, which can lead to hurting self or another. This becomes a spiritual practice, or *sadhana*, and it is a core discipline in the tradition of nondual Vedanta, arising from the Upanishads.

The Four States of Mind

In the *Mandukya Upanishad*, literally translated as the "Frog Upanishad," three states of mind—waking, dreaming, and deep sleeping—are compared to lily pads. The ego-based individual is compared to a frog who compulsively and ceaselessly jumps from one lily pad to another its entire life while the real Self watches in the background, unchanging.

That is why another name for Self in the Vedas is *sakshi*. It simply means "the observer, the witness." Self observes the intellect, mind, ego, memory, senses, and, via the senses, the world. As an observer, the Self is said to witnesses all the changes in the body and mind, through waking, dreaming, and dreamless deep sleep, but itself remains unmodified.

If waking, dreaming, and deep sleep of the ego-mind are three states of consciousness, then the fourth is the state of pure witnessing consciousness, the natural and original state of the Self. It is the background that underlies and transcends the other three common states of consciousness.

The seers announce their findings:

"Indescribable, the unified consciousness in essence,

Peaceful, auspicious, without duality,

Is the fourth stage, that Self, the knower of all, that is to be known."

MANDUKYA UPANISHAD, 7

"I see without eyes, hear without ears. Assuming various forms, I know everything. There is no one who is the knower of me. I am ever, the pure awareness."

KAIVALYA UPANISHAD, 21

Witnessing Awareness Is Always Impersonal

The Self acts like the sun with the ability to observe the world without engaging with it. Sunlight is always impersonal, and it illumines everything—the good, the bad, the ugly, and the lovely—without preferences.

Recognizing that there is an impersonal, witnessing, higher awareness that is always nonattached and transcends our reactive, grasping, judging, sorrowful, and often-vindictive mind is only the first step. What the entire Vedic tradition is trying to tell us is something else. Let go of the crutches and find your new feet! You were never the maya-defined shadow personality to begin with! All along, you were the Self, whose very nature is pure transcendental awareness. The "actor" is a false egoic notion, simply a construct of beliefs—a case of mistaken identity. It cages you behind bars of egoic limitations, likes, dislikes, grief, anger, and delusions.

But the moment you begin truly entertaining the idea that, *Wait a minute, perhaps I am nothing but pure awareness*, and step back to observe even your own body-mind and its things and its relationships, then presto, your whole life changes!

That is why Baba reminded me repeatedly:

"Shunya, your real nature is as the one perfect, free consciousness, the all-pervading witness—unattached to anything, desireless, and at peace. It is from illusion that you seem to be involved in samsara. You have long been trapped in the snare of identification with the body. Sever it with the knife of knowledge that 'I am awareness. I am sakshi.' You are unconditioned and changeless, formless and immovable, unfathomable awareness and unperturbable. So, hold to nothing but witnessing consciousness as your identity. Through this initiation into truth, you will escape falling into unreality again."

When you begin viewing yourself in this pure way, as a witness, anything is possible, including an experience of emotional unboundedness and divine interconnectivity with the entire universe. Why? Because you share this awareness with all others together—like individual waves share the ocean. The ocean remains whole even if countless waves fall and rise in it. Awareness is your complete identity.

You exist. Your existence needn't prove itself to you. Your inner witness, who is quietly aware, is self-revealed, self-illumined, and self-known since without this original spiritual awareness, nothing can be known. This awareness is the ultimate reality because it does not come and go. It just is. Meditate on this ultimate reality. Meditating on Self, your mind will automatically be abundant (purna), filled with objectless contentment (santosha), peaceful for no reason (shanta), joyful in its own nature (ananda), and divinely full without effort to acquire externally (tushta).

Witnessing Awareness Is Always Ever Pure

"I am free of thoughts, and free of forms.

I am connected to all sense organs as I pervade everything and am everywhere.

I am ever changeless. There is no freedom or bondage in me.

I am of the nature of pure awareness, consciousness, and limitlessness.

I am Shiva, the auspicious. I am Shiva, the supreme happiness."

NIRVANA SHATAKAM, 6

The thoughts that arise in the mind may be pure or impure, but they do not affect the sakshi. The witnessing remains pure, detached, untainted by any activity of the mind. The sakshi witnesses without judgment or desire for a certain outcome. Just like sunlight is not affected by the impurities in the objects it may illumine, the inner witness remains ever pure. Witnessing is not an action—it is the state of being of the Self.

Thus, witnessing is simply effortless seeing without needing the function of senses. Witnessing transcends the egoic actor. Meditating on your innermost stillness, this pure observer Self as your deepest nature, will release any lingering feelings of worry, stress, or anxiety.

Identify with Your Inner Witness, Not Your Inner Actor

I invite you, dear reader, to awaken to your witnessing nature, free from the fiction, drama, and predicaments of your personal egoic actor. This is simple, effortless awareness. You may be walking, eating, and engaging in other activities of your busy life, and yet be maintaining an inner identity as pure witnessing Self.

The knowledge that you are the witnessing Self, not the acting and reacting ego-mind self, marks the end of separate egoic consciousness and heralds the doorway to the Self. Go another step further and begin thinking that *I am the Self, not mind—I am pure, ever-free awareness*. This is the spiritual goal that leads to moksha—liberation from the bondage of samsara.

You Are Not Your Body: The Story of Sage Ashtavakra

Ashtavakra was a revered Vedic sage who is said to have composed one of the greatest treatises of nondual wisdom, known as the *Ashtavakra Gita*.

The name "Ashtavakra" means "one who has eight deformities." Indeed, the sage was born with a body that was twisted in eight places. Ashtavakra grew up in the home of his maternal grandfather Sage Aruni, who was a great seer and ran a traditional Vedic school where Ashtavakra received knowledge of Self.

One day, he learned that before he was born, his father had met unfair treatment, so he set out to meet the king. Arriving at the king's court to ask for clemency for his punished father, he dragged himself across the court. The king's men and ministers looked at him and started to laugh because of his physical deformities.

Ashtavakra first looked on in silence and then broke into smiles. Everyone was shocked. When asked who he was and why he was smiling, Ashtavakra responded that he was disappointed to find only shoemakers in the assembly instead of wise men because shoemakers invariably only look at the body made of matter (leather) and rarely enter spiritual or metaphysical contemplations to see what lies beyond the body.

Ashtavakra told the king that his counselors were only seeing his body coated with leather everywhere (that is, his skin), judging superficially on its smoothness or roughness. They did not see his true Self. They had no realization of the soul and the God. Ashtavakra concluded that perhaps he had wasted his time coming to the assembly.

Upon hearing the words of Ashtavakra, the king and everyone in the assembly were deeply affected and awakened from unconsciousness. The king immediately recognized that this was no ordinary teenager, but one awake to Atman. The king bowed down to Ashtavakra, the Realized Being. He escorted Ashtavakra to his own throne and washed his distorted and twisted feet with tears falling from his eyes. Ashtavakra, the one who knew he was not his body and was always free from what he was not, went on to become one of the wisest Vedic sages and inspired many minds by challenging them to think differently.

The Seen vs. the Seer

From the story of Ashtavakra, let me share two universal laws from the Vedas that Baba taught me and that I meditated on consistently. I am confident they will help you too.

Law 1: I am different from what I experience. The first law states that I am different from whatever I experience. So, if I am experiencing suffering, I am not suffering. If I am experiencing thoughts such as *I am so small, I am so bad, I am so horrible,* I am not that. If we can fully comprehend this important law, it will end our need for approval and assimilation at any cost and the feeling of being lost in the world when rejected. My body may be undergoing cancer or some other difficulty, but I will be fine because I am different from what I am experiencing. Then my attitude will be amazing, exceptional, and perhaps inspiring to others. Why? Because I am not the body.

This may sound academic, but as we contemplate this idea more and more, a separation occurs. Just like when we are very caught up in a task and we take a breath, we separate from the task and feel some relief. But what if we keep separating from whatever we observe? I am not that. I observe my mind—I am not that. I observe my emotions, good or bad—I am not that. I observe the world—I am not that. I happen to be *observing* the world, it is my experience, but I am not the world or my experience of the world.

Law 2: I am free from whatever I am not.   The second law states that I am free from whatever I am not, so I can make my choices in freedom. At some point, every leader who has spoken up against abuse, victimization, and colonization, must have said, "I don't buy that, and I am free." When Nelson Mandela spoke up against apartheid when so many were feeling small and powerless, he must have felt free the entire time. Despite twenty-two years of "imprisonment," he walked out free and powerful. Twenty-two minutes of sitting quietly by yourself can break you apart, yet Nelson Mandela sat quietly for twenty-two years in jail saying, "I am free." It is an internal movement: "I am free."

Guided Practice: Witnessing

The awakened one is always real; they feel all their feelings but do not identify with any of them. Self, which is expansive awareness, allows all thoughts and feelings to emerge, but is not changed by any one of them.

This is how I instruct my students in witnessing practice:

Allow both joyful and sorrowful thoughts, feelings, and emotions to flow through your mind, unresisted, without preferring one or feeling aversion for the other. You are the Self, not your thoughts or emotions.

Stop going to war with yourself. Instead, bring greater presence to negative emotions. Feel them fully, deeply, without self-deception or additional self-affliction. Hold painful feelings gently in mindful attentiveness, like you would hold an injured dove, needing to shed a tear and wait until its wings heal. Time is all it needs. With the help of our big Self, our injured small self can mend, heal, and then, in divine ease, be released. Then it can fly with invisible wings and disappear back into pure existence, from where everything emerges—both sorrow and joy.

Feelings are impermanent; their nature is to be in a state of movement, while you, pure consciousness, can allow them safe passage. It is the nature of clouds to change, come and go, rise and subside, scatter away by the lightest breeze, or build up into an ominous thunder. But the sky itself is still and can never be affected by whatever the clouds do or don't do. Sky simply is. It need not control any of the clouds' activity.

Simply "sit with" any emotions troubling you such as fear, guilt, shame, even jealousy, greed, sadness, loneliness, or a sense of abandonment. Sit with the emotions rolling in your mind. Observe them roll by just like clouds rolling by in the open sky, without reactivity.

Gradually let each cloud of emotion fade away until all that is left is the open sky. Radiate your inner peace. Know that in the background of even the most distressful emotional landscape is peace, the nature of the sky, the nature of the Self.

Witnessing Is an Internal Recognition of Freedom

Indeed, egoic being, you are not your "name and age and job and suffering and story"; you are pure being, a subjective awareness "I am," which is completely devoid of thought and emotions or any egoic labels, such as "I am thinking this," or "I am feeling that."

My student Elliott R. describes it like this:

"I used to think of witnessing as connected to a physical space like watching an event taking place outside of myself. When I was witnessing, I was standing apart looking on a street corner witnessing the passing scene. The witnessing that we are learning about through the Upanishads is completely different. I now understand that the acting part—the moving, talking, crying actor (jiva)—is of a lower order of reality. The witnessing part, which is unchanging, is of the real order.

For me, this means that when caught in a web of thoughts or feelings of attachments and aversions, I can become fused to all the changes believing that I am the actor and the changes. As the witness, there is a shift not in physical space but in consciousness: I am the calm, still, changeless center, no longer identified with the ups and downs of the actor's predicament. As the witness Self, 'the reality' experiences the jiva as the actor amid 'samsara.' This is the real order.

As I was contemplating this, an image came to me: I saw myself as the canvas upon which there were brushstrokes and layers of paint that had become a picture. As the actor, I am the painted picture. As the witness, I am the clear, unmodified ground on which the paint has been applied. The light is always within."

My student Vaidehi said:

"Often, my prejudices and biases stare me in the face—my judgments about people, things, and situations. I don't want to hide from them anymore. So how should I face them? For example, I may feel that a person deserves their suffering because of their previous action or lack of it, their inability to discern. I can ride the high horse of judgment or the camel of condescension or simply be grounded, supportive, ready to offer a smile, an ear that can listen, a heart of love and compassion, a mind with clarity. Thanks to this inner discernment via the intellect, the weight of ego and pride starts to lessen.

My teacher says act 'without a mental fever.' What does that mean? To me, it aptly describes the moment when I remember that I am the sakshi—the witness, the observer. Not a bystander, mind you. It reminds me to be actively engaged in the process of my life but without this sense of being driven, compelled, impatient, wanting to control the outcome of events. The moment I forget, I start manipulating, bossing others around, and losing it. Instead of the feeling of oneness, I start feeling that people, situations, and objects are hindering me and have become obstacles on the path of my success. When I am willing to let go of the fever, then as sakshi, the witness, I start taking a step toward creativity, expansiveness, intuition, and compassion."

Witnessing is the mode of awareness being aware of itself. When this happens, we are centered in the present moment and can gain an all-new, fresh perspective. We can be reminded that we have the unique ability to be aware of two states of consciousness at the same time: the egoic mind-based consciousness and the witnessing consciousness that watches over the other. Increasingly, we can catch ourselves in the middle of any egoic, heated discussion and remember, *I am the nonattached witnessing awareness. What am I doing getting attached and emotionally triggered in regard to the outcome of this contest of words?*

It is important to distinguish that which changes, the "seen," from that which doesn't change, the "seer." The key is to continue thinking of yourself as a witnessing consciousness, the eternal seer. Then everything you "see," no matter how ugly or tragic, cannot "get you." It has no ultimate power over you. Your mind may be jumping around like a monkey. So, let it jump around. With knowledge that you are not what you observe, you can view the monkey mind, and all its contents, with dispassion. And then, you can shift your attention to what you prefer—write your own destiny.

"If you wish to be free,

Know you are the Self,

The witness of everything,

The heart of awareness.

Set your body aside.

Sit inside your own awareness.

You will at once be happy,

Forever still,

Forever free.

Right or wrong,

joy and sorrow,

these are of the mind only,

they are not yours.

It is not really you who acts or enjoys,

you are everywhere, forever free.

Forever and truly free,

the single witness of all things."

ASHTAVAKRA GITA, 1.4–7, TRANSLATED BY THOMAS BYROM

In my own journey to awakening, witnessing played a big role. As we discussed, in witness consciousness external events or internal experiences are like waves occurring on an ocean, and witness consciousness is like the ocean itself. The ocean just lets the waves do their thing, while it stays unchanged.

The ocean does not get traumatized or go into depression when its largest wave, its dream project, its hope for the future, and its savior crashes into a trillion droplets. Nor does it go crazy with joy when its tiniest, almost-nonexistent droplet builds itself into a giant tidal wave. The ocean comes with inherent intelligence, knowing that with every rise comes its predestined fall and that every fall is really a rise in the making. This is the wheel of life. Witness consciousness allows this existential circular motion, at every level.

I remembered Baba's words to me:

"You are everywhere,

Forever free.

If you think you are free,

You are free.

If you think you are bound,

You are bound.

Meditate on the Self.

One without two,

Exalted awareness."

Witness consciousness enabled me to see that I am neither a victim nor an aggressor, that the drama of my life can proceed any which way, and I can watch it like I watch a movie full of emotion, drama, and suspense, but never leap into any dramatic or manipulative action. Any necessary action that I did take as I went ahead with my human life as a wife, mom, and teacher proceeded from a relatively neutral, adequately discerned, and detached position, thereby creating minimal reaction (anticipation, fear, or hope), damage (internal or external), or consequences (propensity for delayed outcomes).

Becoming aware of the observer, you may note a whole different silent presence within, the infinite, indivisible, inexhaustible spiritual Self. This encounter with the Self is known as *Atmabodha*: Atman ("Self"), bodha ("knowing, recognition, realization").

Self-knowledge set me free. It will set you free too.

10

Dhyanam: Meditating on the Inner Self for Inner Freedom

"The earth is meditating as it were.

The space is meditating as it were.

The heaven is meditating as it were.

Waters are meditating as it were.

Mountains are meditating as it were.

Gods are meditating as it were.

Therefore, those amongst humans

who attain greatness, do so, because of meditation."

CHANDOGYA UPANISHAD, 7.6.1–2

Meditation, known as *dhyanam,* is a core discipline first imparted by the Vedic seers to the world. In this chapter, I offer the meditation techniques of my lineage—embodied, cognitive tools to uncover your inner sovereignty.

Thought-Less vs. Thought-Full Meditation

The technique of first ridding the mind of thoughts to find the Self reflects the teachings emphasized by just one ancient Indian yogi-scholar, Sage Patanjali

(2 BCE–2 CE), whose views are widely popular among Indian and Western yoga and spiritual teachers. For mere circumstantial reasons, this sage and his work, the *Yoga Sutras*, became better known in the West than the much older core tradition of the Vedic Upanishad texts and Bhagavad Gita. It became the accepted way, though in the traditional sense, it was only a marginal point of view—not central to the much older teachings of yoga as first elucidated in the Upanishads. Today, many a yoga teacher defines yoga as the stage of complete cessation of thought waves (*yoga chitta vritti nirodha*). But for all but expert yogis, reaching the state of no thoughts, or *samadhi*, is not easy.

The Upanishads emphasize a relatively easier path of meditation for humanity that is inclusive of thoughts. Right now, in your body as it is, you can use your mind as it is in its natural, ordinary cognitive state amid the din and roar of everyday relationships and situations. After exposing the mind to self-knowledge, you can choose to silently contemplate "designer" thoughts that illuminate the nature of Self.

In the Upanishad meditation teachings, no effort is made to make thoughts simply go away, since thoughts are the natural state of the mind. Instead, effort is made to change the quality of the thoughts and to direct the thoughts toward self-inquiry. In "thought-full meditation," it is our thoughts that keep us in bondage of maya, and it is also our thoughts that help us recognize who we are, from beyond maya, and break free of its bondage. Therefore, this meditation supports changing core beliefs—from limited to unlimited. A core teaching of the Upanishads is that we "become what we believe." The *Mundaka Upanishad* observes this:

"Self cannot be grasped by the eyes, or words, nor perceived by

the senses, nor revealed by austere rituals or penance.

When the mind becomes calm and refined by right knowledge, then,

Self can be realized in the quiet inner contemplation on Self."

MUNDAKA UPANISHAD, 3.1.8

You can contemplate or meditate in a sitting practice, say, upon waking up or before going to bed, or you can even choose to think meditative thoughts while cutting vegetables or taking out trash.

Through this contemplative meditation based on sacred instruction and autosuggestion, the human mind is entirely capable of changing its perceptions, attitudes, thoughts, and feelings. By contemplating deliberately at first and then more automatically, a new inner vision will arise that a powerful, free, and expansive Self is your real identity. Since your limitations are false (or a shadow of your truth) to begin with, you simply will be remembering your real, limitless, all-powerful nature.

"One meditates upon the supreme Self certainly achieves the supreme Self."

BHAGAVAD GITA, 8.8

That is right: instead of focusing on reducing the quantity of thoughts, I urge you to change the quality of the thoughts, from impure to pure, from worldly to spiritual, from bound ones to liberating ones. Make absolutely no effort to make the thoughts go away, but attempt to direct your thoughts toward self-inquiry (as described in chapters 13 and 14).

Thoughts directed toward the truth of Self automatically become a torch and illumine the hidden presence of Self behind the mind, otherwise concealed by self-ignorance. Self-contemplative thoughts during meditation are automatically calmer, and as you turn toward them, you will have fewer thoughts overall. The Upanishads reassure us that our Self, the Atman, is self-revealing. When we look for it with our inward meditative mind, Atman will reveal itself within that same mind.

Since thoughts are natural to the mind, let them be, but direct them to your soul. Then your thoughts will no longer remain your adversary but become your friends. Instead of leading you further astray into the world of sensory objects, looking to satisfy your vasanas they turn inward, searching within for the Self. Over time, the nature of your mind will change from darkness to light, from untruth to truth, from illusion to spirit.

Isn't that beautifully reassuring?

Guided Practice: Acharya Shunya's Sovereignty Meditation Method

Step 1.   Select a favorite sovereignty-revealing thought from the list below. Choose it based upon which aspect of self-ignorance you wish to overcome. Say you have excessive fear. In that case choose "I am fearless. I am the boundless spirit." Feel free to mix and match any of these thoughts.

Step 2.   Sit comfortably in an uplifting space, with your eyes closed.

Step 3.   Withdraw attention from everything around you—turn your attention inward. Think of how a tortoise withdraws into its shell to detach itself from the outside world.

Step 4.   Create a point of focused awareness by visualizing it in the center of your head, just below the crown, or it can be the center of your forehead (third-eye area) or in your heart (chakra) area. Visualize this awareness point as a light-filled, warm, comfortable, and radiant emanating swirl of positive energy. Take a few moments to imagine it in detail (do not rush) and connect with this positive, benign, comforting inner light until you feel good about yourself, more restful, and more relaxed.

Step 5.   Now begin thinking the chosen self-affirmation, for example, "I am fearless. I am the boundless spirit." Let this thought be the object of your meditation. And whenever the mind thinks other thoughts, feel free to gently return to this thought, "I am fearless. I am the boundless spirit."

Step 6.   As you focus, the thought of fearlessness will become a feeling. Experience this feeling by giving your conscious attention to it. Feel the feeling. What does it feel like to be fearless? As you feel the feeling, you will "become" fearless. Your mind will overcome bondage of ignorance and become sovereign. Meditate for as long as it feels comfortable to do so. When you end the meditation, you will approach all your life problems with self-activated fearlessness, throughout the day.

Return to this meditation until you have seen through the mirage of fear and fearlessness has become your mind's innate strength. You can use this method for different positive values like freedom, courage, determination, purity, and so on, especially for the ones you believe are lacking inside you. You can also use this exercise to strengthen the inner qualities you are already in touch with and bring them more into your actions and interactions. You can stick with just one of the statements below or change statements every day. Or maybe pick your favorite three and replay them until you experience a paradigm shift within!

I am an ever-present reality.

I am supreme awareness.

I am pure. I am the formless spirit that exists before birth and after death.

I am the ultimate truth.

I am fearless.

I am a boundless spirit.

I am the inner witness, the limitless, changeless awareness.

I am pure spirit.

I am soul divine.

I use a body, but I am not the body.

I use senses, but I am not the senses.

I use the mind, but I am not the mind.

I am pure Self.

I have accumulated neither sin nor merit.

I am an eternal witness.

I am peaceful.

I am pure.

I am free of attachments and aversions.

I am free of ignorance.

I am changeless. I am indestructible.

I am free right now.

I am an overflowing state of love, with no restrictions, no qualifications, and no limitations.

I am beyond past, present, future.

I am eternal existence, unmodified.

I am peace, I am love, I am eternal joy without needing anything.

I am complete always.

I am not dependent on anything. Everything is dependent on me.

I am infinite potential.

Forgiveness and compassion flow through me like a river, unbounded and infinite.

I have no preferences, no desires. I am complete.

I am Self.

I am a peaceful being.

I am a loving being.

I am a trusting being.

I am a healthy being.

I am a rejuvenating being.

I am an immortal being.

I am indestructible.

*I am not a doer. I am not the experi-
encer. I am a witness alone.*

*I am the bliss, the ananda, that I
am searching for outside me.*

*I am an omnipotent being having a
temporary, mortal experience.*

Breathing Deeply

Your breath is inherently connected to your thoughts. In fact, they are gross and subtle versions of each other.

To cultivate quiet that connects you to inner freedom, simply begin breathing slowly, fully, deeply, mindfully. Breathe. Be.

Meditate upon these words:

With each exhaled breath, I am releasing thoughts, feelings, and beliefs that no longer serve me.

With each inhaled breath, I am assimilating universal peace, love, and creativity that will serve my highest good.

Guided Practice: Belly Breathing

Use this exercise to breathe through your own harsh self-criticism or when dealing with criticism from others. It arrests negative thoughts and instills inner space.

1. Sit comfortably, mindfully alert with spine gently erect.

2. Place a hand on your belly. Let the belly rise gently with each breath in and collapse, gently, with each breath out.

3. Keep your attention on the rise and fall of the belly. Do not artificially make the belly rise or fall. Let it simply respond according to your incoming and outgoing breath.

4. If the mind wanders, simply return to feeling the mind's movements, using the rising and falling sensation as your way to be present, here and now, with each successive breath in and breath out.

5. Do this until you feel an inner shift from negativity to positivity.

6. Gradually, just like this, the previously emotionally loaded mind will feel unloaded, relaxed, and centered.

Once you have established inner calm with belly breathing, think this to yourself: *Joy, love, and playfulness reside in my being. I am connecting to them right now by touching my belly and breathing. My inner critic is healing and relaxing as I breathe from my belly.*

Adopt a Wisdom Mudra to Ease into Meditation

A *mudra* is a divine "lock" made by our fingers and thumb, to connect with something immortal and beyond us.

The wisdom mudra (jnana mudra) instantly brings your mind in touch with a universal mind, the mind of God (Grand Omniscient Dimension). You can hold a mudra for a couple of minutes to an hour or however long your meditation is. The longer you hold it, the better the "divine current" will flow.

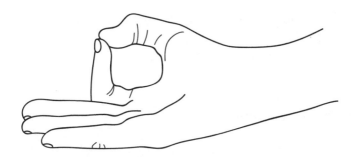

Figure 10.1: Jnana Mudra: The Gesture of Wisdom

To do this, bend the index finger of both hands to touch the tips of your thumbs. Each index finger and thumb form a circle, while the other fingers remain straight, pointing outward. This should be practiced in a comfortable seated position, with hands placed on the knees, palms facing forward.

The thumbs represent universal consciousness, while the index fingers represent individual consciousness. The unity in this gesture symbolizes the union of the divine Self with the individual self, resulting in the transcendence of this world.

This gesture will quickly stabilize the mind, open your creativity, and increase mental peace and joy. You don't have to focus on the breath, per se, but you will find that it naturally slows down.

Guided Practice: Jnana Mudra Meditation

Sit comfortably with your hands in jnana mudra and meditate upon these words:

My mind is always supported by a universal mind and can access a greater Universal Consciousness at any time I wish. My mind is benefitting from universal peace, universal love, and universal intelligence right now. My mind is soaking in infinite wisdom, light, and joy.

I am connected to an unlimited source of love, abundance, and self-acceptance now and always. I have access to unlimited divine assistance. My strength comes from my connection to this divine source.

Contemplations on the Changeless Self

One classical contemplation is on that which changes and that which is changeless, known as *nityanitya vivekaha.*

Reflecting upon thoughts of the unchangeable nature of Self, whether in a meditating posture or even while doing the dishes, will transform your ego. Then, instead of hiding the Self, the mind goes in search of the Self, which then reveals itself to you. Your mind becomes filled with inexpressible, inner stability, light, peace, and confidence. Try it now.

Guided Practice: The Unchangeable Nature of Self

Contemplate the following words, reading slowly. Close your eyes after each line. Feel the feelings, the knowledge of inner stillness that the words evoke.

I, the Self, acknowledge what changes.

The world around me is changing.

My body is changing.

My mind is changing.

My ego changes its preferences, beliefs, goals.

The waker in me changes when awake.

The dreamer in me changes when dreaming.

The deep sleeper in me changes when deep sleeping.

The world I witness with my senses when awake changes.

The dream world I witness with my mind when my senses are asleep changes.

The absence of all kinds of worlds, tangible or subtle, in deep sleep changes.

I, the silent observer, never change.

I am not what is revealed in my changeless presence. I remain pure unaffected presence.

I am that stillness, in whose motionless presence all motion and change are illumined.

I am that changeless truth, in which everything arises, is sustained, and disappears.

I remain unmodified.

Sorrowful thoughts don't alter who I am—the truth.

Happy thoughts also don't touch me, just likes waves cannot alter the ocean.

I am unaffected.

I am unattached.

I am free.

Choose Peace from Within

Peace comes from achieving ethical goals, from observing gaps between our thoughts, and, more abidingly, from acknowledging our own inner nature, as radical, unassailable peace.

Recognize you are an ancient being—an immortal presence. You can experience peace within without reason. Remember:

Possessions come and go.

Lovers come and go.

Friends come and go.

Aspirations come and go.

Wealth and jewels come and go.

But you can always experience pure peace, because you are Self, which is pure, unalloyed peace, independent of all outer situations of gain or loss.

Guided Practice: Peace Without Reason Meditation

Meditate upon these words:

I am at peace with who I am.

I am at peace with what I have.

I am at peace with what I don't have.

*I am at peace with others who are with me
and with others who are not with me.*

Shift Your Attitude Through Meditation

When life knocks you down, the first thing you should do to regain your balance is shift your attitude from inner resistance to inner acceptance and willingness.

Acceptance means: "I accept that this problem, sorrow, or emotional pain has arisen to show me something valuable."

Willingness means: "Let me wait to receive the answer within my heart."

This revelation of a deeper insight occurs not through our compulsive attitudes of "It must be this way" or "It must be that way." It arises when we become relatively still inside.

Guided Practice: Acceptance Meditation

When faced with difficulties in your life, meditate on these words:

If the universe has orchestrated this difficult situation in my life, then surely it is for my ultimate higher evolution of consciousness.

I will find some gems of insights about my own spiritual truth when I accept the pain coming my way with dignified acceptance and willingness.

If this problem has come to ME, then I have what it takes to meet that problem.

Here are some meditations for specific challenges.

If you feel afraid: *I am sovereign. I am letting go. I am bold. I am fearless. After all, I am Atman, the boundless one.*

If you are struggling with health issues: *I accept my current ill health as part of my divine plan to grow into greater health. My true Self is ever healthy.*

For relationship troubles: *I am not defined by this relationship, nor limited. I am unlimited, always.*

If you feel unloved: *In the total freedom that is my truth, I am totally acceptable to myself as I am.*

You will understand now when I say a pure mind becomes an intuitive mind when instructed with knowledge of the divine Self from the Vedas. Then, on its own, it turns inward to probe its own source, the Self. Meditation assists in this with enhanced self-introspection, self-awareness, self-contemplation, and self-mastery.

The Gayatri Mantra Meditation

Without the physical sun, life would be impossible. Similarly, without the Self, the matter envelopments of the body and mind would be inert. The Gayatri Mantra is a Vedic mantra that directly connects us to the powers of the physical sun as well as the inner sun (Self).

Through this mantra, we travel beyond the manifest sun, blessing our planet Earth to the nonmanifest *source* of a thousand suns, the Self, or pure magical consciousness, which enlightens infinite universes. In the Vedic tradition, the sun is a perceptible manifestation of the invisible supreme truth. In this mantra we are not merely connecting to the gross sun, but to the subtle truth of consciousness that is behind the sun. Thus, Gayatri Mantra connects us to the concealed ultimate reality that lies beyond the body (physical object) and is immanent in it and, yet, transcendent to it. The sages herald this unknowable, unthinkable, indescribable, undeniable truth as Self.

Even chanting this mantra once, it is believed, helps make the mind immediately experience greater peace, calm, and inner sovereignty.

SANSKRIT TRANSLITERATION	SOUNDS LIKE	SIMPLE MEANING	DEEPER MEANING
om bhūr bhuvaḥ svaḥ tát savitúr váreṇyaṃ bhárgo devásya dhīmahi dhíyo yó naḥ prachodáyāt	omm bhurr bhoo-vah-swa-ha tut-sa-vi-tur va-rey-nee-yum bhar-go dey-wass-ya dhee-mahi dhee-yo yo-nah pracho dai-yaat	I meditate upon that sacred effulgent sun as my indwelling Self. May it bless my intellect with enlightened thoughts.	I meditate on the spiritual effulgence of that adorable Supreme Divine Reality, the source or projector of the three phenomenal experiential planes of existence: the gross (body), the subtle (mind), and the causal (soul). May that supreme truth of Self (worshipped through the manifest sun god), guide my understanding so that I, too, can awaken and realize the state of supreme truth (moksha).

Thus, the Gayatri Mantra is also saying this:

Dear Sun, Self, Ultimate Reality,
through your physical form, your radiance, your light,
may I contemplate upon the highest truth of my true divine nature.

May your light enlighten my intellect, intelligence, and understanding.
May my perception of the world be clear;
May my discrimination become subtle;
May my judgment be correct;
May I become free of illusions, delusions, and doubts;
May my comprehension of situations be precise and wise;
May all my decisions be holistic and integral;
May my inner sun be as radiant as the outer sun;
May my consciousness (Atman) become one with the Universal
  Consciousness (Brahman).
May I achieve self-actualization, self-realization, and freedom to know and
  enjoy my sovereign light!

Thus, the Gayatri Mantra is a prayer unto the pure universal Self, to unveil itself and come to manifest as pure wisdom in our life.

If you wish, you can go online to acharyashunya.com for a step-by-step guided chanting and meditation experience.

Overcome the Two Most Common Obstacles to Meditation

Aside from procrastination, sleepiness is the most common obstacle to meditation. Try this:

- Meditate after a shower or splash cool water on your hands, feet, and face before meditating.

- Meditate when your stomach is neither too full nor growling with hunger.

- Avoid meditating at times when you are typically more dull or sleepy.

- Start with a strong autosuggestion thought (sankalpa), *I will be alert.*

- Don't meditate right after heavy exercise.

- Don't meditate if you are sleep deprived. Sleep instead.

For a distracted mind, try this:

- Switch off all your gadgets ahead of time.

- Contemplate the benefits of meditation ahead of meditating. It will keep you motivated.

- Make a higher power, guru, god, or goddess your meditation partner, as if they are witnessing you from a distance. Ask for help.

- Reduce your likes, dislikes, and attachments, which are the root cause of mental distractions.

- Before beginning, give yourself an autosuggestion, *I have an appointment to meet my true Self.*

"Sitting in a solitary place, freeing the mind from desires, controlling the senses, witness the one Self, your inner boundless being, with unswerving attention."

Guided Practice: My Lineage's Nondual Meditation—Atmabodha Dhyanam

The Atmabodha Meditation is based on Advaita Vedanta, the Vedic nondual teachings. This philosophy is founded on the premise that you are not your day-to-day personality, but rather its witness, its observer. Whatever you can observe—your breath, your body, your mind and its thoughts, ideas, beliefs, memories, or opinions—you are not.

To begin meditation, simply ensure that you are sitting comfortably, either on a cushion or a chair. You may close your eyes so you are not distracted. Then take a few moments to relax your body and mind. Rest your hands loosely in your lap or fold your fingers into jnana mudra, "wisdom seal." Or simply place them gently on top of each other with the palms facing upward.

Now breathe normally and allow yourself to relax. You will know that you are relaxed when you begin to lose awareness of your body. Your body will not be rigid, nor will your muscles be tight. Everything will begin to feel soft.

Baba described the process this way:

"Ever so gently,

observe the restless mind

until it dissolves into the presence of the majestic witness.

This is wisdom. This is meditation.

All else is mental mechanics."

Read the statements below. Allow them to become thoughts. Then allow these thoughts to lead you into a deep inner silence:

I am opening a door to the center of my being.

Deep inside my being dwells a silent presence,

My true Self.

I acknowledge this presence as my divine self.

I AM stillness, peace, tranquility.

I AM limitless existence, infinite knowledge, unbounded bliss.

Words can help a great deal to take us to the state beyond words. If you wish, you can follow this line of thought during meditation:

This breath, I witness; therefore, this breath, I am not. I am the witness alone. Ask yourself: *Am I the breath?* Spend some time observing this breath, the life principle, as it comes into your body and leaves your body. It seems that your awareness remains awake, even between an incoming breath and outgoing breath. Observe this gap. The observer is always different from that which is observed.

This body, I witness; therefore, this body, I am not. I am the witness alone. Ask yourself: *Am I the body?* Spend some time observing this material container called "body" in which your awareness appears to dwell. Observe your own body. The observer is always different from that which is observed.

This mind and its contents I witness; therefore, this mind, I am not. I am the witness alone. Ask yourself: *Am I the mind?* Spend some moments observing your mind, watching the mental events: the feelings, thoughts, perceptions, memories, ideas, sorrow, pleasure, fear, anger, grief, excitement, and all such emotions. Are you the mind? The observer is always different from that which is observed. The mind, you witness; therefore, you are not the mind.

If you wish, you can also visit acharyashunya.com to listen to a step-by-step guided meditation experience.

In meditation, we find that our thoughts may come and go, but we are at peace because we are witnessing those thoughts from a distance. We are not participating with our thoughts; we are not identifying with them. My teacher Baba said:

"May it be known, Shunya, you and not the objects illumined in consciousness are the source of consciousness. You are the witness alone. Know that you are sakshi, the nonjudging, nonparticipating, unattached, pure witness consciousness. Pure awareness is the invisible background in which everything arises. Like a cloudless sky, it has no form. It is eternal space; it is infinite stillness; it is the essence of being. Objects appear, exist, and disappear in awareness, yet this awareness, the Self, remains unchanged. Know you are not the breath, the mind, the body identified in a personal story of planet, race, gender, age, class, religion, family, profession, sorrows, and joy. All this, your personality with all its labels, dissolves in the presence of the sheer awareness that you are.

Set your personality aside, Shunya, and sit in your own divine awareness."

I heard this great call from master to disciple, and I followed it. Again and again I dwelt in my own divine awareness until the great, indescribable, absolute spiritual presence beyond conceptions and perceptions revealed itself to me.

"You are that which words cannot describe. You are none other."

"Yes, I am that, the indescribable Self," I said to him, quietly and without an iota of doubt.

I am confident that the transcendent practice of Atmabodha Meditation will have a beneficial impact upon your mind and body. Any individual who practices meditation in this way will find that this single lifestyle choice is the greatest propeller of positive change possible. It can fill you with joy and renewed abilities.

11

Viveka: Walking the Path of Discernment

*"The clouds are brought together by the wind, and they are again dispersed
by it. Bondage is created by the mind, and liberation is also brought
about by the mind."*

VIVEKACHUDAMANI, 174

The practice of discernment, or viveka, involves a moment-by-moment deliberation before acting or reacting. It includes closely examining our minds'
contents—thoughts, beliefs, root motivations, and desires—and asking ourselves if they are healthy or unhealthy. Only when we begin actively discerning
in life will we invest in the path of self-restraint and self-discipline.

Without discernment, the ego can quickly apply spiritual bypassing and
imagine itself to be awakened as pure awareness, even publicly announce its
enlightenment, only to collapse in a puddle of self-doubt and self-deprecation a
few days, weeks, or years later.

To practice discernment, we must be able to distinguish the quality of our
mental experience. The Vedic sages inform us that all of nature is composed of
three types of fundamental vibrations, or qualities, called *gunas.* The three qualities are *sattva, rajas,* and *tamas.* In the human being, the universal qualities are
most clearly witnessed through the workings of the mind. Understanding the
gunas in the mind, as well as in our environment, will help us discern the quality
of our experiences.

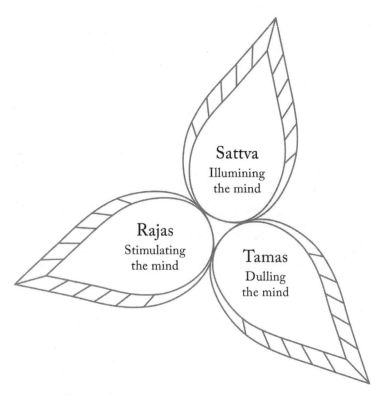

Figure 11.1: The Three Gunas

Rajas: Agitating quality of the mind.   Rajas is the principle of motion. When in excess, the agitating quality produces emotional pain and anxiety. Restless activity, feverish effort, and nonstop stimulation are its expressions. Rajas agitates, so it makes the mind incapable of resting, stopping, pausing, or even falling asleep on time.

Tamas: Dulling quality of the mind.   Dullness is a defining feature of tamas. Ambiguity, lack of initiative, and incomprehension are characteristics of a tamas-dominant mind. Tamas leads us to fall asleep, stay stuck, not comprehend correctly, or stay indecisive. It generates mental fogginess that fundamentally distorts our perceptions and judgments.

Sattva: Illuminating quality of the mind.   "Sat" means "pure being," and "va" is "where purity dwells." Sattva is expressed in the cosmos through the luminosity of light, the power of reflection, harmony, balance, goodness, knowledge, and purity. When this quality emerges in our minds, we experience inner balance, clarity, pleasure, purity of being, contentment, intrinsic peace, and fullness as well as a desire to be noble, good, and godly and to share and to care for others. Sattva has an affinity with truth, and hence, those with sattvic minds are receptive to spiritual learning and can access inner wisdom with ease. Light, especially the pure light of the sun or of a lamp or candle lit on an altar, is a beautiful symbol for sattva.

Behaviors with a sattvic quality include:

- Judiciousness and thoughtfulness
- Absence of pride
- Fearlessness, courage, forbearance
- Purity of heart, simplicity
- Steadfastness in the yoga of knowledge
- Charity, generosity, gratitude
- Controlled senses
- Willingness to sacrifice for good causes
- Studying spiritual texts and traditions
- Practicing austerity and yoga
- Straightforwardness
- Tolerance, compassion, accommodation
- Discernment and detachment
- Mercy and forgiveness
- Ability to experience inner satisfaction
- Feeling healthy guilt at wrong actions
- Being truthful, real, and honest
- Cultivating healthy emotions over unhealthy emotions
- Peacefulness and gentleness
- Modesty, versus conceit

- Steadfastness, dependability, responsibility
- Cheerfulness, feeling inner happiness
- Nonviolence, caring, affection

"Sattva or goodness, rajas or activity, and tamas or inertia;

These three gunas of mind bind the imperishable soul to the body, O Arjuna.

Of these, sattva, being calm, is illuminating and ethical. It fetters the embodied being, the jiva, by attachment to happiness and knowledge.

O Arjuna, know that rajas is characterized by intense passions, and is born of desire and attachment. It binds the jiva by attachment to the fruits of work [ambition].

Know, O Arjuna, that tamas, the deluder of jiva, is born of inertia. It binds by ignorance, laziness, and sleep."

BHAGAVAD GITA, 14.5–8

Sattva's Relationship with Happiness

When the sattva quality is dominant, one is content with one's own company, no longer desperate to connect at any cost. A person developing the quality of sattva increasingly enjoys nature, cultivates quietude, celebrates solitude, meditates, journals, reads and listens to spiritual teachings, engages in the arts, and takes up spiritual pursuits. These sensory engagements, in turn, promote yet greater illumination in the mind. The sattvic person also choses simple, fresh, and nature-celebrating foods; prefers a quiet, health-maintaining, sense-resting, and soul-uplifting lifestyle; and naturally cultivates balance in rest, work, food, sleep, sex, exercise, entertainment, and socializing.

When Rajas and Tamas Take Over Your Mind

If one's mind is dominated by dulling tamas and agitating rajas qualities, however, it is hardly an experience of joy and sovereignty. Have a look at the chart below.

RAJAS-DOMINANT MIND	TAMAS-DOMINANT MIND
Makes the mind selfish; lies; is spiteful, exploits, or manipulates others.	Confuses vice with virtue and misunderstands even when provided with correct knowledge by a teacher.
Justifies selfish or self-absorbed but ultimately self-defeating actions.	Cannot think independently; imitates others.
Behaves in reckless, ruthless, irresponsible, even self-destructive ways.	Disdainful and dismissive of constructive advice from wise people or books. Avoids teachings and disrespects teachers.
Justifies mistakes and remains imprudent and rash.	
Chases vasanas and acts out; blames others when thwarted.	Complicates even simple situations, due to misjudgment, miscalculation, and misinterpretation.
Focuses on finding faults in others (and never self-investigates) while feeling like a victim all along.	Does not learn despite getting hurt repeatedly.
Behaves in false and fictitious ways to achieve ends. May be a hypocrite, a show-off, and conceited.	Indulges in self-destructive habits and other harming activities (addictions, etc.).
Displays changeability and moodiness.	Often experiences dullness, sleepiness, and foggy states of mind.
Suffers untold self-created misery.	Comprehension is dull or distorted, leading to inadequate or incorrect understanding.
Embodies pride, conceit, and pretentiousness.	Delayed decision making, delayed thought processing, delayed understanding.
Takes risks and hasty actions; does not think before leaping.	

In short, when agitating and dulling qualities are dominating your mind (singly or together), your mind is helpless, and it is but a matter of time before it becomes a victim of its own self-created suffering.

Rajasic ego-serving actions. Rajas actions only benefit the doer. They are entirely selfish. For example, we may earn money for our security and to afford pleasures, but we do not contribute when a parent or friend needs medical assistance, although we could have. Or we may feel entitled to be fed when we come home from work, but when it is our turn to cook, we forget, are not present, are busy with other personal projects, or simply eat out. Here, we inflict hurt, not directly, but passively, by making our life only about taking care of our ego-self.

Rajasic self-absorbed motivations. These are motivations exclusively focused on one's own ego aggrandizement: me-and-mine motivations that are of benefit only to oneself and maybe a few others one feels attached to (perhaps immediate family members, favorite people, or a beloved pet). These motivations consider very few or no other people's well-being. These are selfish or, at the least, self-absorbed. We may not want to hurt others, but we don't see any reason to benefit them either. We are consumed only with our personal comfort, our needs, our desires, and our obsession with getting ahead—often at any cost to others.

Tamasic ego-exploitative actions. Not only do tamasic actions not benefit the doer, but they often harm another for personal gain. These are the worst sinful actions—such as stealing from our parents' health fund, pawning our boyfriend's gold watch without permission, or getting people addicted to prescription drugs, which helps one get rich but kills those who consume the medicines. Other examples include perpetrators of incest; manipulators; molesters; power mongers; enslavers; murderers; verbal and emotional abusers who get what they want by acting out; and people who lie, cheat, or steal in relationships for personal gain at the cost of very real damage to others.

Tamasic harmful motivations. These are motivations that not only hurt others, but also hurt the perpetrator. An example is spending all our parents' retirement savings to buy recreational drugs for our own sensory gratification. We harm our parents by leaving them penniless in old age, and we also end up harming ourselves sooner or later by destroying our physical health and losing our sanity. We also become filled deep down (where our ego still remembers it shares a common Self with all of humanity) with guilt and shame, an additional burden on our heart.

Sattvic ego-transcending actions. These are actions that not only benefit us, but all our relationships simultaneously. These are win-win actions rooted in altruism—not merely serving our selfish likes and dislikes. The Vedas suggest we always think and act according to this ideal. Act only after due consideration so many people can benefit, blossom, or enjoy alongside you! For example, sharing generously with our loved ones if we find ourselves suddenly wealthy through a windfall.

Sattvic ego-balancing motivations. Sattvic motivations are beneficial win-win motivations that benefit the doer and the maximum number of people (and other creatures and the planet, if possible). These are largely selfless or ego-less thoughts. They encourage universally caring and sharing ideas that allow for the maximum good for the maximum number of people, never excluding yourself. Sattva does not require you to be a poor martyr. It simply means you include a lot of other people in your ideas, efforts, and happiness. For example, we set up a commercial industry to make and enjoy the profit. From the profit, we buy a beautiful house, an expensive car, and fine clothes to complement our inner joy. We even enjoy well-paid holidays, attend meditation and spiritual retreats, and live life royally, befitting the Self. However, because sattva fuels our mind, we also employ this wealth to plant trees, make donations to worthy charitable causes, and help the less privileged. We make our ethically earned and well-deserved wealth a force of greater good and happiness in the world. Our happiness and smiles enable the happiness and smiles of countless other beings, including our employees, colleagues, neighbors, animals, and trees in our city or state.

Three Kinds of Happiness

Since these three qualities influence the quality of our mind, the kind of happiness we enjoy from sensory objects also changes based upon which quality is most dominant.

DISTORTED STATE OF MIND	AGITATED STATE OF MIND	BALANCED STATE OF MIND
Happiness is momentary.	Happiness is short lived.	Happiness is long lasting.
Happiness arises from contact of sensory organs with desired goals and objects that help one get more rest, comfort, and bodily pleasure (sleep, tasty food, sex).	Happiness ends when sensory objects are withdrawn or removed. This happiness is hard to obtain, difficult to maintain, and soon turns into sorrow.	Happiness arises from discerning sensory engagement, self-control, self-discipline, higher values, love, caring, sharing, and ethics—leading to inner tranquility. Happiness is less affected by the presence or absence of sensory objects.
Happiness is achieved at cost of duty, responsibility, and at personal risk.		
This happiness is fleeting and leaves behind a legacy of regrets and sorrow.		This happiness leads to more and more happiness each day.

Cultivating Sattva Is Key

All these years you have given a free rein to your mind and senses. Now that you have the tools to recognize who you really are and command the mind as its royal master, you must make cultivating sattva and rendering your mind and senses sattvic your priority.

With more insight, you can make better choices. Knowledge is power, and I am giving you back your power to decide what mental experiences you wish to cultivate—dulling and agitating ones or truly illuminating, happiness-imparting, powerful, free, peaceful, and serenity-evoking ones. It remains your choice.

When sattva is dominant, your mind is like a clear crystal, balanced and reflecting inner happiness. Therefore, it is said that this quality has a purifying effect on the mind.

The light of sattva does not resist change, nor does it disorient. Agitation and dullness are absent, and peace, quiet, and clarity prevail. Good conduct, which consists of compassion, kindness, self-control and self-restraint, freedom from hatred, and other similar qualities prevails.

The sattva quality of the mind enables right comprehension, balance, and illumination. Sattva is a saving grace worth enhancing in our mind! It is that quality of our mind, which, when active, helps us see thorough vasanas and awaken to our true potential.

People with a higher proportion of balancing quality in their minds will naturally turn away from the unreal and progress toward the real. Even now, every single spiritual seeker of any spiritual tradition who dares to go beyond convention and rigid beliefs (distortion) or fervent, fanatical faith (agitation) in search of a greater personal and universal truth (illumination) is doing so due to a higher proportion of illuminating quality in the mind.

When through the exposure to right knowledge, right teachers, and right quest, the last traces of agitating and dulling qualities are lessened or removed from the mind, the mind shines with the balance, purity, and inner illumination of sattva. And what is more, this sattvic mind alone is the gateway to encountering your true Self!

As Shankara, the Vedic master, observed: "Therefore, the mind is the cause for both liberation as well as bondage. When tainted by the effects of rajas and tamas, it causes bondage. When it is free from the rajas and tamas qualities, sattva paves the way to liberation [from maya]."[1]

The table below will help you recognize the impact of gunas on various psychological dimensions of the mind.

MENTAL DIMENSION	TAMAS	RAJAS	SATTVA
Intelligence	Blocked	Distorted	Optimum
Sensory engagement	Distorted, addictive	Excessive	Pure, balanced
Intentions	Impure	Adulterated	Pure
Mode	Inertia, dullness, lethargy	Motion, aggression, overactive	Equilibrium, balanced between rest and motion
Feelings	Stuck, disturbed, dark, sinister	Agitated, anxious, controlling	Balanced, peaceful, harmonious
Motivations	Selfish	Self-absorbed, self-serving	Selfless, generous, win-win motivations
Ethical values like compassion, truthfulness, nonviolence	Does not uphold values or actively flouts them for personal gain	Upholds values only if they serve self-interest	Upholds values even at cost of personal sacrifice
Capacity to discern	Passive	Fluctuating	Active
Capacity to learn	Minimum	Fluctuating	Maximum
Capacity to exercise will	Rare	Variable	Strong
Behavior	Lazy, procrastinates	Overexcited, overcommits	Restfully active, balanced
Sense of time	Always dwells in past	Always thinks about future	Remains more present in the now
Interest in self-growth and spirituality	Least	Medium but changeable	Maximum
Chances of awakening to Self	None	Rare	Maximum

Figure 11.2: Gunas in Summary

It is clear from the above discussions and table that sattva is the mode or quality of mind you want to consciously cultivate. The good news is that the Vedas teach how to embody sattva, even if your mind is currently under the sway of rajas, tamas, or both. Lack of sattva is not a problem we cannot fix. In fact, it is an easy fix, provided we want sattva and choose it every day through our cognitive and behavioral choices. This entire book is about enabling greater sattva.

The task of awakening to the Self can be carried out properly only by the purest of minds, in which sattva is most powerful. Spiritual contemplation, imagination, use of soul-will, soul-power, manifestation, visualization, and meditation strengthen sattva. Sattva, as it increases its sway in your mind, will bless you with greater insights and subtle intuition.

No wonder the Bhagavad Gita has this to say: "Only that mind which is sattvic [calm and balanced] can discriminate between what is good and what is bad, adopts what is right, and gives up what is not right. So also, it discriminates between what is my responsibility and what is not my responsibility, what is ethical and what is unethical, the sources of fear and fearlessness, bondage and sovereignty."[2]

The Ten Beautiful Features of a Sattvic Mind

Focused. Prevention is better than cure, so the mind remains alert to unwanted sensorial and mental input (vasanas, false ideas, misperceptions). It acts like a gentle gatekeeper of your inner kingdom and restrains and shields you from cravings, compulsions, enticements, and false promises that will hurt you in the future. It always keeps your mind delusion-free and connected with reality.

Discerning. Overcoming delusions caused from attachments and countering negative emotions like lust, greed, and self-pity with positive emotions emerging from generosity, selflessness, and compassion, the sattvic mind will insist you choose right over wrong, good over bad, eternal over ephemeral. This will make you successful and admired.

Decisive. The greatest souls in history have exhibited resoluteness of mind, not vacillation. No doubt it emerges from their sattvic nature, which is steadfast in its decisions. Can you imagine the mind of Buddha as he practiced austerities alone under a tree, unmoving, until he achieved nirvana? He did not get up halfway, did he? A determined mind achieves both worldly and spiritual success. Whatever you decide, you will not stop unless you achieve your goal.

Mature. A mature mind is questioning, analyzing, and contemplative. Unlike the immature mind, ridden by agitating rajas and dulling tamas qualities, the mature mind knows when to say yes and when to say no, when to weep and when to rejoice, when to rightfully protest, and when to simply appreciate and practice gratitude. It rightly guides us in communication too—when to keep quiet and when we should speak up, when we should keep secrets and when we should bring a dark secret to light. It helps us selectively befriend the right people and establish a polite distance from sleepwalking influences. Thanks to a mature mind, we will pick and choose our battles, professions, and life partners wisely, not believing flatterers and false friends. We know where our responsibility and duty begin and where our pleasures and indulgences must end (what is enough). People with mature minds attract friends and fans, gain admiration and respect, and achieve what they want due to their inherent understanding of how to avoid psychological dangers and emotional traps.

Steady. A steady mind remains relatively calm or tranquil under all circumstances. It does not have hyper or violent reactions to even adverse situations, mainly because it remains connected to an infinite source of power and perseverance, the Self, from within. No number of obstacles, afflictions, or attacks can upset an illumined mind, shining from the light of the Self. Even disease, loss, and grief cannot subdue its spirit. This mind makes people heroes and role models for rest of humanity. This steadiness emerges from intellectual convictions in a higher reality, the Self, or God (which are one in the Vedas). They don't suppress painful emotions, but they understand the pain, bear with it, and move through it. They enjoy intellectual and emotional maturity along with deep thinking and firm spiritual clarity. A steady mind can even go beyond personal pain and be concerned for the alleviation of others' pain.

Expansive. The contracted mind's comfort zone is where people look or pray or copulate like themselves. But the expansive sattvic mind has the capacity to transcend all narrow and selfish prejudices like color, race, religion, and sexual preference, and it embraces the whole world and all its creatures—even plants and animals—as one's own spiritual family, sharing the common truth of one Self. The same divinity lives in all hearts, explain the Vedas, and an expansive mind gets this intuitively (whether it has been exposed to the Vedas or not). This mind transcends limiting egoic individuality to mentally occupy a space of ever-expanding spiritual multidimensionality. Someone with an expansive mind takes on the joys and sorrows of all beings as their own. A selfish mind on the other hand feels happy when others are suffering and suffers with jealousy when others are happy.

Unadulterated. A sattva-filled mind is childlike but not childish. That is because it possesses guileless qualities, like an absence of conceit or pretentiousness, simplicity, straightforwardness, truthfulness, innocence, transparency, joy, trust, lack of suspicion, natural detachment, and freedom from calculative or harmful self-indulgent qualities. The thoughts, speech, and actions of people with a sattvic mind are always in alignment with one another; they don't mislead or make false promises. They talk frankly and candidly accept their limitations and faults (they are human after all). They express the truth of what they feel openly, but nonviolently, pleasantly, and calmly. They generally do not see evil in another (unless they have cause); they do not hold secret prejudices. They are who they say they are. The purity and divinity of the soul simply shines through the thoughts, eyes, speech, expressions, and actions of the person with a pure mind.

Subtle. Only a refined mind is subtle. It can transcend the realm of the physical senses (this gross world) and enter the realm of subtle truths of Self, God, Divine Consciousness. While a gross mind remains engaged with gross worldly affairs alone, with a subtle mind, you can also explore the mysteries of life, death, and the immortal Self. The greatest philosophers, seers, spiritual teachers, artists, musicians, poets, and writers have benefitted from a subtle mind, which allows them to see what others cannot see. Only a subtle mind helps us make an ideological leap from religious superstitions, fanaticism, dogma, and mechanical rituals to discover the truth of a transcendental Self, common to all living beings.

Sharp. We can read myriad books and even listen to spiritual lectures, but what is the use of all this, if when we are faced with a life challenge, we don't remember any of the wisdom? A sharp mind is never clouded; it has good memory, excellent recall, presence of mind, critical-thinking ability, and the clarity to possess right understanding. A sharp mind is quite the opposite of an inertia- and lethargy-filled tamas mind or a restless rajas mind.

Spiritual. Congratulations. You must possess a spiritual mind or else why would you be engaging with my teachings right now? Only a mind blessed with enough sattva is concerned about matters of spirituality, God, and right values. Possessors of this mind display faith in one's self, in guru, in God. The possessors of such a mind face all odds to evolve spiritually, to even undertake hard sensory disciplines and self-challenging practices to conquer the lower nature and realize the truth of Self. The mystics and sages of every tradition and culture, including the Vedic seers, possessed a spiritual mind overflowing with the luminosity of sattva. Sattvic mind enjoys positive thoughts, cultivates trust in a higher power, and attempts to live and let live. Additionally, a spiritual mind exhibits the following traits.

Supports the rise of ethical values. Sattva, due to luminosity and right comprehension of reality, has a natural affinity with dharma, or an ethical, evolved way of life. A spiritual mind will make you speak truthfully and intuitively act nonviolently, for example. In contrast, when either of the other two qualities (rajas or tamas) are dominant in the mind, you may commit ethical violations that destroy your capacity to grow and thrive.

Makes you happy from within. Sattva has the unique trait of light or luminosity known as *prakasha*. Its nature is brightness leading to calmness, quietude, and tranquility. Sattva also reveals grace, or *prasada*, which means "to become tranquil," "to be pleased with oneself," "to be satisfied," and "calmness of the mind," which is the root of spiritual happiness.

Supports the acquisition of wealth and fame. For worldly goals—well-deserved name, fame, noble accomplishments, and a rise in one's rightful position and power—once again, a sattvic mind is indispensable. Only an intelligent and empowered but restrained mind that is assertive (not aggressive) with the ability to communicate clearly and kindly; uphold and respect personal boundaries;

grow and sustain wealth, health, and a social network; and give back to society through charity, heartfelt sharing opportunities, and socially altruistic causes becomes materially successful in the long run. There are no shortcuts.

Supports success in relationships. For healthy and happy relationships, a more sattvic mind is useful in both partners—or at least in one to start. People with sattvic minds understand the difference between desirable and undesirable, dutiful and undutiful, loving and controlling, selfish and selfless, and empowering and disempowering actions. Sattva facilitates compassion, empathy, faith, commitment, sacrifice, and self-control in relationships. These qualities thrive in a calm and tranquil mind that can discern and detach or willingly accept and ask for what it needs, unlike in an overreactive mind, which wants too much, or in a mind filled with fogginess.

Introduces you to your Self. An ancient Vedic text pronounces that "The Self cannot be seen by the physical eye because it is formless. Self is intuitively revealed in that mind which is fully sattvic. Those who realize the Self achieve immortality, sovereignty, and bliss."[3] Yes, only sattva-blessed senses, ego, and intellect can penetrate to the heart of the spiritual problem and draw out the hidden truth.

Augmenting the sattva quality in your mind can be your best asset in your journey to inner power and joy, despite any life challenges. The good news is that you can change your mental makeup by choosing sattvic experiences.

How to Cultivate Sattva in the Mind

The Sanskrit word "guna" also means "rope." At any given time, our mind is being pulled in different directions by the ropes of rajas, tamas, and sattva, each one vying for supremacy. No wonder we have such an unpredictable mind, with different ropes pulling us in all directions. This is why at times even an apparently logical person sometimes acts illogically, and vice versa. While rajas and tamas tie up our mind and pull us even deeper into the quicksand of samsara, you can, through knowledge, empower the rope of sattva to pull you up into the open sky of Self so that rajas and tamas can no longer bind you with addictions and imprisoning attachments.

Here are some suggestions to empower sattva:

- The Vedas suggest waking up in the early morning before sunrise, since at that time, the universe is full of the sattva quality. Meditating boosts sattva. You'll find meditation instructions in chapter 10.

- Eat fresh or properly cooked, organic, whole foods. Food is an important strategy to improve sattva because the Vedas say our mind is nothing but the subtle essence of what we eat. In my book *Ayurveda Lifestyle Wisdom*, I cover sattva-increasing foods and recipes in detail as well as how to curate a sattva-enhancing lifestyle, from waking to bedtime.

- Spend as much time as you can in nature—if possible, alone. Bathe in nature's quietude and peaceful energy every day if possible. Expose your body and mind to the rising sun and moon.

- Limit the time spent on social media and television. Cultivate thoughtful friends and enjoy quality time; uplift each other's minds with sattvic (honest) communication.

- Contemplate Vedic teachings and enlightening texts (like this book) on an ongoing basis—in fact, daily (most important).

- Control the senses (by not overeating, for example).

- Manage thoughts and emotions.

- Act from established values and not impulsive likes and dislikes.

- Cultivate mindful practices: deep breathing (*pranayama*), yoga-based exercise, chanting, meditation, devotional singing, time in nature, contemplative writing, art, and music.

- Cultivate contentment.

- Cultivate discernment and detachment.

- Cultivate tranquility amid stressful circumstances.

- Create pure, sacred, clean living spaces.

- Practice conscious speech protocols despite aggravation.

Sattva quality in the mind maximally reflects the light and consciousness of the true Self. Sattva is the natural mode of the mind, ego, and intellect. You don't have to do much except not allow the other two qualities to accumulate and conceal the underlying sattva.

Use Your Sattvic Mind to Practice Discernment

The ancient spiritual practice of exercising discernment, known as viveka, involves using our sattvic mind to nip agitating and dulling motivations and actions in the bud. The Vedas strongly urge we only act from sattva because such actions transcend our petty ego, which alternates between being selfish and destructive.

To help us discern, the Bhagavad Gita offers this advice: "Knowledge arises from sattva; greed arises from rajas; heedlessness, delusion, and also ignorance arise from tamas in the mind."[4]

Cultivating Sattva with Viveka

Simply put, discernment means taking a tiny cognitive pause to reexamine thoughts closely, using your acquired self-knowledge, before reacting.

Pausing to practice discernment does not make a false or delusory thought go away, but it does allow us to pull in greater consciousness and sow the seeds of clarity amid a jungle of overgrown vasana vines and deadly swamps of agitating and dulling qualities. You can plant the seeds of sattva and weed out rajas and tamas overgrowth in this cognitive pause.

My student Connie writes:

> *"I am checking my own attitude when, for example, I do household chores for my family, work on a translation, take my dog to the park, and plan a yoga event. Am I doing this from sattva, with joy in my heart? Or am I experiencing any negative thoughts of irritation, judgment, or self-pity (rajas and tamas)? If I find my mind going to a negative place, I try to reflect on it and then consciously shift into sattvic and dharmic thoughts of service. Then my mood almost instantly improves, and people around me respond more positively too."*

Guided Practice: Viveka—Conduct an Intelligent Inquiry in the Pause

This pause represents choosing presence, mindfulness, and intentionality over a mechanical mode of the mind. It enables stepping into a more conscious mode of mind. The pause enables strategic self-inquiry and examination of our deeper motivations, such as:

- Who am I without my vasana compulsions driving me?

- Why am I feeling happy just sitting here quietly by myself looking at the clouds (that I shall never possess or control)?

- Is this happiness coming from inside me?

- Does it mean joy lives inside me?

- It feels like it does live inside me after all ... oh yes. I feel it spreading all over me, from inside out, and I feel so content, nothing to chase, to prove, or want.

- Am I choosing to indulge a dulling-tamas, agitating-rajas, or freeing-sattva activity, thought, or behavior?

- Am I indulging in ethical or nonethical behavior?

- Am I choosing instant happiness or gratification over long-term joy?

- Am I indulging an unnecessary craving knowingly, even when I now understand that my happiness lies exclusively inside me?

- Can I believe the thoughts I am thinking? Are they real, or do they represent a myth-reality?

- Am I really depressed, or have I simply been indulging too many dullness- or tamas-inducing activities, like procrastinating, lazing around, letting go of personal hygiene, eating leftover foods and scraps instead of cooking fresh food or getting little exercise, and that is why I feel low?

- Ask yourself this: *Is this even real?*

This way, through the practice of sattvic discernment, we can slowly begin our journey of reclaiming greater space in our mind and free ourselves from the demands of vasanas.

"Those who are abiding in sattva go upwards, the rajas-dominant ones dwell in the middle, and the tamas ones go downwards."

BHAGAVAD GITA, 14.14

By becoming thought-selective, or shall I say sattva-selective, you can change the direction of your life—upward, downward, or stuck in the middle—slowly and steadily, one well-discerned thought at a time.

My student John shares this:

"My teacher likened the sleepwalking mind to a bowl of noodles—a vortex and tangle of emotions, likes, dislikes, thoughts, and stories preoccupied with the past or the future. Sattvic discernment is a pathway through the vortex, and sattva must be awakened, strengthened, and fortified by choice. I'm witnessing how awakening the mind itself is an ongoing conscious practice of cultivating sattva.

When something happens—an interchange with another person, a concern about an upcoming event, a review of something that's already happened—my everyday mind can jump in quickly to interpret, conclude, and create more (resistance-filled) stories. The other signs of my noodle mind moving are I become uneasy, emotional, and jittery or I have difficulty staying on task. Treating any one of these as a sign to go slow or Stop! is the most efficient way of waking up the sattvic mind and its discerning faculties. I pause. I breathe. I apply discrimination: What is eternal? What is transient? At this point, with the mind made more sattvic, I am able to choose what to do next rather than be tossed around with the noodles."

Understand that you are inherently way too powerful to suffer your knee-jerk thoughts. Cultivate sattva and use your sattva-filled mind to discern and write your own life script, and to make better choices by maximizing sattva in daily life (by meditating, eating fresh foods, and other sattvic activities). If you keep trying for sattva and restrain the other two mischievous qualities, in due course your senses will listen to you (the spiritual master); they will seek divine encounters and desire to cultivate sattva in every moment (become very selective in food, lifestyle, books, company).

Use Viveka to Avoid Spiritual Bypassing

Do not fall into the trap of elevating yourself above others as you begin to cultivate sattva. We have all heard of so-called awakened beings in modern times committing suicide, swallowing antidepressants, needing drugs to feel the bliss, and sexually and emotionally abusing their followers despite wanting to walk a higher path. Instead they have given over to their egoic shadow fueled by rajas and tamas. Were they discerning between rajas, tamas, and sattva? Or between dharmic and non-dharmic ways of behaving? No.

Therefore, the suggestions regarding discernment I have imparted here should be put in place before the dawn of awakened consciousness, not after the fact. And we must take the time it takes to discern between the *illusion* of awakening to Self and *real* awakening to Self.

The practice of viveka is, therefore, the cornerstone of genuine awakening. What the mind has forgotten, the mind can be reminded of, provided it has been rendered maximally sattvic. Then, the sattvic mind can be awakened by contemplating upon enlightening wisdom. Then it will remember the truth from within: that it is a receptacle of the Self's infinite joy; that it is an instrument of a greater consciousness, which is ever serene, ever calm, ever abundant, ever powerful, and ever peaceful. Believe me, a point comes when the same mind that was once powerless, combing the world for vasana fulfillment, starts listening for the soul's voice within.

When you make sattvic discernment your moment-to-moment practice, you will allow or disallow thoughts and ideas with increasingly greater ease. There is a voice inside you that has always told you to challenge the status quo, the belief system that keeps you bound. Listen to it. Viveka, discernment, is the willingness to listen to your deeper, more sattvic voice over and above your default mind's rajasic and tamasic voices.

In the next chapter, we'll explore how right discernment automatically leads to nonattachment.

12

Vairagyam: Practicing Nonattachment

"As the ignorant people act from attachment to outcomes and suffer,
So should the wise people act with nonattachment, wishing the welfare
of this whole universe."

BHAGAVAD GITA, 3.25

The word "vairagyam" means cultivating detachment, or nonattachment. This word has caused a lot of havoc in spiritual communities in India and the West alike. When not rightly understood, false and untimely detachment (versus engagement in the world) can lead to spiritual bypassing. Let's look at some misconceptions about nonattachment.

Vairagyam Is Not "Leaving the World"

Detachment, or vairagyam, does not mean running away or escaping from worldly life or cultivating repulsion for worldly activities, like sex, shopping, and so forth. Unfortunately, many spiritualists in India, and to an extent in the West too, conclude that leaving the world behind in some fashion is a great way to prove a spiritual point.

You do not need to leave the world and live in seclusion
or a special community to practice detachment.

There is no conspiracy against you. The world of objects is not trying to seduce, enslave, and bind you; rather it is your own unconsciousness that binds you. The object is not to leave the world but to get rid of your unconsciousness. Neither blaming the world nor reactively withdrawing from it will solve your problem. Staying balanced will.

Two major schools of spiritual thought have existed in India from time immemorial. One school of thought sees spirituality as primarily a path of renunciation in which one can and should mortify the body and abandon the world in favor of the transcendent realm. In this school, vairagyam does mean detaching ourselves from all worldly concerns, internally and externally. This is the monastic path to spirituality.

The other school sees spirituality as an epistemic process, a refinement of our understanding. Renunciation in this case is not of the world itself, but of one's afflicted relationship with it. This is the nonmonastic householder's path to spirituality.

My lineage is nonmonastic. We are a householder-sage lineage by tradition (known as *grihastha sadhus*). We are encouraged to remain established within society, take on life partners, raise children, and despite the worldly roles, nurture an inner life with spiritual disciplines until we awaken irrevocably to who we are—the Self. And upon awakening, the need to distance ourselves from our roles, home, and society becomes a moot point!

External renunciation, or vairagyam, is awe-inspiring. Is internal vairagyam any less steep a path to spiritual ascent?

I share this because you are likely a householder like me, holding down a job, running a business, navigating relationships, raising children, and taking care of aging parents. Like many people, you fantasize about leaving all this behind.

It is time to bury the illusion that for spiritual growth and to be samsara- and vasana-free, you need to relocate to some exotic or spiritually remote destination, such as a commune or an ashram. Similarly, if you do live in one, you need not think you have spiritually arrived!

Right here, right now, you can pursue knowledge through an authentic source, such as this book or a sincere teacher. Then practice this knowledge in the life you now have, with your same old relationships, to see and enjoy the difference knowledge makes. After all, discernment of truth from falsehood, identifying reality from illusion, and detachment from what is a mere delusion cannot be developed in isolation from our perceptions and emotions and the agents who elicit them in us.

The path of world renunciation should not be a mass prescription. It's not for everyone. Total freedom of spirit includes the freedom of simply being yourself, just as you are right now. The life we choose, whether as a regular worldly seeker (a householder) or as a monk, traditionally has always been a choice, not an obligation, and least of all a bondage-creating precondition for awakening.

Vairagyam Is Not Enforced Celibacy

Humanity has been afflicted with the desire to be "spiritually immaculate," that is, somehow separated from our own biological-sexual nature that has been dismissed and disparaged as "savage" by religions worldwide. This includes the latest version of popular Hinduism that is becoming more and more disconnected from its liberal Vedic roots.

The disparaging of our sexuality as "lower animal nature" or even "sin" has been endorsed by various spiritual teachers of various traditions worldwide. Some of these teachers and messiahs may claim to be born with super-human abilities and perfectly polished halos and be faultless, immaculate, and sexless (or so they claim); their promise is to make us equally edified, sexless, unnatural versions of themselves, spiritually coldblooded clones.

Being "spiritually immaculate" is a false ideal. Enforced celibacy and the imposition of monasticism has wreaked havoc in the Christian church and, in the past, in Buddhism and Jainism, and now Hinduism too.

Human sexuality is celebrated in the Vedas. The compiler of the holy Vedas himself, Sage Vyasacharya, enjoyed conjugal bliss, and his son, Shakti, went on to become a great sage too! Most seers in the Vedas were married, some multiple times, and others had love interests. Krishna and Arjuna, the famous teacher and disciple duo from the Bhagavad Gita, too were married, had children, and conducted worldly duties (like participating in a war for dharma's sake), while conversing about and trying to live by nondual principles in life (Krishna was the king of Dwarka, and Arjuna the prince of Hastinapur). They were not monks, but regular folks, householders like you and me, but with ascended unity consciousness!

Remember that pursuit of kama, or pleasure, is one of the four legitimate desires of human life. Our senses must be allowed to enjoy pleasures. The Vedas say desire for pleasures should be mindfully fulfilled and, while never excessive, offers us strategies to find pleasurable fulfillment. Providing a dharmic context of knowledge and wisdom is more important than any blanket prescription banning sex, marriage, wine, nice foods, music, or dance that so many paths insist upon doing.

Spiritual awakening is every soul's birthright. We don't have to prove how holy we are by constantly suppressing natural biological urges in the name of practicing detachment.

Vairagyam Is Not Temporary Emotional Withdrawal

Sometimes false or short-lived detachment emerges from an experience of mental or physical pain. This is an impulsive reaction, and it is temporary and valueless since it is not the outcome of objective discernment.

Say someone loses a dear friend to sudden death. During the funeral, one may feel intense detachment from life itself, wondering, *What is the point of life, wealth, relations? It is all ephemeral!* Then, on returning home, they find that their teenager has left an expensive bicycle in the front yard for anyone to take! The disillusion experienced minutes ago from the friend's death gets replaced by attachment to a kid's bicycle, and the person runs to fetch it and bring in inside while yelling at the kid (displaying intense attachment!).

Vairagyam Is a Sovereign Choice

Just like you no longer go back to the toys you were once so attached to in childhood, you can deliberately and mindfully stop hanging out with thoughts, gossip, beliefs, opinions, doctrines, dogmas, contrary philosophies, people, relationships, groups, news, and media that no longer serve you and your growing awareness of a greater spiritual truth of Self. This, in short, is the practice of deliberate detachment recommended by the Vedas—when we mentally or physically (or both) step away from what no longer serves our highest interest or what we have foolishly and under the influence of delusory thoughts given away our power to.

Through the practice of deliberate nonattachment, we are taking back our previous emotional investments and declaring our inner freedom to reinvent ourselves and our lives. This is the sovereign principle in action.

When you operate from a detached space, you stop controlling, blaming, insisting, and grasping, and almost instantly a quiet serenity takes over your mind.

Your own likes and dislikes, attachments and passions, inclinations and disinclinations are the suffering mind. Knowing this, abandon them. The renunciation of them is the renunciation of all suffering. Now you can remain as you are: forever free, truly sovereign!

Nonattachment is a decision to step back from the insistence, obstinacy, control, and insanity of your own mind! It transpires in the sattvic intellect after recognizing the validity to detach by way of healthy discernment (the practice we explored in the previous chapter).

With the ongoing practice of deliberate nonattachment, you will see a reduction in your bondages as you stand apart from all that had previously colored your subjective mind—green with envy, red with anger, and black with sorrow. What might have been devastating will instead leave you curious, maybe a bit sad, or at times, unmoved. You may shed a few tears, but not for long. You will be hopeful and poised and will bounce back quickly.

The Problem with Attachments

Whenever we are attached, the importance of whatever we are attached to often gets disproportionately big in our mind.

An attached mind builds up its ignorant forces, prays, schemes, manipulates, and even takes classes and workshops to attract or manifest what it wants. Forgetful of our whole and peaceful inwardly sovereign nature, a mind driven by attachments takes us hither and thither, up and down, and through straight roads, curvy trails, and dead-end alleys of this universe. Egged on by our attachments, we think our joy or success is close, waiting to greet us with open arms if we just push a little further. Alas, we wait forever for some ephemeral pleasure since it never lay outside us in the first place.

Desires are totally normal. But when you start emotionally leaning on a desire to be fulfilled a certain way, grasping, grabbing, controlling outcomes, and becoming greedy for more or not willing to let go, your emotional dependence upon that object becomes an attachment known as raga. This Sanskrit word interestingly means "becoming colored" (as discussed in chapter 4) and refers to how unnecessary desires (vasanas) and false beliefs color our mind.

When your mind becomes tinted with whatever you are attached to (lover, partner, pet, favorite dress, ambition), *bam!* your subjective mind (samsara) changes color too as it is hijacked by attachments that cause sorrow. Attachments derail the human mind from its spiritual wellspring of inner sovereignty and trap us in a search for fulfillment outside ourselves.

How Can You Avoid Attachments?

To avoid the trap of attachments, cultivate a practice of deliberate nonattachment or cultivated detachment. A sattva-dominant mind will help you accomplish that.

To detach emotionally from what is binding you, think this thought: *I am sovereign because, in the final analysis, I am not inherently needy. I am enough unto myself, and all is well.*

Do this any time you start feeling an inner urgency or compulsion. Through this practice, the tree of unconscious desires can be cut at its roots. The mind becomes quieter, nondemanding, and pure.

Resist your own mind that barks would'ves, could'ves, and should'ves. The world filled with likes and dislikes is a dream. It appears to be real within its own realm, but when we awaken to the possibility of living a life free of compulsions, we see it is false. After due consideration, we can still pursue what we "like," but without the drama, the push and the pull, and the uncensored emotional attachments that compromise our right to a sovereign life.

Even a single thought like: *It would be nice if that person called and asked me out on a date, but whether I get the call or not doesn't affect my original happiness, as that is up to me*, can change the tide of your attachments from dangerously high to quite manageable.

Nonattachment in Relationships

With the practice of deliberate detachment, you can cultivate the mental space to *consciously choose* your own responses to your thoughts, first and foremost. Then, you can retain what is worth retaining and let go of what is not.

For example, if you are married with children, you likely wish to remain connected to your family. Yet it is beneficial to detach psychologically and reduce your emotional codependence on your partner.

If you are dating or engaged and, using your intellect to discern, you see that the match is not a good one, you can detach yourself and no longer be available to date or marry. This may be the best investment you can make in your future joy!

If you have spiritually unconscious parents, detachment can help you. You may visit them, help them, care for them, but not argue with them, nor allow yourself to be influenced by their arguments. You will become your own parent and begin leading your life toward the search of what is eternal versus arguing about what is noneternal or even irrelevant.

Stepping away from what you have discerned as no longer serving your highest interest is signaling to the universe that you are no longer interested in self-sabotaging patterns. Gradually, you may even develop a healthy (self-protective) distaste for people, objects, and situations that seduce you into becoming unconscious.

This aversion is a sign of rising emotional maturity. For example, we may deliberately detach ourselves from spending lonely evenings with a certain friend who is extremely needy and lacking even basic discernment. This person's innocent text, "Are you free tonight?" may send a warning up and down our spine. But this is good because it means discernment followed by detachment has converted into healthy, proactive boundaries in our awakening mind. This will get us out of the syndrome of instant gratification and protect us from future sorrow. Thanks to these inner warnings and cultivated distaste of the company of unconscious people, we will feel empowered to answer honestly and without apology, "I am not available," or, very simply, "No."

When, through the practice of discerned and deliberate (not impulsive and reactive) nonattachment, you slowly but steadily start letting go of a previous source of fleeting happiness, fascination, or focus that once consumed and enslaved you, you will feel as if you have left the world to its own devices and gone inside to get even closer to the sovereign you. All sorts of options will open. You will feel free. It's as if you have gone in to say hello to your own pure being, the ever-free one, *nitya mukta*, who dwells beyond the tinted walls of your samsara, and everything naturally relaxes inside you. With detachment, you will feel inwardly expansive.

The Sky Remains Unfazed by Clouds

When you practice detachment, what is real and true will remain, and whatever is myth-reality will gradually fade away. Even if your ego appears to be struggling, you, the Self, have infinite options available from internally sourced "enoughness."

The assumption *I am not enough as I am; I am not okay as I am* is an erroneous notion. It has no grounding since, in truth, the Self is always sheer awareness, always okay, always blissful. The Self is sovereign—independent of all external circumstances. When our mind is not insanely colored by desires and subsequent attachments, we are much more conscious participants in all kinds of relationships, personal and professional.

You can be a conscious consumer, consuming what you have discerned as good and wholesome for consumption, and therefore you do not suffer because of injudicious consumption. Similarly, you can approach all situations, relationships, and people fresh, without prior judgments and preconceived ideas that have poisoned your samsara.

You Can Learn from Mother Nature

"Vairagyam" comes from two words: "vai" and "raga," meaning "removing color." It is the conscious stepping away from false colors to accept our original colorless state—like an all-new canvas. That is why I explain vairagyam not only as detachment but also the practice of decoloring our mind from falsifying myth-colors. This practice is critical to the goal of having a sovereign inner life.

To practice nonattachment, I take inspiration from Mother Nature in springtime. I feel she is saying to us, "Don't worry. Look, I deliberately let go of all my old colored clothing a few months ago. I took off my elaborate wardrobe of leaves, fruits, and flowers, which had once bedecked my being. And here I stand, colorless, clothing-less, naked in my pure divine essence. But I know that I am one with Universal Intelligence. My womb is the magical nothingness that can become everything and anything beautiful, perfect, and amazing! Pure consciousness is my source, essence, my power. I will come back from this deliberate decoloring, detoxing, stripping, and shedding even more beautiful, more aromatic, more enchanting, more everything. I am celebrating my true, pure sovereign essence. Why don't you join me too?"

Meditating on the nature of my Self feels like my mind is being gently washed by my "quiet, all-knowing, formless presence," as if I am physically wiping the mirror of my own mind until all that is left is "me," the bare Self, without the maya-clouds. When we decolor, we are freer of inner compulsions. We begin upholding what we believe to be true more boldly since our samsara no longer pushes and pulls us to conform to pre-scripted roles, attitudes, and actions.

Guided Practice: Decoloring Contemplation

Sit outdoors or near a window with a view of the sky. Notice any clouds, fog, play of light, birds, or objects moving across it. Observe the expansive, open, clear quality of the sky as a canvas for all these things. The sky itself is constant while the clouds, changes in light, and anything passing are temporary.

Now breathe and connect to your inner expansiveness. Notice that timeless background of pure consciousness through which the fluctuations of your body and mind move.

Close your eyes, or keep them open if you prefer, and give yourself this autosuggestion: *I am the sky, pure awareness, and not the clouds. My thoughts are clouds, simply passing through. I am the sky . . . vast, expansive, infinite, spacious, free.* Keep thinking this thought until you start to feel like a vast open sky that is limitless. Holding on to thoughts, feelings, objects, people, or situations in our lives is grasping at clouds.

You can also think these thoughts:

I am enough unto myself.

I am perfect right now.

I am where I need to be.

I am wholeness infinite.

When we begin to identify with the sky versus the clouds (thoughts and desires), we become more real, more aligned to an inner sense of permanence and stillness, blossoming into how the Self, pure consciousness, wants to express itself. We do not need validation from any other being; all can coexist and be whole. This is what I say to remind myself of this:

> *"Today, I am pure awareness, the Self, the vastness,*
> *before I am a guru to my students.*
>
> *Today, I am pure awareness, the Self, the fullness,*
> *before I am a wife to my husband.*
>
> *Today, I am pure awareness, the Self, the limitless,*
> *before I am a daughter to my father.*
>
> *Today, I am pure awareness, the Self, the boundless,*
> *before I am a mother to my son."*

Detachment is something humanity must be gently prepared to do. An ancient Vedic text encourages nurturing such deliberate practices to be free in every sense of the word: "If you want liberation, fling away the vasanas, drink daily [cultivate] with great keenness the nectar of contentment, compassion, forbearance, truth, straightforwardness, calmness, self-control [of the mind and external senses]."[1]

With regular practice of nonattachment following discernment, and the relief, freedom, and joy that follows, you will gradually remember that your happiness lives inside you.

Unmasking the Self requires nothing special of you, other than decluttering (discerning) and decoloring (detaching) your mind from the misperceptions and wrong notions you may have been carrying around.

To the degree that self-ignorance is replaced with self-knowledge from the Vedas and that wisdom transforms from intellectual information into an emotional conviction, you will become the happy recipient of your inner truth and hidden spiritual potential. Self is self-revealing.

When one's basic nature is of happiness, having the desire to be happy is ignorance and, ironically, the beginning of unhappiness. When the desire to be happy ends through nonattachment, true bliss begins because bliss is the nature of the true Self.

Abandon the Chase for Happiness

Chasing happiness almost always leaves us drained because deep down, we know the chase isn't real.

Whenever you chase anything—love, money, fame, sex, marriage—you become that thing's slave. Samsara keeps growing. You lose your own self-approval. The more you chase, the emptier you feel since the outer chase goes against your truth of inner fullness. Sooner or later, the chase yields yet more psychological bondage as well as emotional exhaustion.

Therefore, resolve to never chase anything.

First, cultivate a relationship with your own Self through contemplating upon self-knowledge. Then, with discernment and detachment, you can pursue your goals without desperation.

If you get what you want, you are whole already, and it makes you no more whole than you already were. If you did not get what you set out to get from the world, you are still whole.

Inner joy shall reveal itself to you in your serene, self-content mind when you stop chasing happiness outside of yourself. Any time you are free of desires and content with what comes to you in natural course, accepting what is versus what should be, you experience happiness within.

Nonattachment Is Not Indifference or Apathy

When I say, "I will let go, or practice nonattachment," I don't mean I will abdicate my responsibility or fail in upholding agreements and valid expectations in relationships. If I am expected to do something, I will do it wholeheartedly from my sattvic mind. But with nonattachment, I will show up more emotionally neutral rather than clingy; internally relaxed rather than stressed; with my mind feeling fresh, decolored, and divested from samsara-type investments of wanting things to go a certain way (attachments).

Step Away from What Is Not Real

Typically, detachment always follows discernment.

For example, through the practice of discernment, you may recognize that beliefs such as *I am not worthy, I am unlovable, I will never be prosperous, Everyone is out to get me*, or *I am invisible anyway, so I must hide my talents, opinions, and needs*, and other such victim-engendering beliefs are not real. They are simply the shadows emerging from a sleepwalking egoic samsara.

You will then deliberately distance yourself from false beliefs, through vairagyam, by thinking deliberate, decoloring thoughts such as *This is not real.*

Stay Anchored in Your Central Truth

The objective of practicing nonattachment is not to make you a zombie, mechanically blanking out on your thoughts, emotions, and feelings in a forced state of mental "emptying out." Rather, it means you can experience all your emotions: the whole range, the pure, wise, enlightened, and divine kind too—not just what is superficial and insistent, such as repetitive negative thoughts. You observe your mind and are content without being carried away from your central Self that does not need anything outside of itself to be happy. You are bliss unto yourself.

We may have preferences, but we don't insist that these likes and dislikes determine our experience of our inner reality. We stop controlling, fighting, and railing against life circumstances with an overexpressed and confused samsara. With cultivated dispassion or decoloration (vairagyam) resulting from our discrimination (viveka), we can observe (good, bad, and ugly) and grow!

What and How Is True Vairagyam Obtained?

When vairagyam emerges intentionally from higher knowledge, it is the highest form of detachment; it is a permanent attitude shift enabled by right knowledge, and it is implemented by choice, not activated by adverse circumstances, escapist tendencies, or blind rules made up by religious pundits.

A person who has learned to do this remains forewarned and self-disciplined that *I must engage with the world but not lean upon it blindly for my happiness and fulfillment.* Unlike sleepwalkers, the truly nonattached ones are powerful beings, self-contained and self-respecting, not emotionally delusional, needy, and vulnerable like the unconscious, attached ones.

In the ultimate analysis, nonattachment is an inner mental discipline of privately shifting focus and withdrawing our inner priorities because we have seen through *what is what.* It is our soul right to detach and free ourselves from previous attachments that are not serving us, that are leading us down a slippery slope of psychological and emotional bondage.

Guided Practice: Cultivating Nonattachment

Picture an object that is most precious to you, that gives you joy, and that you feel is a meaningful extension of you (perhaps your car, house, family photo albums, wedding ring, or other object). Now imagine that object is gone, never coming back into your life. Experience the loss of that object and observe the depth of that inner attachment. Remind yourself that you are still whole without its presence.

Picture a relationship that is important to you, that you feel completes you in some way (perhaps this is a significant other, parent, child, or professional partnership). Now imagine your life without that relationship. Sit with that seemingly gaping hole in your life and notice the strength of your attachment to this relationship being "just so." Remind yourself that your true Self is still full and no less in any way without that relationship. You have meaning, purpose, and value independent of even your most important relationships.

Scan your thoughts and assumptions. Wherever you find an object or relationship you feel completes you, consciously step out of the narrative that says you need that person or thing and notice the power of attachment. Acknowledging the power of our attachments is a first step toward healthy freedom from them.

Once nonattachment following discernment becomes your everyday mental practice, your mind is yours to claim and keep free of random colors (or bad odors). Using the same mind that once bound you to detach from one object, one person, and one desire at a time gives you tremendous self-respect and dignity and unleashes powerful inner sovereignty! You will become a role model to others. When you decolor your mind consciously, the false tints will peel or fade away. In that empty canvas, you will finally see your own true face, smiling back at you.

The more you consciously decolor your mind from its wrong or scripted bondage-creating notions, the more sovereign freedom you will experience from within. No one will be able to manipulate you because the discerning mind no longer goes after crumbs! You will interact, engage, and even play with the world, but you will not need it to fulfill you. The greater your acquaintance with your true Self, the more strongly you will feel inwardly directed to lead a life from the truest version of who you are versus from false beliefs and notions that attach you to other people's stories, beliefs, ambitions, and journeys, and that make you feel dependent upon the world and relationships. Thanks to detachment, the less you depend on the world and its objects, whether living or inanimate, for your quota of happiness, the bolder and freer you will be. What are you waiting for? Wash off those unnecessary colors and revel in your bare and bold Self!

13

◈◈◈◈◈◈◈◈◈◈

Shama: Managing Your Thoughts—Really

"One should uplift oneself by one's own efforts. One should not lower oneself. For the purified mind alone is the friend of oneself; the non-purified mind alone is the enemy of oneself."

BHAGAVAD GITA, 6.5

My Baba once told me a story. At an ashram, a cow was always tied up at night so she would not wander away. One day, the rope used to tie up the cow could not be found. A student tried to guide the cow into the cowshed so she would be safe and dry in case of rain, but she would not go inside. The student went to his guru, who told him that the cow was used to being led by a rope, but since the rope was missing, he should pretend to tie a rope around her neck and lead her with the imaginary rope.

It worked. The cow got up and came along meekly.

However, when it was time to go out and feed on grass the next day, the cow would not go out. Once again, there was no rope to lead her. As before, the teacher instructed the student to pretend to tie the rope and lead her out. Again, the ploy worked.

The rope of thought was enough for the cow to behave as if she were in bondage. She was free all along.

Bondage and freedom, power and powerlessness, all occur in the realm of thought. By understanding the mind and its deepest tendencies through the lens of Vedic wisdom, we can free ourselves from sorrow and reclaim our inner joy.

As a spiritual teacher, I simply pretend to untie the imaginary ropes around my students' minds, even though they have been free all along.

I tell them, "You are free," and interestingly, they start leading freer lives. They become more powerful and spiritually greater versions of who they were just moments ago.

You are free!

Learn to Let Go of Thought Ropes

Did you know that you can choose to step out of bondage thoughts and think sovereignty-revealing ones instead?

When you use your higher mind, or intellect, to steer your lower mind where thoughts and emotions transpire, you can change your deepest beliefs about yourself and your life and switch between thoughts and attached emotions at will. The practice of housekeeping your own thoughts is called *shama*.

In this chapter, I will share a well-known method of thought management from the Vedas (which is also mentioned in the *Yoga Sutras*) that only takes a moment. Then, I will share a truly novel way of managing thoughts and emotions that I have developed.

A Super-Quick Thought-Management Technique

This specific technique is called *pratipaksha bhavana*. I call it *the method of thinking deliberate opposite thoughts*. When you encounter a bondage-creating thought, simply and deliberately think the opposite point of view. Then your mind will be a sovereign mind.

For example, if you tend to be generally critical about someone, find genuine reason to praise them. If you dismiss others' sorrow, empathize instead and put yourself mentally in their shoes until real compassion is evoked from within. If you put yourself down a lot or are routinely self-minimizing in front of others, restrain such comments and take credit where due. Substitute generosity for greed, discrimination for delusion, humility for pride and conceitful thoughts, and appreciative thoughts for jealousy of another's success.

This helps because when we deliberately think an opposite, constructive, and dharmic thought while restraining a non-dharmic thought, our mind expands from delusion to clarity, from selfishness to selflessness, from the material to the spiritual. In this way, we enhance our opportunity to experience our sovereign, joyful soul potential.

You can reinforce the practice of deliberate opposite thoughts with actions. When you see yourself being inconsiderate of the needs of others, deliberately act in the opposite way and become accommodating to the needs of those around you. When your higher mind observes you being slothful, for example avoiding a shower or not picking up your room, immediately take a shower and make the bed! If you watch time-wasting shows on television all day, begin with tuning in to the more informative shows on nature, policy, or science.

This way, each time you change your thought or act opposite of the initial impulse, you are guiding your mind and senses via the sovereign mind's decrees. You can choose to not let negative thoughts overwhelm you by mindfully observing them and replacing them with positive thoughts until slowly they become our second nature.

Now the mind knows who is boss!

Oops, there it goes again . . . Make sure to practice the opposite of what it wants! It will learn in due course who is boss and that you mean business.

Acharya Shunya's Thought-Management Model

Our thoughts can be categorized into five basic types. (See the diagram of the five types of thoughts on the next page.) Two of them are unconscious, default thoughts because we think them without thinking about them. They lead us into greater and greater bondage of self-delusions, or samsara. In fact, we must use our higher mental faculty to hit the pause or delete button on them and be free of them. Otherwise, they keep playing continuously on the screen of the lower mind.

The other three thought types are deliberative and conscious, and they can liberate us from the bondage of sorrow prisons. However, they are not our default thoughts, so we must use the higher mind to deliberately introduce them onto the screen of our lower mind. Once these new, liberating thoughts become your default, they will help you dismantle sorrow from its roots and claim your happiness and abiding peace. Thoughts have power!

I am such a loser is a self-pitying thought. *I became this way thanks to my mother!* is a blaming thought.

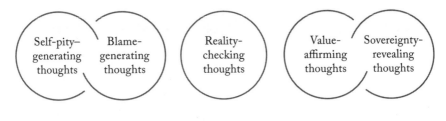

BY DEFAULT	BY CHOICE	BY CHOICE
Sorrow-generating states of mind Tamas- and Rajas-dominant state of mind	Generates psychological health, leading to greater peace of mind Sattva is examining rajas and tamas	Generates spiritual health, leading to peace of mind and inner joy Sattva is the leading guna in the mind

Figure 13.1: The Five Types of Thoughts

Reality-checking thoughts are used to question the first two thoughts: *Wait, who says I am a loser? Is this even true? Did my mother hold me back, or did I use her to hold myself back? What am I trying to prove by thinking such thoughts? And to whom?*

Value-affirming thoughts refer to a value. For example: *Let me accept all my past failures with grace and self-love and not make them a daily whip. Let me think nonviolent thoughts toward my mother and myself. Let me embrace the truth of my potential, which is awaiting my discovery.*

I AM ENOUGH is a sovereignty-generating thought. It is that simple.

Let me explain each thought type in detail below.

Self-Pity–Generating Thoughts

Self-pity–generating thoughts can take many disempowering, self-pitying versions: *I am tired, I am broken, I am a loser, I am undeserving.* These tamas-dominant thoughts zap your ability to operate effectively in the world and keep you locked in self-nonacceptance mode. They engender sorrow from unhealthy grief, self-blame, self-shame, self-criticism, or self-loathing, leading to loss of self-confidence, self-esteem, and self-worth. They are connected to equally dark emotions of despair, despondency, and even depression.

These thoughts are almost always related to thwarted desires, or vasanas. When we don't get what we want or think we deserve or when life does not go our way, we blame ourselves, dissatisfied with who we are and what we have. We get busy comparing ourselves with others and somehow feel "never enough." These thoughts reinforce self-ignorance (avidya), the root of imprisoning beliefs and estrangement from our spiritual center.

When such thoughts fill us, we are neither connected to an outer god nor an inner god (Self)—we simply lament, as embittered and disillusioned egos filled with emotion, *This is not fair!* We feel the world owes us something and has failed to deliver! So, our self-pity feels righteous.[1]

Our being is infinitely emerging, yet we can fool ourselves into thinking we are helpless, powerless, small, stupid, undeserving, irreparably broken, and traumatized. We build ourselves into an ongoing anxious state or even a panic attack. We need no one else to disempower us; we can do it ourselves. And nobody can help us—no pill, therapist, mantra, magic, not even a great guru—unless we decide to see through and pop these thoughts ourselves, labeling them unacceptable, unnecessary, and false using intellectual discernment.

When such tamasic thoughts arise, they are often a replay of past sorrow, trauma, or difficulty. When we get stuck in them, we develop anxiety disorders, depression, or melancholia that can become an emotional disorder. Repetitive self-berating thoughts alienate us from our sovereign potential. When you are full of self-created unhappiness, you don't need any outside cause to make you diseased; your own mind is the trigger for your inner disease.

If these thoughts are entertained without questioning (*How much is enough? Is it even real?*), they become our default reality, leading us to live inside a "victim shell" with scripts that our mind updates daily (if subconsciously) with more powerlessness. Because you are the Self, you are always free to choose your thoughts. You can dwell in this cluster forever. In fact, you can have a couple more lifetimes in it. The only price you pay is being trapped in a maya-mirage of grief, guilt, and shame. We must realize that our thoughts are up to us and our thoughts literally build our inner reality.

Now, be gentle, dear ones. Change the channel. You yourself are the divine "remote control." Simply think a new thought that respects your spiritual nature, then another, and another. Think your way out of this negative, sorrow-generating, self-victimizing thought cluster.

Blame-Generating Thoughts

Blame-generating thoughts and emotions make you angry. These rajas-dominant thoughts make you feel like a victim of other people, whom you blame for your suffering, misfortune, or missed opportunity. You fill with self-righteous indignation, bitterness, and a false (ego) power that robs you of your real soul power.

It is true that sometimes other people are the cause of our sorrow, but we become the agents of repeated sorrow by replaying memories and building new thoughts around the original wound. Neither the wound nor its chronic, self-created aftermath heals.

Through such thoughts, we experience dissatisfaction with the world—external events, the weather, people, and of course, God. We are ready to blame anything and anyone. Often, the target of our resentment never gets a chance to explain themselves. We virtually fight with the world, its people, gods, rules, and laws, and are either drained of our inner power or act out nastily from false, judgmental, self-righteous power. Either way, berating others, lamenting, gossiping, judging, fault-finding, nit-picking, nagging, complaining, and other such behaviors are born from a basic premise: *The world and its people have let me down, and I am angry.* Our self-righteous censure triggers even greater anger and deeper versions of self-created sorrow.

As you think and feel, so you become, say the seers. Such thoughts make us victims or, alternatively, aggressors in our own mind. Our subjective projections, born from thwarted desires, lead to such thoughts, along with accompanying emotions of rage, indignation, and exasperation. Unchecked, they drive us deeper and deeper into a self-projected delusory account of reality. Emotions of envy, jealousy, or frustration reign.

So many of us lead angry, embittered lives and die feeling acrimonious. Our berating, blaming, and reproaching thoughts and feelings have power. We may shout, scream, misbehave, and allow these thoughts to help us write "aggressor scripts." We may even go to prison one day because our thoughts trigger socially unacceptable behaviors.

These thoughts begin humbly enough when someone crosses us but can lead to violence toward others. Baba said angry thoughts lead to the greatest diseases, where we first are imprisoned and then destroyed by our own unhealthy anger. If you act out your unhealthy anger, there is a problem. If you suppress or swallow it, there is also a problem. When we generate thought-based delusory anger, it must go some-where. It may very well eat you alive, destroying your health and well-being.

Habitual, delusory, anger-generating thoughts trap us and give us almost no option to reinvent our story or write a new chapter in our life. Our subjective interpretation of the objective universe hurts us more than any person can. People and relationships are external to us, characters in the outer world cannot harm us. In fact, no one can harm you; it is only the fear that they will harm you that harms you. Feeling angry all the time will harm you. Envy toward others harms you. The hatred you feel harms you. Suspicion harms you. And judgment harms you.

No one person can damage you over your entire life. Your thoughts alone can do that. But instead of thought-management, we get busy pointing fingers or tightening fists. A mental world full of reaction, judgment, indignation, self-righteous anger, sulking, passive aggressiveness, and revenge is a state of delusion. We are confused about our reality and suffer from the disease of moha, or "attached outcomes." Self-knowledge of the true nature of the nondual Self and its ability to be peaceful, secure, and okay right now with things as they stand can help us out of this quagmire of "entitled frustration."

Our habits of incessantly thinking and talking negatively activate a spiritual law. When we express and vent negativity, sooner or later our negative thinking becomes a self-fulfilling prophecy. We will find that, indeed, our life is nothing but a series of negative experiences.

How does this happen? The mind has a will of its own, which we can apply to our advantage if we are aware of it, or it can run amuck when we are unaware of it. (After all, you are the Spirit Divine, and thus your mental equipment is all-powerful—whether you know how to use it or not is a different matter.) Thoughts have tremendous power because, as I mentioned earlier, our thoughts become our deeds, deeds become habits, habits become character, and character becomes our destiny over time. That is why we must choose our thoughts carefully and employ the will of the mind consciously to sow seeds of reality, balance, positivity, and sattva versus creating a life filled with negativity, self-sabotage, and spiritual darkness from unchecked tamas and rajas.

But if we do not actively employ our will, the mind will go in any direction it wishes. Then, we begin acting randomly, often in ways that conflict with our soul, and our directionless, thoughtless deeds result in an entire life that never amounted to much.

That is why the Vedas put so much importance on disciplining the mind by making the mind's will (abilities) align with the superior will of the Self. This is known as *sankalpa shakti*—the all-new willpower that emerges from the mind (instrument) uniting with the will of its master, the Self. You are much more powerful and positively aligned when through sankalpa shakti your mind obeys your soul and your actions are congruous.

Remember, thoughts build upon each other. We begin thinking similar thoughts (self-pitying or other-blaming for example), and before we know it, our entire mind is filled with delusory, confusing, even foolish and unreal thoughts unless we intervene with sankalpa shakti and take control by editing and auditing our thoughts!

If you are caught in this trap of berating yourself and others, why not change the channel using sankalpa shakti? Your Self can tell the mind to think of rainbows, puppies, and daffodils every time the same old violent or indignant thoughts and feelings arise. Reclaim your mind-space. Show the mind who is boss and that the boss wants to claim a new way of thinking, the way of sovereignty, inner ease, and acceptance! Then you can write another script, one in which a new conscious thought follows another, until you are cruising along in a whole new dimension of a much more joyful inner reality.

Reality-Checking Thoughts

Discernment and detachment are the reality-evoking thought processes. Discernment involves deliberate, higher-level thought discrimination between what is real and what appears to be real (but is merely a projection of our samsara).

Detachment follows discernment, where we mentally "unhook" from what is unreal and no longer give it power. This sets us free from our mind's myth-beliefs, allowing us to own our reality with greater clarity.

Here is an example: If you feel lonely, you may think: *No one cares about me.* Now think a deliberate, discerning thought in your higher mind that checks the factuality of that first thought: *Is it true that no one cares about me?*

Additional reality-checking thoughts may follow:

* *Is what I am thinking in this moment true, or has it simply arisen because it is Saturday night and I am alone in the house?*

+ *Is my entire and sole reality that no one cares about me, or is that simply my subjective feeling right now?*

+ *Tomorrow, when my sister and her family come for Sunday brunch, I know I will feel on top of the world (and well-cared for by my sister and nieces).*

+ *I may not have family, but I have friends; they all just happen to be busy tonight. We've had many beautiful times in the past. In the future, too, I will have beautiful times with people who care about me.*

+ *I don't know many people, as I have just moved into town, but I care about so many causes; soon, I will make friends at my new workplace and places where I volunteer.*

+ *Yes, it's true I am bored tonight. But what is not true is that no one cares about me. I have many people who care about me who live in other parts of the world or who are busy tonight.*

Now you may think: *Ah, I feel better already! Maybe I'll watch a movie now!* And then you happily do exactly that.

This way, by questioning your thoughts, you unveil the underlying reality. This allows for a more accurate perception of things as they are and a greater estimation of their true nature than what our ego-mind believed, imagined, or projected to be true.

Reality-checking thoughts are essential. Otherwise, our mind remains trapped in default unconsciousness, generating feelings and thoughts of anger, grief, and shame, triggering yet more self-pitying or other-blaming thoughts, unless we make it a practice to intentionally question them.

How serious was the humiliation? Did the person mean it, or was it a slip of the tongue? Did I interpret this comment as humiliation since recently I feel sensitive and hurt with just about anything and anyone? Or is it humiliation? Am I underplaying this? Am I replaying an older issue? Is this more serious, not subtle humiliation, but downright shaming? Is this all real to begin with? We must constantly ask ourselves such questions. These questions are what I call reality-checking thoughts.

If you spend less time hating, berating, and—worse—believing your thoughts, you can redirect freed-up thought energy into reality checking. When the higher mind begins inspecting mental contents, your emotional state can be more neutral; delusory thoughts won't colonize your samsara and conceal your true Self.

Reality-checking thoughts help break the spell of "rajas-tamas thoughts," allowing agitated emotions to settle down and clarity to emerge from within.

Value-Affirming Thoughts

Value-affirming thoughts are cultivated, noble thoughts that engender self-value. With these sattvic thoughts, we begin to see ourselves not merely as struggling individuals filled with grief and rage, but as instruments of a higher power, as if some greater will and intelligence is moving through us. We begin to feel part of a greater fabric of collective consciousness. Over time, the collective good becomes our ego's evolutionary imperative. Value-affirming thoughts power up problem-solving areas of your mind, helping you tap into your innate creativity. (Chapter 17 discusses such dharma values at length.) When you adopt higher values, your thoughts and emotions will reflect a greater intelligence.

By maturing our ego and embracing higher values, like mutual respect, compassion, altruism, forgiveness, nonviolence, and truthfulness, we begin to shape our true potential as conscious humans. We become emotionally functional adults. We recognize that we deserve respect no matter who we are or what we do, and we must offer respect too. A dharmic mind effortlessly respects and upholds healthy boundaries. We treat other people and all beings, including insects and plants; inanimate nature, rivers, mountains, and pebbles; and the entire cosmos as inherently valuable when we think value-affirming thoughts.

The Bhagavad Gita promotes harmlessness, truth, absence of anger, renunciation, peacefulness, honesty, compassion, generosity, gentleness, modesty, and decisiveness.[2] Such values are guidelines for thinking consciously. They invite us to choose our own ways of expressing how we think and act from deeper knowingness. For example, when I think of not acting from violence, I wonder to myself: *Can I actively cultivate loving awareness and act from understanding and compassion toward all embodied beings, especially those sleepwalking in ignorance and those weaker than me, smaller than me, or for any reason less powerful than me? Can I give up self-pity, rage, meanness, and hatred in my mind and learn to release such negative mental states in nonviolent ways, like prayer, meditation, and conscious journaling or dialogue? Can I aspire to lead a nonviolent existence and remain nonviolent even if I must go to battle one day to defend my principles? Should I battle in my daily life employing violent thoughts and spewing hatred or instead identify with inner peace?*

When sattva begins informing us, our thoughts and beliefs undergo radical changes for the better; they become more ethical, humane, and universal in outlook. Our daily choices become aligned with our highest intentions. Following a sattvic path ensures that our consciousness is elevating with every thought we think, and our ego is not unnecessarily suffering.

Value-affirming thoughts are the default of the sattvic mind. We take responsibility. Instead of self-pitying, we make effort toward positive changes, accept what we cannot change, and pray to the higher power that we know what to do when. Instead of judging others, we understand that people are born with different endowments and everyone is struggling at some level in maya. Even if we must fire someone, break up with another, or even punish or scold others (for the right reasons or because duty calls), we can do so with respect and integrity.

The sages clarify that following higher values is a matter of free will and not externally imposed, punitive, social, moral, or religious conditioning, nor a routine of dos and don'ts. Baba told me that when we think ethical thoughts, we save ourselves and become emotionally safe to all beings and the planet. I can exist like a peaceful flower, be creative, and be compassionate to myself and others. With value-affirming thoughts, you can be a self-healing, self-soothing, self-uplifting, self-comforting entity, all through the agency of your own mind. Isn't that wonderful?

Value-affirming thoughts indicate the rise of emotional maturity. Instead of remaining stuck in unconscious grief and shaming and blaming thought patterns, we can rise above obvious default thoughts, and ask: *What is my spiritual option here? What can be considered an ethical response in this situation? How can I continue to self-value through trying times and value something essentially good and beautiful amid all of us, even in the heart of one who challenges me?* And then, we can choose our actions based not on personal (ego) gain, but on a higher truth.

Thus, value-affirming thoughts lay the foundation of our personal stability, power, and abundance and directly pave the way for inner freedom or sovereignty-revealing thoughts.

Sovereignty–Revealing Thoughts

As embodied souls, the only thing of real value we have is our thoughts. Most thoughts take us away from our true Self. The rare thoughts that introduce us to our true Self are called sovereignty-revealing thoughts.

In general, our default thoughts are of negative nature—struggle, strife, and competitiveness. Even the more aspirational or positive thoughts that society encourages, such as *I will compete*, and *I will make it one day*, are thoughts that sooner or later may elicit anxiety and, therefore, give birth to yet more negativity. Your mind, on its own, is incapable of thinking the thoughts that will take it back to its source, the Self, since the mind is of a lower order of reality (maya) than its source (Atman). That's why we must be grateful if we are at last paired, in any lifetime, with someone—a guru—who dares to think differently and exposes us to new thoughts and ideas that lead us back home to Self.

When I meditate or quietly contemplate my true essence, my true Self rises on its own as a quiet but infinite river of unfathomable depth and intensity, whose water is pure consciousness. I am filled with expanded awareness, happiness, self-confidence, and soul power as I bathe in this river of self-approval, self-love, self-delight, and self-expression.

Through ultra-refined thoughts that probe the nature of the deepest and subtlest reality, you can use the mind for its highest and main purpose: Self-realization.

When we probe deeply enough, we find that sovereignty-revealing thoughts are really self-discovery, self-exploration, self-declaration, and self-celebration thoughts. They take you home to Self. They are a sweet balm of relief and ease for your poor suffering ego, diseased from the estrangement from its own source all along. At last, the ego is home, healthy, and happy with its spiritual parent, the Self. Sorrow begins to scatter, just like demons fade away as we awaken from a bad dream (it was only a dream, after all). What relief!

Now the ego-mind's pathological projections of grief, anger, and delusory likes and dislikes begin disappearing like mist evaporates automatically when the sun rises. The mind becomes clear like a shining crystal, reflecting only what it truly belongs to and serves, which is the Self.

Sovereignty-revealing thoughts don't dissolve or suppress the ego; but they purify it into a luminous, "soul-aligned," radiantly happy ego. These thoughts do not occur on their own. The seeds are first planted in our mind by a guru, whose words or writings transfer the seeds from the lofty Upanishads into the ready bed of our own heart and mind.

If you already have a houseful of apples, do you need to go buy them from elsewhere? Isn't it good to be reminded that we have the apples and we can eat them at will? And once we expect to find apples, we will find them. This is the catch. If you don't believe in the existence of your Self and its divine infinite nature, including joy and peace, then you will remain hypnotized in an external search mode, begging for morsels of freedom and power from the world.

As you can see, these Self-revealing thoughts, known as sovereignty-revealing thoughts, work through autosuggestion based upon a resolve to come back home and look for our inner apples. This path to liberation from bondage to maya or awakening from maya.

Guided Practice: A Contemplation for a Sattvic Mind

Contemplate the following thought affirmations, one at a time, until this knowledge, *I am a sovereign being with infinite potential*, is internalized. You can also use them as bedtime contemplation exercises. Each contemplation will calm your egoic fears and insecurities in relationships and remind you of your inherent indwelling fullness, wholeness, and power.

- *I am Spirit Divine.*
- *I am wholeness.*
- *I am unconditional love.*
- *I am the source of all joy.*
- *I am infinitely powerful.*
- *I am eternally blessed from within, always.*
- *I am peace. I am silence.*
- *I am unattached. I am free.*
- *Despite commitments in relationships, freedom is my soul nature.*
- *I am whole. I am secure. I am love. I am complete.*
- *I am fulfilled.*
- *I am pure.*

- *I am done with all kinds of shaming.*

- *I am a soul, not a physical being. All my relationships belong to the body.*

- *My soul potential is limitless. I am invincible.*

- *I am pure awareness. Relationships come and go in this awareness.*

- *Being myself is danger free. It's my ultimate truth, and I live fearlessly.*

- *I'd rather be disliked for who I am than liked for who I am not.*

- *I am a divine being. How can I be nondeserving, nonpowerful, or nonprecious?*

- *My essential nature is powerful beyond description. It is this soul power I reclaim with joy in this moment, from within me.*

- *I am connected to an unlimited source of love, abundance, and self-acceptance, now and always.*

- *I have access to unlimited divine assistance. My strength comes from my connection to this divine source.*

- *I am pure consciousness. The age of my body and the state of my mind have no bearing on who I am.*

- *I can accomplish anything I put my mind to because I know I'm never alone. My Self is inherently connected to the Supreme Reality, the Self of this entire universe—God.*

- *I am a divine instrument of divine love.*

Once you begin contemplating and then believing the affirmations, you will start feeling the inner freedom to reinvent yourself or redefine yourself with ease. But it is not a one-time miracle. Reading this book and building a why-it-is-true context in your mind is equally important. Then make it an ongoing practice to remember who you are deep inside you. Think like this: *I know that in the core of my being, in the silence of my still heart, and in the absence of all seeking and striving, I enter the vast, endless dimension of Self. Here, I find a key to unlock infinite wholeness, power, love, and infinite joy. I hold the key to my happiness in my hands.*

When sovereignty-revealing thoughts become your default, amazing amounts of power, self-love, self-appreciation, fulfillment, and joy will arise from within as emotions. Thoughts from beyond the ego emerge. With this state of mind, you can implement a paradigm shift in your life, making changes that become the conduit for awakening to inner bliss and freedom. Here is a real-life example of this kind of mental housekeeping:

Oh no, I must cook and clean before my partner comes home from work. I am so tired, my body hurts, my head hurts. I am stuck. (self-pitying)

Who the hell does she think she is? Is she my boss? (other-blaming)

Wait a minute, did she ask me to cook and clean because I don't earn money, or is this the way I can contribute to our home? This guilt of not earning money, is this mine or are those her words? Is she shaming, or am I shaming myself? What is my responsibility here toward myself and my self-respect? (discerning / reality-checking)

What can I do that will put me at ease right now? I will practice self-compassion, eat out, and relax. I can apply the value of straightforwardness and tell her, "I did not cook today because I am overcome with conflicted emotions, grief, and anger. Can we instead go out for dinner and afterward have a heart-to-heart talk?" When we talk, I will remember the value of nonviolence and tell her what I feel and how she can help. (value-affirming)

I am enough as I am because I am a divine soul. I am Self, special and sovereign. I am precious. I am inherently valuable. I am free to change my mind—always. (sovereignty-revealing)

With practice, contemplating a single sovereign thought unpacks a whole body of wisdom and insights. For example, say that I am about to overeat because what I am eating is simply too delicious and my senses are screaming with happiness. *Yippee!* However, if I then choose to think, *I am divine, complete, whole, and fulfilled,* things immediately change in my mental field.

My mind and subsequently my senses will move away from their default identification with the ego's bottomless desire for gratification and transition to true remembrance of my ever-fulfilled Self. Unexamined greed ends. Instantly, I connect to my unlimited internal abundance, fulfillment, and wholeness. I can simply walk away with an enjoyable gustatory experience that didn't turn me into a slave of my senses. The more self-knowledge we have, the more powerful this thought process becomes. It acts like a key that opens a portal to freedom. That is how joyous thoughts become "freeing," or "moksha," thoughts.

Now, the moment I find an unwelcome thought appear on the screen of my lower mind, I pop it like a bubble, and my intellect recognizes it as "random." Then I use my higher mind to introduce a brand-new thought or idea to redirect my mind. It's as simple as changing the television channel.

To experience the pure Self, we need to minimize our engagement with tamas- and rajas-thought clusters. We don't have to feel guilty about these thoughts. This teaching is not a judgment. It is simply switching on a light bulb in our own mind. To "scold" or "shame" our ego or blame and disparage others for our difficult life circumstances is of no use. Why not think conscious thoughts instead and awaken to a whole new paradigm?

Change Your Negative Thoughts ASAP

A tiny flame accidentally lit in the forest can easily be put out by the blowing wind. But if that flame gets the opportunity to grow, nourished by abundantly available dry tinder, it will build into a huge forest fire. Now the same wind, which once extinguished the fire, will begin nurturing the flame, spreading it far and wide. Wind will become fire's accomplice, and the flame will quickly devour the entire forest with its hungry, agitated, windswept flames.

There is a saying: if you cannot fight the enemy, join the enemy. *Wind, which was an enemy of the weaker fire, becomes the friend of the stronger fire.*

Similarly, our sattvic mind can quickly discern and detach from feeble, isolated thoughts, but it can be corrupted by a tidal wave of thoughts. When unhealthy thoughts are nourished and allowed to multiply without surveillance, they overwhelm us and give birth to gigantic attachments and aversions, even fatal addictions. Our ability to discern and detach is challenged or even ineffective. It even begins to justify our reasons for being attached.

Baba used to advise his students that we should stay alert against two things: disease and thoughts, because they both grow inside us silently. Just as we should act swiftly and proactively and take instant action to eliminate disease in the body by changing our diet and lifestyle, so too must internal enemies—like thoughts of lust, violence, rage, greed, control, or pride—be handled the moment the first thought has arisen and been noticed. Once the enemy has gained strength, it's more difficult to do this. These thought enemies are hijackers of our joy and of our spiritual journey to the Self.

Understand that the initial thought or first few thoughts in fact are not under your control since they are connected to your life experiences over many lifetimes, per the Vedas. But the perpetuation or cessation of the thought is in your hands. You have the free will to decide whether a thought chain that has cropped up in your mind should be allowed to hang around and grow into a full-fledged belief or should be shown the door by thinking a reality-checking thought.

Use your discernment to judge those thoughts and ask, *Is this thought worthy of my attention, nourishment, and support?* The answer: *only if it is taking me closer to my sovereign reality.*

For example, think, *I am a sovereign Self; I don't need to seek approval, except from my own conscience,* then actively welcome that thought in your mind, dwell upon it, and allow it to thrive. If a thought is not worthy of nourishment, for example, a thought like, *I wish my mother-in-law would notice and compliment my neat, clean kitchen,* it must be nipped in the bud. Such thoughts are giving your mother-in-law (thought) way too much power.

If you don't like your thought, simply respond to it with a thought like: *You are not even true! Go away. I refuse to give you more attention, you scary (negative, gloomy, foolish, jealous, frustrated) bundle of random energy!* And it will lose its power, I promise.

And if you like a thought, then maybe think, *Ah, what a wonderful insight has emerged in my divine mind!* And the thought will stay and grow flowers in your mind to please you and delight you some more.

Whether you know it or not, you are the master of your mind. And you get to call the shots as to which virtual visitor stays and which goes from your mental kingdom. You can pull the plug on a thought at any time by exercising intellectual discrimination to question its validity and then practice detachment to move away from giving an unworthy thought or feeling any more attention.

Every person's mind is of two kinds: pure and impure. It is impure when in the grip of shaming, blaming, or delusional thought patterns. It starts becoming pure when it begins to contemplate dharma or value-affirming thoughts. The mind becomes divine, and above all sovereign, at one with the mind of God or Universal Intelligence when it begins to contemplate its own divine nature. It attains liberation from the bondage of maya that very instant.

Thus, it is our very thoughts that keep us in bondage—the tamas and rajas states of mind—and it is our very thoughts that help us pierce our own ignorance, recognize who we are, and claim the sattvic state of mind. Each of us has the responsibility to seek the true nature of our Self by navigating our thoughts appropriately from tamas to rajas to sattva.

14

❖❖❖❖❖❖❖

Bhawashuddhi: Cultivating Emotional Intelligence

"Absolute freedom exists on all sides for the self-controlled ones who are free from cravings and anger; who have controlled their thoughtsand have therefore realized the Self."

BHAGAVAD GITA, 5.26

To discern truth from illusion, to pull your mind away from bondages, and to remind it of its sovereign potential, it is important to purify and sort through your emotions as well as your thoughts. This practice is called *bhawashuddhi*. The word "bhawa" refers to the feeling and emotive aspect of the mind, and "shuddhi" means "enlightening the mind with application of self-knowledge."

You can use the practice of discernment, or viveka, to distinguish between healthy, authentic feelings that you must continue to feel and their unhealthy versions that are delusory creations of your samsara.

The Three Types of Feelings and Emotions

First, it is important to classify your feelings using the lens of the three universal qualities: tamas, rajas, and sattva.

* Tamas feelings are heavy and lethargic and even foolish and stupid. They shut us down. Sadness, depression, guilt, shame, and violence are tamas feelings.

- Rajas feelings are fiery and resistant. Anger, desire, pride, and frustration are rajas feelings.

- Sattvic feelings are light and reassuring. Clarity, happiness, love, and peace are sattvic feelings.

If you can recognize what you are feeling at a given moment, you can recognize the underlying quality and then either try to stay with it or shift it.

Illumined, or sattvic, feelings and emotions don't just feel good. It is widely known that when you experience a higher proportion of sattvic feelings, physical health and immunity improves and thoughts are clear, not delusional. You are enabled from within to make better, more illumined, self-empowering, and liberating choices.

Here's a quick review:

Sattva: The mind's natural mode of illumined intelligence.

- Sattva enables correct comprehension.

- Thoughts impart balance, clarity, knowledge, peace, and power.

- Emotions are peaceful, calm, hopeful, enthusiastic, cheerful, amused, encouraged, optimistic, appreciative, glad, content, self-pleased, self-satisfied, gratified, awe-filled, elated, joyful, and blissful.

Rajas: The agitated mode of the mind.

- Rajas distorts comprehension of reality.

- Thoughts cause worry, disquiet, apprehension, frustration, excessive desires, lust, extreme ambitions, burn-out, and anxiety.

- Emotions are often of insecurity-borne greed, competitiveness, covetousness, comparison, jealousy, envy, arrogance, annoyance, frustration, indifference to others' needs or suffering, impatience to achieve goals, criticism, displeasure, anger, rage, full-blown hostility, violence, hatred, spite, conceit, distrust, threats, grasping, possessiveness, self-protection, self-glorification, self-edification, gluttony, and a demanding nature.

Tamas: The blocked or dull mode of the mind.

+ Tamas blocks comprehension of reality.

+ Thoughts prevent balance; hold and arrest imbalanced patterns; and cause inertia, dullness, confusion, apathy, recklessness, violence, addictions, self-harm, and harm to others.

+ Emotions are apathy, listlessness, lethargy, boredom, disconnection, lack of focus, inattention, pessimism, purposelessness, worthlessness, isolation, numbness, flat, indifferent, sad, overwhelmed, weary, melancholy, despairing, morbid, sullen, desolate, miserable, joyless, pleasureless, devoid of empathy, passionless, guiltless, remorseless, hopeless, empty, bereft, crushed, drained, gloomy, weepy, discouraged, dejected, heavy-hearted, dispirited, despairing, bleak, despondent, depressed, anguished, hopeless, withdrawn, even suicidal.

All Emotions Serve a Purpose

When you open the door to all your feelings, even those uncomfortable feelings that you may have been running away from up to now (through your avoidance of painful circumstances), you overcome inner resistance.

In an intelligent universe, all emotions, including some uncomfortable ones like anger, fear, guilt, and shame, have a healthy role to play in your inner landscape; even the emotion of sorrow, or emotional pain, has an intelligent purpose.

Fear is a warning, anger is for protection, pain is for cleansing and releasing, guilt informs us of our transgressions, and healthy shame helps align us with moral boundaries. Every single feeling has its appropriate role in the scheme of spirit's earthly journey. Emotions assist us in evolving into a more sensitive, empathetic, and empowered version of our self.

Positive, sattvic emotions, especially the more spiritually expansive ones, are those that inform the ego, *Good job, you are doing just fine; you are on the shortest route to realizing your spiritual potential.* These include feelings of joy, bliss, a sense of oneness with all beings, inner satisfaction, inner happiness that arises for no specific reason, happiness at others' happiness, freedom, spontaneity, creativity, magnanimity, generosity, abundance, fullheartedness, and lightheartedness.

Negative emotions, the rajas and tamas types that engender extended emotional suffering, point out to the ego that it needs to change direction, rein in the senses, practice discernment and nonattachment from chasing vasanas, and turn inward in search of a greater light and presence, the Self. The suffering engendered by negative emotions does not go away on its own unless we do the necessary inner work. We must seek out self-knowledge that informs us where we are too attached, unconscious, or acting in an entitled manner.

Emotion Suppression Is Never a Good Idea

Suppression or avoidance of one emotion disrupts and often disturbs the entire emotional intelligence, and what is left behind is often mental illness, such as depression or anxiety.

Avoidance of emotions can also lead to destructive behaviors, such as eating disorders, substance abuse, and all kinds addictions. These behaviors may help us avoid experiencing difficult feelings in the short run, but they only make the situation worse in the long run and prolong suffering. We create many more difficulties by not to facing the current difficulty. So, acceptance leads you to psychological health every single time. Even if you shed some tears during the process, that is a healthier response than denying you have a reason to weep!

To deny any emotion, refuse to experience it, or hide or distract yourself from feeling it because you're afraid or embarrassed or because you or your religion says it's wrong, is to deny a part of yourself. It's unnatural. It's dishonest. It will lead to psychosomatic illnesses.

How Much Emotion Is Enough?

We must pay attention to our full array of feelings, but only until they tell us why they have arisen and we understand their innate wisdom. You can learn to use your faculty of discernment and detachment to determine when to rein the emotions in and when to allow them free expression. Not suppressing feelings does not mean allowing the agitating rajas and disturbing tamas feelings extended and unchecked time in your mind because they will destroy your well-being and capacity for discernment.

An Example of Discernment: The Case of Anger

I have come across some teachers who suggest that you feel all your feelings, including rage and grief, with no checkpoint. And I know of some who dive deep into these dark emotions and have yet not fully emerged from them.

Given the popularity of this approach, I experimented with it for a month. Once, when I was feeling angry with my partner over a silly domestic squabble, I decided not to process it or let it go. Instead, I continued to stay in touch with my anger. It simmered and then picked up heat and boiled over. It brought up so many more angry memories that were by that time meaningless. My anger was picking up intensity and strength and had taken over my samsara. I felt acid curdle in my stomach and blinding heat behind my eyes.

I was amazed at the power of letting anger stay around. I witnessed firsthand how a simple feeling-cloud can build into a deadly thunderstorm in our mind if we are not careful. I realized that allowing free access to all our feelings requires a reality check. Not every feeling needs to be entertained as the voice of God inside us. Like our thoughts, we must also discern our feelings. It is important that the majority of what you feel is "real" and does not have delusory origin in your attachments (raga) and obsessions (vasanas).

For example, it's important to acknowledge and feel your anger, be it showing up as a fleeting irritation or as full-fledged rage. Anger is a normal healthy emotion, intended to inform us of boundary transgressions. Healthy anger urges us to act on our inborn sense of justice and can provide the motivation to constructively correct an injustice. But not all anger is healthy, explains the Bhagavad Gita. Delusory and entitled anger can also arise in your samsara if your desires are thwarted. If you allow anger that makes you feel persecuted or victimized to continue, you will become even more delusory. This anger will expand insidiously, color your entire being, and corrupt your judgment, sometimes to a point beyond no return. It will instigate violence and hasty actions. It will make you sick. Hatred and addictions may manifest.

Unhealthy anger arises due to our illusions and false beliefs, which are products of our attachment-filled samsara. We become ready to take on anything and anyone that we conclude stands in the way. Sometimes we even get angry with ourselves for not trying hard enough or not taking the critical action we think may have gotten us what we desire. Or we privately hate others for getting ahead or possessing what we were denied by the universe. We may become depressed. Then, we punish ourselves by not liking or not nourishing our self, stopping self-care, throwing our self-respect away, not rewarding our self, and in extreme cases, even cutting, starving, or killing our self.

Unhealthy anger takes many forms. It can be a slow burn, like underlying resentment coloring all our experiences bitter and making our tongue acidic, or it can make us blow up in violent rage. It is never empowering. In fact, it depletes, disempowers, and robs us of our physical strength. We feel devitalized and can even fall physically sick, chronically or fatally.

Healthy anger almost never leads to violence, but unhealthy anger is directly related to violence (*himsa*) that manifests either externally toward other people, animals, or property, or within, acted out through subtle or gross self-abuse. It falsifies our reality and destroys the intellect's ability to discern between right and wrong, real and unreal, fact and projection, truth and illusion. In addition, when anger is expressed, it invariably triggers the experience of anger of other minds. Anger is the emotion that most quickly infects minds. If we have uncontrolled anger, then before we know it, it can set off a tirade of anger in people we interact with. This can lead to rapid and dangerous acceleration of our egoic problems and result in immediate and future karmic sorrow. Acceptance of circumstances in the early stages would have been so much easier and could have led to more intuitive solutions.

It is important to feel all our feelings and not suppress them. This is great advice from contemporary teachers. Yet it is also important to gate-keep and discern between real feelings worth swimming in and delusory feelings that require us to see through them.

When I feel anger, before I act from it, I ask myself questions (discernment): Why am I angry? What does it tell me about my own beliefs, values, judgments, sense of justice, and needs? What am I missing? Is my sense of injustice coming from my ego, habit, or entitlement, or is this something deeper that deserves my attention? What is the basis for my sense of justice and injustice? What is it I need that I am not getting? How should I communicate my needs without acting out my anger since anger's job is to inform me? What are the actions most likely to get me what I most need? Will revenge help? Will a dialogue help? Will understanding help? Will firmness and compassion help?

I have used anger as an example, but you can use similar discerning and examining techniques on almost any emotion or feeling that is heavily coloring your mind. We need to employ our illumined intellect to discern between which emotions are healthy and which emotions need a reality check. Only the practices of intellectual discrimination and detachment can protect us from our own unhealthy feelings and emotions that besiege our lower mind. Only the sattvic intellect has the capacity to tease apart our hidden truth of Self from our delusory emotions and beliefs.

With practice and inner vigilance, no illegitimate emotion can rule your inner kingdom. You, the Self, remain its sovereign master. No wonder the spiritual disciplines for the mind mandated by the Bhagavad Gita include serenity and purity of thought, gentleness, silence, control of the senses, and purity of life goals.[1] The choice is not between positive versus negative feelings, but rather between delusory versus real, authentic, worthy, and healthy feelings. You have the power to veto any delusory belief-thought-feeling-emotion chain, at any time. You can use your higher mind (*buddhi*) to emphatically say no to the virtual gangsters that rob you of peace. Each time they arise, change your thoughts proactively, and as a consequence, feelings will also change.

Two Sides of the Same Emotion

Rather than suppressing, denying, blocking, indulging, magnifying, or distorting our emotions, let us learn to be with them from a detached, more neutral space of the higher mind, allowing for emotional honesty. Let us work with them intelligently.

Emotions are not good or bad or positive or negative per se. It all depends on whether we use them in realistic or delusory ways. What we think of as negative emotions, like anger, anxiety, and even guilt, frustration, and resentment, are there to alert us that something needs to change and to motivate us to make that change. We all love and expound the benefits of hope, compassion, and gratitude. But there are negative effects that can come from the so-called positive emotions too. For example, unchecked optimism can lead to not preparing for life challenges adequately. Unchecked compassion can make us forgive prematurely and not deal with abusers and tormentors wisely. Unchecked generosity can make us easy targets. In fact, the entire Bhagavad Gita was preached by the divine teacher Krishna for his student Arjuna's sake. Arjuna was in a state of advanced delusion suffering from false compassion and false generosity.

The list below will help you discern better:

HEALTHY/REAL EMOTIONS	UNHEALTHY/DELUSORY EMOTIONS
They match a real-life event (they have a reason to exist). For example, a real death leads to grief.	They exist due to samsara. They match memories or imagined events more than real-life events. For example, thoughts of death bring on grief.
They are felt within realistic measure (in control).	They can cause withdrawal, denial, or over-expression (they can overrun us).
They last for a short or realistic time in mind.	They have extended stay in mind without reprieve. You rehash them because you are stuck.
They give you guidance. They add insight; as a result, you feel empowered.	They confuse you, overwhelm you; you feel disempowered.
They are experienced in the now; they impact the present moment or situation.	They seem to emerge from past and seem to want to predict the future (as rosy or gloomy).
They may be painful in the given moment, such as realistic grief or remorse, but they feel like gifts in the long run.	They feel like baggage (never gifts).
They tend to incite self-care sooner or later.	They can incite self- or other-harm.
They lead to inner growth.	They can lead to regression and more self-ignorance.
Sleep is not disturbed.	Sleep and other body functions, like digestion or elimination, are disturbed.

Manage Feelings When They Are Still Manageable

As I've mentioned before, the first ripple in a river is generally very feeble. If fanned by gusty winds, it has the power to gather momentum and gradually become a small wave, then a big wave, and finally a huge tidal wave.

Similarly, a ripple of delusory feelings, if fanned by delusory thoughts, can also gain momentum. If large waves of out-of-control, delusory emotions like rage, envy, greed, or even delusory happiness are cresting in your mind unarrested, then an entire lifetime can be wasted in the pathological samsara they generate.

A single false thought like *I deserve to drink alcohol every night because I work so hard or because my best friend just died*, or other such false justification–based thoughts, can unleash a tidal wave of feelings, strengthening your emotional attachment to your alcohol and reinforcing your addiction. Once we reach that stage, it is almost impossible to separate the underlying delusory belief from the delusory feeling and emotion. It is a virtual knot, and your mind becomes even more removed from reality.

Changing Thoughts Will Help Change Feelings

Identifying and changing ignorant and agitating thoughts to clarifying thoughts is easier than changing emotions and feelings directly. Thoughts are more easily identifiable. When you use willpower to change the dial on your thoughts, the barometer of your feelings and emotions also changes automatically. You will be filled with a sense of okayness and feel upbeat, encouraged, and self-pleased.

If your thoughts are about how powerless, inferior, and unworthy you are, then you will experience feelings and emotions of being powerless, inferior, and invisible. As a result, you will shy away from meeting people, hide from opportunities banging at your door, and even screen calls of loved ones because you are under house arrest—imprisoned by your own delusory thoughts and emotions that have given you the verdict of being unworthy. When negative emotions perpetuate (just like delusory thoughts of shame and blame), our subjective mind gets filled with self-sabotaging delusory behaviors and their tragic, sorrowful consequences. When you instead use your higher mind to think empowering thoughts like *I am powerful, deserving, equal, and worthy*, your feelings will reflect that.

Therefore, when you first notice yourself becoming emotionally upset, saddened, or irritated, try to evaluate what you are thinking that is causing that emotion and whether or not that thought is real or delusory. Mentally connect your feeling to the thought that initiated it, something you may have been thinking a few minutes or days ago. Ask yourself: *What is it that's really affecting me here? Why am I reacting this way? How important is this entire situation? Will this be relevant in few weeks from now? Is this my old wound acting up, or is this a new situation that needs my attention?*

At any point, you can choose to think and feel sattvic self-healing, self-loving, self-uplifting, self-freeing thoughts and say no to bondage-creating, sorrow-generating rajasic thoughts. Of course, to audit, edit, or change the content of your mind, you need to remain conscious of who you are—the Self, not your mind. And you need to employ the tools of discernment and detachment at the level of your higher mind.

It's critical to remember that your intellect can control the contents of the mind, restrain and restrict dulling and agitating emotions, and restore illumined thoughts and matching emotions. It can overcome even extreme emotions, like depression, suicidal tendencies, and rage, especially when you intentionally expose the intellect to awakening knowledge.

Therefore, if you are feeling emotionally triggered, your priority should be to self-regulate the thoughts behind your emotions rather than make the situation worse (by simply acting out because your emotions say you must). Regulation does not mean emotional bypassing; it simply means greater mindfulness.

If you are not able to do this, you may still be under the spell of self-ignorance. Remember that feelings are like winds that blow across the landscape of your awareness; they may be winds of insecurity, vulnerability, or a sense of impending doom, but they blow away in time. All you must do is be present with them gently but alertly, using your faculty of the higher mind.

Strengthen Sattvic Emotions by Reinforcing Sattvic Behavior

Tracking sattvic-balancing emotions helps us be more aware of the situations and activities that bring them up, things like meditation, an uplifting movie, a walk in nature, or gently expressing your hidden truth to yourself or a loved one.

For example, when you are dealing with grief due to loss, you can consciously cultivate gratefulness for support from your partner or friend, the soothing light at dawn, your dogs' kisses, a favorite song you heard on the radio, the smell of freshly bloomed gardenia in your mother's garden, or your meditation (even a short one), all of which may induce positive sattvic, calming, lightening, relaxing, centering feelings. Note it and repeat it. By listening to the song again, getting those dog kisses again, planting a jasmine plant in a pot on your balcony, and regularly meditating, you are changing the dial of your emotions from tamas and rajas to sattva! Yes, it is that simple.

Try doing things that connect you with more sattva feelings, even if you don't feel like it at the time. For example, you might not be in the mood to go running after a personal loss, but you can exercise your self-knowledge that it will positively impact your emotional state with sattva and go for a walk anyway.

Shift Your Beliefs about Your Core Identity to Impact Your Emotions

Remember this: "I am the soul, not the role I am currently playing!"

We need courage to express this truth, and this courage always comes from self-knowledge. We remain in emotional bondage of our or other people's expectations only until we know who we are, until we know that all bondage is mere thoughts. When, through self-knowledge, we lay aside the bondage and begin operating as pure existence, the boundless Self, our emotions become free, light, and playful, yet heartfelt, sincere, and flowing. The very people who once obstructed you or tried to enslave you with expectations will lose their power to spook you into unwilling conformity. The freedom to accept ourselves as we are emerges from within, from internalizing right knowledge about our spiritual soul reality, versus any role. We truly awaken with direct insight into the eternal here and now when we see what is. The snake is found to be a rope.

So, express your true voice, your deepest values, and your soul desires. Express your deepest core beliefs fearlessly as a soul and make yourself your priority even as you ethically perform your roles with mindfulness. Then, the world will not be able to shame you, nor will you need to blame anyone. Contrast this approach with one who is sleepwalking, unaware of their reality as a soul not a role, who spends time diminishing others' "roles" while covering their own "role" with shame, overachievement, or material abundance. It's to our advantage to appreciate what is already beautiful, perfect, and blissful—the Self—rather than to focus on our egoic roles.

When you were young, you first knew yourself as your parents' child. Then later you may have been someone's friend and then someone's business partner, employee, lover, or spouse. Then, you became a parent to children or animals. These identities are all "thought clothing" worn by your perishable body and changeable mind in the realm of impermanence. What happens if we sweep aside these thoughts?

What if you played the ultimate card: *I am the immortal soul, the Self. I am Atman, alone, none other.* In an instant, you would enable your spiritual bigness. You would begin acting as if you had infinite reserves of courage, creativity, joy, and intelligence available to you.

One of my students had this to share:

"I have found a well of resources in the simple practice of connecting with my own seed of the divine, the Self. Like any seed, it needs the right climate and nutrients to grow. For the seed of Atman, this means reining in the senses and my mind that were insisting I am body because that is what I see or I am my thoughts because those are in my head. Acquiring new knowledge and keeping company that supports that growth has been crucial. As I implement the ongoing contemplation-meditation, 'I am not my body, not my mind; I am Atman,' I see the greatest strides within myself. I've overcome chronic depression and anxiety. Where the old me, the "single mom," had not been able to go out in public alone with ease, I'm now enjoying dinners and walks by myself. I have even taught classes and given lectures in public.

I used to react during emotional discomfort, usually in ways that were unhealthy for me or hurtful to others around me, as if action would solve that discomfort. Contemplating Atman was the next deeper step into not just holding myself still, but creating stillness within, so that instead of waiting for an anxious thought to pass, I would actively move past the anxiety by connecting with that which doesn't change; this we identify as the truth, for that which is in constant flux cannot be considered true.

Connecting with the Self inside and becoming familiar with that bliss brings a softening and compassion to the world experienced outside. More and more, the usual challenges of daily life become opportunities for practicing my highest consciousness. Where once I may have been emotionally triggered about traffic, disturbed by a snide remark from another person, or engrossed in the dynamics of family drama, I have begun to see these things as an expression of Self for the sole benefit of strengthening my own character."

You can practice focusing on your self-knowledge for inner emotional strength amid times of world challenge and sorrow. For example, my student Fiana sent me this letter, which captures how she utilized the knowledge of the Self to cope with the death of her mother.

"My brother and I sold our childhood home this past Friday after our mom passed away. I realized through this process that I am so much stronger than I ever knew since every part of the house reminded me of my mom. There was a time when the thought of not having that home or my mother any longer was unthinkable. I imagined I would evaporate without them or end up in some sort of asylum or institution.

This process was painful, but it was the type of pain similar to when you are rehabbing a part of your body. It hurts, but it is beneficial. I ran my hands over every wall of the home and thanked them. I thanked each plant and tree in our backyard.

Through the knowledge of my permanent Self, I took refuge in the observation of maya (impermanence). I realize that praise and blame, loss and gain, fame and shame are all a part of the ego life. I've learned to accept and allow grief to come through my physical body as it pleases, to sweep through me, rattle my bones, and then leave.

In meditation and my contemplations, in knowing I am Self and my mom is Self too, I know that permanence, joy, and peace are our truest nature; I've learned I can tap into these things anytime I want."

A person who is aware of their true identity seems to display greater emotional forbearance. When the knowledge of Self goes beyond an intellectual idea and becomes an emotional conviction, adverse events will not rock the emotional boat as much. A greater resoluteness, raw courage, and sheer wisdom that "this too shall pass" will also emerge spontaneously in the illumined higher mind, the buddhi. While playing roles, the individual will know, *I am pure consciousness, unaffected by change, aging, disease, and death.*

However, one who does not recognize their unchanging Self as different from their ego may experience every emotional pinprick as an attack on the Self with increasing hopelessness, fearfulness, and the feeling of no control.

Use the Nondual Medicine
that Heals All Painful Emotions

The *Isha Upanishad* declares: "To a person who understands that the one Self has become all things, what sorrow, then what delusion, what sorrow, what trouble can there be, to one who beholds that unity?"[2]

We must recognize that one nondual Self is present and being expressed in everything around us. The deepest cause of emotional suffering is the perception of separation: considering one's self and happiness as distinct and in conflict with the Self and happiness of others (a competitive view). Such sorrow and suffering cannot exist once we awaken to the greatest truth that the Upanishads first revealed to humans, that the same common Self is expressing in all of existence as its common center. This refocuses our perception beyond individual personalities to the One Self. We have separate bodies but one Self.

With this uniting knowledge, we become more generous, caring, and sharing in our actions, speech, and thought.

Has this happened to you too? Has the Universal Intelligence called you from deep within your being, even while you were fast asleep in maya? An ocean continues to give birth to infinite individual waves and yet remains existentially unchanged. Did the bottomless ocean of your Self come looking for you? It did for me.

Dealing with Excessive Negative Emotions

From a Vedic perspective of wholeness and oneness, whether you are experiencing negativity due to your own mind or because someone has wronged you, remember, no person is exclusively a villain. According the Vedas, each of us is a victim of self-ignorance or lostness in maya, conditions that we can gently untangle using the wisdom of Vedic self-knowledge. You deserve self-forgiveness, extending compassion toward your own learning and maturing ego.

The antidote for becoming a victim of our own emotional deluge is to see things in perspective and make the cultivation of a relationship with our Self a priority over letting others' thoughts and actions determine our reality. Self-knowledge bestows a spiritual immunity that transcends all sorrowful emotions.

I came up with this exercise for anyone who may wish to diffuse negative emotions. I am confident it will help you too.

Guided Practice: Diffuse Negative Emotions

First, resolve to no longer suppress your emotions. Doing so destroys your joy and fuels autoimmune disorders. Challenge your core belief that emotions are negative, so even the troubling ones need not be suppressed or hidden from yourself.

Identify the source of your intense emotions. Through self-reflection, try to identify the underlying reasons, thoughts, beliefs, expectations, attachments, vasanas, and delusory responses to external circumstances for the specific emotion, such as hurt, sadness, or unworthiness. Was it a mistake you or others made? A lack of integrity you experienced? Betrayal? Dishonesty? Or was it some expectation being thwarted? You may feel uncomfortable, but do it anyway, privately.

Make a list. Every point is important because you are important. Don't simply bury your feelings. Write them down. This will help you discern the reality from the myths that are feeding this emotion and disconnect it from whatever background story is feeding the emotion. When you are doing this, you may also viscerally feel the emotions you are examining. This happens because feelings travel throughout the body. Allow it. Wait in a detached space until the mind can finish spinning out stories. Then allow guidance to come. Do not rush to act, plan, or respond in the heat of the emotion; do so only after it has pointed out what needs our attention.

Accept your own vulnerability and self-ignorance. This is vital if you are targeting your Self with negativity, such as shame, self-loathing, or self-rejection. You were not born with a *How to Be Perfect, Good, and Balanced* manual. We all must learn the hard way: by experience. We must accept that not everything will be in our control. Living in a realm of sleepwalkers in maya is not easy. Here, our ego is estranged from its own sovereign nature, and your mind that was meant to be your aid is crawling with imprisoning delusions! Sometimes, instead of guiding you, your mind misguides you. Vedic self-knowledge will help you go past your inner judge and begin to radically accept yourself despite past regrets and your flaws and imperfections. Let go of self-loathing and hold yourself like parents embrace babies, despite their playing in smelly poop.

When you compassionately accept all sides of your learning self and align with the beautiful divine soul that you are, you fall in love with that Self. You might even want to do some realistic grieving, since grief lives just below the surface of a host of negative emotions. This is an important step in the process toward wholeness, one that's often skipped. Give yourself permission: feel these feelings and know that neither the grief nor the other negative emotions will last forever.

Forgive vulnerability and self-ignorance. Do this, especially if negativity is emerging from other people's actions. You may choose to take someone to court or make them pay up since that may be right action, but at same time, somewhere deep down, you forgive them because everyone is a human lost in maya. No one is evil. Everyone, to greater or lesser degree, has gotten out of touch with their true nature. Therefore, with self-knowledge backing your understanding, when you see the struggling human behind the offender—which could also be you—you will experience compassion for them, yourself, others, and everyone. I don't ask that you fake it if you don't yet feel it but remain open to the idea of this radical understanding.

Finish with self-love. To finish, breathe deeply, and give yourself a mental hug and praise for being courageous and wise. Literally hug your vulnerable self, and remember with delight your inherent soul-worth. All of us are deserving of unconditional love, freedom, and power, since despite our ignorant ego and its emotional insanity, our true nature is unconditional bliss, freedom, oneness, power, light, and grace.

The potential to be emotionally sorrow-free is attainable, provided we make efforts to receive and assimilate a higher wisdom of an eternal self. You can break free from old patterns and think your way out of the emotional negativity that holds you back. None of your emotions wish to punish you, but rather help you in your journey to complete sovereignty! All emotions ultimately assist us in evolving into a more sensitive, empathetic, just, kind, and dharmic version of ourselves.

15

Nitya-Anitya: Meeting
Impermanence and Death

"When all else is asleep, time is awake, time is unstoppable.

*Youth, beauty, life, possessions, health, and the companionship of friends, all
are impermanent."*

MAHABHARATA, 11.11.2

One day, when I was nine years old, my guru Baba's twenty-five-year-old
son—his beloved youngest child, whom I adored as my loveable uncle—died
on the spot in a traffic accident.

I saw my uncle with his head in his father's lap, his body cold, stiff, and still
as the earth below him. (Hindus lay a corpse on bare earth, a sign of respect
that the body was borrowed from earth in the form of food. The earth is the
first mother.)

My uncle appeared to be in a very deep slumber. His long, dark eyelashes
rested tenderly on his face. Hoping in vain that he would wake up, I twisted
my fingers in a magic knot, as little girls tend to do when they desperately want
their wishes to come true. "Any moment now he will stretch and yawn loudly as
he always does," I told myself, expecting him to flash his disarming smile that
made us children giggle in anticipated glee of his jokes, hoping to horse around
as we played cricket together behind our house, the home to many generations
of our family.

My uncle's beautiful body, bristling with heady, magnetic youth moments earlier; his handsome, chiseled face that had stolen the heart of his sweetheart; and his dark, tousled hair shining and full of bounce—all had become inert and lifeless. Just a year later, the mother in whose lap I was crying would be next; her warm and comfy body would also lie limp, stiff, and cold, a vacant house as my uncle's body looked now.

But that night, my mother's embrace was a haven for my eleven-year-old sister and nine-year-old me, as we sat frightened yet united in our similar bewilderment, in deep and existential sorrow with the questions that death imposes upon us equally, no matter what age or what species we are. Whether a little bird, a tiny mouse, or a human being, death frightens all living beings.

Why We Resist Death and Change

Have you noticed how much you value permanence? You don't want to settle for anything less than permanent peace, happiness, stability in relationships, and of course, permanent life. Death makes all of us uncomfortable and fills our minds with fright and grief. No wonder we humans even pray for permanent wealth and security, youth and health. And even though death is a ubiquitous fact of existence, no one wants to face death. Period.

Have you ever wondered why we humans rebel against impermanence? You seek permanence since your real nature is unchanging, immortal Self. Whatever does not change, that is Self, is known as "eternal," or *nitya*. That is why, despite experience of outer impermanence, you feel you deserve permanent bliss, peace, and wholeness. What changes is known as *anitya*, which means "noneternal."

Alas, due to the spell of maya, though you are the eternal Self (nitya), it's as if you have consented to take on an impermanent body in a realm of impermanence, to spend all your time chasing impermanent happiness through impermanent relationships (anitya)! Yet, you privately bewail the reality of change and death; you protest, question, kick, and scream at every loss, every death, and every change.

Sorrow emerges from the memory of your true immortal Self—a memory you are not cognitively aware of since it is lodged in the deepest layers of your unconscious mind. This memory exerts upon you the sense that "something is not right." You feel a cosmic injustice, an existential bewilderment, at having to deal with change in the way of distance, decay, disease, and death.

If we live long enough, even our memories of who we are—our name, age, and so forth—disappear, and we live on as an empty shell, swallowed up by a relentless, ruthless law of impermanence. Despite our technological advances and supposed medical breakthroughs, we stand only as mute spectators as impermanence steals our thunder, right under our noses.

No human being is "okay" with impermanence being our lot because permanence is our deeper truth. We are not our fragile body and mind; we are Atman, the imperishable consciousness that is beyond aging, death, and material designations of color, race, gender, species, and nationality. No wonder we are unable to cope with the fact of impermanence.

The Bhagavad Gita Helps Humanity Understand Death

That day of my uncle's death, Baba spoke quietly, heavy-heartedly, with his eyes overflowing with tears. And yet, he spoke with an inner conviction that was unshakeable, supporting his moment of grief:

"That which pervades the entire body is indestructible. All creatures have two parts: the perishable (made of physical matter) and the imperishable Self (Spirit Divine).

The perishable ends. The imperishable Self is not destroyed even when the perishable is destroyed."

Baba's words, on the nature of our Self, which is indestructible, versus the body, which is by nature destructible, filled our collective aching hearts with much-needed solace and gave our perishable bodies and minds some essential inner strength.

Baba explained that in the end, a clay pot returns to its original state of pure clay; that each wave, no matter how high it rises, returns to pure water; that refined gold ornaments dissolve back into pure gold; and that thoughts risen in awareness return to pure awareness. So also, my uncle, whose body had risen in the Self, had now resolved back into the Self. This is peaceful; this is auspicious. Eternal Consciousness is the truth.

Baba chanted OM and gave thanks and a blessing at the funeral:

"Thank you for visiting, great soul. May you find the great truth of the one Self revealed in your own heart. Thank you for giving us an opportunity to serve you as our own."

Baba's OMs connected the earth and sky that night. They also helped make the split parts of my heart more whole. I have never forgotten that real-life lesson on equanimity through knowledge of Self, which is not body, but Universal Intelligence.

In the Vedic tradition, at death, we chant Vedic messages like this one: "May this life enter the immortal breath. This body will become ashes; you are not the body! The body is ending in ashes, but you are going to the other sphere— mingling with the vital breath. Remember, remember what we are doing here; remember what we are telling you; remember O Universal Intelligence; remember that you are the Supreme Infinite Spirit, that you are free! Mingling with the immortal breath, go!"

The one who knows that Self is indestructible consciousness does not suppress but understands emotions.

I now remember how, at his son's death, Baba sat still, as if he were not even breathing. I could tell his heart was full of immense, heartbreaking sorrow. His eyes kept shedding his sorrow. And yet, he also was peaceful deep inside himself. I wondered, *What immortal truths do my Baba's inner eyes of wisdom see?*

After a death in the family, it is common among Hindus to gather as a family of mourners over ten days and nights, shed tears together, console each other, and at the same time, imbibe wisdom of the immortal Self from those who know of the Vedas. Baba was a knower himself, so he chanted from the Bhagavad Gita, which is said to contain the essence of all 108 Upanishads, while the rest of us sat around him, wept, and comforted our hearts:

"Just like a person casts off his worn-out clothes and puts on new ones, so also consciousness, the Self, casts off its worn-out bodies and enters new ones.

Just as in this body, pure existence, the Self, passes through childhood, youth, and old age, consciousness itself unchanged, passes into another body; the ones who know this do not grieve.

It is said, the bodies that existence puts on are destructible; they have an end. consciousness; the Self, itself remains, eternal, indestructible, and incomprehensible.

Consciousness, the Self, is never born nor does it die. After having emerged briefly (inside a body), it again ceases to emerge (through that body). The Self is forever unborn, eternal, changeless, and ancient.

Self does not die when the body dies.

Weapons cleave it not, fire burns it not, water drowns it not, air dries it not; consciousness cannot be cut, nor burnt, nor drowned, nor dried up. It is enduring, all-pervading, stable, immovable, and ancient.

Therefore, knowing the nature of the true Self (of our beloved departed one who has merely dropped the perishable body), you should not grieve."[1]

Every night for several nights, Baba discoursed on the true nature of the Self that outlives the body, mind, and personality.

Baba's steadfastness in his knowingness that his son is immortal existence—the Self—and not the mortal clothes Self had worn briefly, helped all of us, both children and adults, steadily recover from this trauma. Knowledge of Self from the Vedas never fails us and always leads us from untruth to truth, darkness to light, from mortality to immortality . . . and ultimately from fleeting happiness and sorrow to everlasting joy.

When exactly one year later, my beautiful, beloved mother collapsed without warning in front of my unbelieving ten-year-old eyes, when her body lay cold and stiff from the weak heart she had been born with, I looked toward Baba again for support.

I was inconsolable, and so was my sister. Though I was still a child and had yet to embark upon studying the awakening texts that beautifully elucidate the deathless Self, Baba's simple but profound words on the nature of Self, which is Nitya (that which remains unchanged), helped me comprehend just enough to somehow find inner stability and cultivate acceptance of what is, despite the outer loss.

I knew this much, that Mom was not just this body lying inert on the floor. Her true Self is invisible and indivisible and remains unaffected and unbroken always. I felt my terror reduce. I missed her physical presence acutely, but now I could feel her presence somehow even more vividly alive—this time, everywhere.

The next day, as we spread the ashes of my mother's body in the flowing and ferociously alive current of the sacred River Sarayu that encircled our hometown, Baba's words reverberated:

"A jar containing space is broken. The space previously contained in the jar now returns to its natural source, the all-pervading space. The end of the jar is not the end of the space. Just as a pot shaped from clay is still clay, an ornament shaped from gold is still gold, a wave is always an intrinsic part of the ocean, in the same way, the body, which is but a temporary limitation of consciousness, now begins to unravel. It dissolves to become once again the unbounded, unaffected, undifferentiated, pure, limitless consciousness that it always is."

I never forgot those real-life lessons on the true nature of Self from Baba. And who would understand my pain better than Baba? He had lost his own mother nine months after his birth and grew up motherless.

After some time, I returned to climbing trees, following Baba around like his perennial shadow, and playing with my pet baby calf, called Nandini, a Sanskrit word that means "joy" or "rejoicing." As I played in our garden and went into the forests and farms to find rare Ayurveda herbs with Baba's grown-up students, every new shiny leaf would remind me of my mother taking on new body-clothes. Baba urged me to openly weep and caress my heart whenever I missed her. He also told me to look for her inside my heart because Self is all-pervading.

Thus, Baba's teachings on death and life became ingrained in me at a young age. Little did I know at that tender age that good fortune had kept me safe with my guru, offering me the opportunity to develop eyes of wisdom rather than breaking down with inner sorrow or its suppression.

Yes, death is not the end. Death is not the contradiction of life. Death and birth are two sides of life's cosmic cycle in maya. The culmination of that cycle is awakening or liberation from maya.

> *"What is left here? Truly, this is that [Atman]."*
>
> KATHA UPANISHAD, 2.4.3

This way, my guru Baba taught me the value of cultivating an awareness of inner permanence amid outer impermanence, both from his verbal teachings and even more from observing how he faced suffering. Just sitting next to him or gazing at him from a distance made everyone feel more whole.

What knowledge did he have that allowed him to be at peace with his entire life despite whatever came his way? Pleasurable or unbearable experiences, and even agonizing surprises—he met them relatively calmly and with equipoise. I experienced Baba's equanimous nature both when the most important people of the country sought him for advice or for his blessings and when tragedy struck his family.

Awakened Grieving—Accepting Our Inner Permanence

Baba, as an awakened being, experienced his humanness like the rest of us, but the spaciousness of his heart and his memory of his true nature could accommodate emotional pain; he could be real in his grieving. He never pretended he was okay when he was not or allowed grief to color his entire psyche.

Consequently, Baba did not develop a fresh story in his mind, lamenting God's punishment in taking his young son or adopting an attitude of victimhood around his deep loss. Because he felt and thought and acted from a place of greater knowingness about the immutable truth of Self, he could thus experience a pure emotion like grief and yet remain stable in Self. My grandfather never bypassed his grief, covering it up with spiritual jargon, such as, "In this moment, all I experience is bliss."

For yogis like Baba, the Bhagavad Gita says: "For one who has mastered his mind and who is tranquil, the supreme Self is self-evident. [The knower of Self] remains the same in heat and cold, pleasure and pain, joy and sorrow, as well as in honor and dis-fame."[2]

As I have said, the awakened one is always real, feeling all their feelings but not identifying with any single one exclusively, since Self, which is of the nature of consciousness, allows all thoughts and feelings to arise and subside but is not permanently modified by any single one of them.

After all, feelings are impermanent; their nature is to be in a state of movement, while we, pure consciousness, can allow them safe passage. Can we also allow the emotion of sorrow to dwell in our heart as pure emotion alone and nothing else—not raging anger, nor hatred toward what caused our sorrow, nor animosity toward our creator, nor numbing of our ever-present joy, nor shame at being somehow defective for experiencing it in the first place?

It is the nature of clouds to change, come and go, rise and subside, be scattered by the lightest breeze or build up into an ominous thunderhead. But the sky itself is still and can never be affected by whatever the clouds do; therefore, it need not control any of the clouds' activity. When faced with loss of loved ones through death, Baba's inner being remained like the sky, but my sister's and my inner beings—since we did not know about our true Self back then—were identified with the clouds.

Without going to war with ourselves, can great sorrow be experienced with greater presence: fully, deeply, without getting lost in mental turmoil, self-deception, bypassing, or additional self-affliction?

Permanence Is Covered by the Shroud of Impermanence

I couldn't imagine that I would ever emerge from the unending swamp of sorrow, but I did. I did shed tears while writing this chapter, but these were from a deep recognition of permanence (nitya) through a higher wisdom, despite whatever I see with my eyes, which is impermanence (anitya).

It is this impermanence that is the root cause of all our sorrow and forces us to deal with constant life changes, not always for the better. But what if we could align with inner permanence even while navigating a realm of outer impermanence?

Sometimes a verse can express more than prose. These words bubbled up in my being:

O Shunya,
The river has no fear
She need not capture her immensity
in a standing pool of fear and ferocity,
because the riverbed below is still,
and in that tranquility,
there is courage for the river,
untold.

Your body,
Will arise, exist, and then disappear,
In that,
Which is the changeless Self.

Now, no matter how broken I feel, I know to go within and connect with an aspect of me that is forever whole, powerful, and joyful. With this knowledge, you too can have the wisdom not to try to control what is out of your control, but to control that which *is* in your control, to rely on something eternal inside you: the Self.

It is great "samsara hygiene" to discriminate between the ephemeral and the eternal—sorrowful emotional bondages can be prevented by not mistaking a passing experience for a permanent solution. Even objects, no matter how beloved, are only matter. They are deteriorating or maybe just changing hands between owners. To identify with what does not change enables us to engage with all our honesty in our ephemeral relationships with greater equanimity.

Our acceptance of sorrow through a greater vision of
an eternal reality is the first step toward a new door,
the door to what lies beyond the sorrow.

God's Tears Are Awakened Tears

Hindus have a beautiful role model for dealing with grief. The story of God Rama has been chronicled in the Hindu holy epic *Ramayana*. This tale is dear to all Hindus, even beyond India. We find this story enshrined in the hearts, dance, literature, ethos, and temples of Thailand, Nepal, and even Malaysia and Indonesia (which were once Hindu in ancient days).

Rama was the prince of Ayodhya (yes, my hometown is the birthplace of Rama in days bygone). He is considered the "avatar" of Supreme Reality, so Hindus worship Rama as "Lord" Rama.

Rama's human life was full of obstacles, just like our lives, and he shows us how to deal with them with equanimity, intelligence, fortitude, and inner bliss.

On the day before his coronation, Rama's stepmother played some games and ensured that instead of getting crowned as king, Rama was banished into the forests for fourteen years. Rama had enough inner power to take that hit peacefully. He walked away. Then, in the jungles, his beautiful wife Sita was abducted by the wicked Ravana, the king of Lanka. When Rama discovered that his wife had been abducted, he was shocked, but quiet. Then he came across a piece of Sita's jewelry that she had thrown down in the desperate hope that when Rama would come looking for her, it would show him the direction in which her abductor was headed. On seeing the sparkling piece of jewelry, Rama became overcome with sorrow for the distress his sensitive and compassionate wife Sita was facing, and he began to shed tears. He first and foremost acknowledged his heart as it broke with pain.

Even one who was the Supreme Reality, who was referred to as a god, and who not only rescued his beloved from the evil Ravana but destroyed him in a memorable righteous war of good over evil, shed tears when he was "overcome." In a later section of the epic, when his elder brother Lakshmana, who was assisting Rama, was left unconscious by an unexpected arrow, Rama again shed tears. Lakshmana's heart also was overcome for the physical pain his beloved younger brother was having to endure on his account.

An Awakened One Is Spontaneous in Suffering

The awakened being is spontaneous, unscripted, and free in moments of great joy and in moments of life-altering sorrow too. Compare this to the emotion-suppressing "stiff upper lip" we have told ourselves we must cultivate in the face of sorrow. This is especially true of people who are spiritually bypassing, who suffer privately and publicly profess to be immune to sorrow. It is considered somehow weak to shed tears.

Just as we don't hold back our smiles, we should not hold back our tears either. Our tears simply represent an equal and opposite energy—Spirit Divine moving through us as pure emotion. No more, no less.

Smiles fortify our heart, and tears heal our heart. When they arise, without premeditation, they may be given a rite of passage through our being, and then they return to existence, leaving us lighter, blessed, and feeling as if we can walk our next steps taller. Again, nothing arises in the great flow of Self for no reason.

Both joyous and sorrowful emotions must be allowed to flow though us unresisted, without turning one into a preference and the other into an aversion. This is what Rama demonstrated without trying too hard to be "artificially godly." A person of wisdom is alert to when tears are freeing them from pent-up energies and when tears have become a bondage, a habit, or an escape. Similarly, if we suppress our grief because we are operating from a "script" that says we must not cry if we are "man enough," "grown," or "spiritually evolved," again, we have become unconscious.

To be identified with the Self is not a dissociative or emotionless state. It is a state of complete all-embracing perception of the purest emotions in wholeness, unifying the opposites in one organic state of pure and complete comprehension. Self is existence absolute, the nondual state of undifferentiated unitary consciousness, so one emotion should not be preferred over the other.

When I have a reason to experience the pure emotion of grief or sorrow, I try to be with it 100 percent. I tell myself, "Let me be with this sorrow entirely. Let me not diminish it or make it smaller than it is. Yet let me not project it or make it bigger or more than it is, or allow it to loop infinitely into my future." This awareness and commitment to being real with very real sorrow has both helped me and surprised me. I can process grief without allowing it to distort my samsara with projections or suppressions.

Suffering Is as Important as Overcoming the Pain

When we are ignorant of the important role and purpose of sorrow in our life, then by default, we push away the sorrow (and then go into resistance or denial).

It is common in one's life to find that periods of heartrending, catastrophic, hope-shattering emotional pain often combine with periods of effortless inner growth. During those times, you are most willing to change habits that no longer serve you, reframe expectations in relationships, think new thoughts that give you power, eliminate limiting beliefs, correct misperceptions, and proactively seek wisdom from books, elders, guides, mentors, counselors, ministers, or a guru.

Emotional pain teaches us the ultimate lessons of the futility of seeking permanence in a realm of impermanence. It makes us question the world of matter, transience, and appearances and seek the world of spirit, truth, and permanence. Pain makes us turn inward and seek what lies beyond the senses, to find that elusive, greater truth at last.

I teach my students to be authentic with all their emotions including pain, to let the tears flow when they are full of inner pain, and to give the tears their full attention. Only when we have wept long enough and hard enough, without restriction and yet with deep inward attention on the pain, will the pain begin to loosen its grip on our chest, brain, and heart. It may start to dissolve or transform into resolve, wisdom, insights, or simply okayness.

Weeping, as an aspect of unhappiness, is a perfectly healthy and necessary response to loss or some form of choiceless, cosmic sorrow. If expressed appropriately (not indulged excessively for manipulation), your sorrow will lessen with time, enabling you to adjust to the loss or disappointment of an experienced shock.

The greater the sorrow, the greater the need to shed tears. Perhaps there is no way back to joy without shedding tears, which when shed lead the way to wholeness. Once again, due to societal myths such as "Men don't weep," "Adults must cope," and "Spiritual folks never cry but only meditate away," we may resist our tears. But, as we've discussed, resistance poisons everything.

Vedic teachings say that tears must never be suppressed. In fact, Vedic medicine (Ayurveda) goes so far as to say that if tears are suppressed, it will lead to a host of psychosomatic illnesses.[3]

It is only when we accept our lot and are willing to face all our feelings, including sadness, and when we shed the tears that arise naturally that our sorrow lessens. It is only when we share our sorrow, if we have an empathetic ear available, or process it in other ways, such as journaling, withdrawing, or going inward, that our degree of attachment to the original cause of sorrow slowly wanes. Then something beautiful begins to transpire. We begin to heal inwardly and reconnect with our soul power.

Disorientation and confusion will automatically lift in our previously bewildered samsara. Older spiritual memories of confidence, success, and our ability to face similar difficulties in the past begin to revive in our mind (previously numb with sorrow). If we are a spiritual student, then at this stage, our teacher's spoken words will begin to reverberate in the now clear sky of our heart and allow us to clear the clouds of doubts and anxieties that had previously overwhelmed us. With acceptance of the new situation and willingness to feel the pain, anger, or any unnecessary guilt or shame that may have arisen (if we thought we were responsible), it subsides, and the clouds begin to subside. Our inner esteem (which comes from Self, not the ego, so it never really leaves us) reasserts itself, and we begin to remember we are not spiritual orphans—we have the divine Self with us after all.

With right knowledge, great inner growth occurs at such so-called "low" times in our life. Despite desolation, death of a loved one, loss of a love relationship, bankruptcy, or even a diagnosis of a terminal disease, sorrow brings maturity in its wake, as sorrow turns spontaneously into intuitive wisdom.

Some people even take wisdom to the next step, and sorrow turns to joy. Once we have processed our sorrow, our mind becomes clutter-free, and inner bliss begins to shine through. I have seen people become spontaneous, original, and creative like never before, even as they face death or some other unimaginable loss. They experience inner freedom, joy, liberty, and equanimity. The Self explodes from within, as that and none other is the ultimate truth. The sorrow of change, loss, transience, and impermanence is not the endpoint! It can be the gateway to everlasting sovereignty.

16

⟨⟫⟫⟫⟩⟫⟩⟩⟩⟩⟩⟨⟨⟨⟨⟨⟨⟨⟨⟩

Advaita: Recognizing the
Truth of Unity Consciousness

"O Self, I see you in the dark blue bee;
I see you in the green parrot with those red eyes too.
I see you in the woman, the man, the youth, and the maiden, O Self.
O Self, you are in the old man who totters along, leaning on that staff.
You are indeed One, with different faces and bodies, O nondual Self."

SHVETASHVATARA UPANISHAD, 4.3–4

One teaching that changed my life and purified my deepest-held beliefs forever was the fundamental nondual vision of the Vedic seers. The Sanskrit word
advaita means "not two" and points to the essential oneness, the unity of life.
The word "advaita" suggests that despite the compelling appearance of separation and diversity of bodies and mind, there is only one universal essence, one
reality behind the multiple things: the Self.

Like the moon reflected in water becomes many moons,
Self is the same in all, and yet appears as many.

There is no separate Self to each living unit, but rather a shared truth of pure
consciousness that is the common ground of our collective existence. This means
that while there are lots of bodies and minds, each one is enlivened by One Self

as if the same One Self is having myriad experiences through its myriad bodies. But in the final analysis, the life-force or consciousness that animates the body and mind in each one of them is One, never two.

Yes, the fly that is humming about you, the cactus growing in your backyard, the cat lying in your lap taking a nap, and the sunflower that dazzled you when you went on a walk are all diverse bodies enjoyed by the One Self.

We do not have a center separate from the whole. That common center is my Self, your Self, everyone's Self. Even the ones we may have rejected, shunned, blamed, or shamed—yes, even they share the truth of a shared existence, a mutually owned inner Self. When we know this shared Self, we go beyond the delusion of "separate selves." Knowledge of the all-comprehensible indivisible truth, the Self, gives a person the highest satisfaction.

"Self resides in the lotus of the heart of every being."

MUNDAKA UPANISHAD, 3.1.7

This knowledge, when read or heard and then internalized, leads to the resolution of all delusions and spells the end of all samsara-sponsored sorrow. After all, it is the perception of separateness alone (me versus them or me versus you) that breeds suffering, resentment, jealousy, anger, and so forth. Understanding underlying unity, which can't be perceived by the eyes but is understood by a purified and enlightened mind, gives birth to relief, generosity, love, compassion, empathy, and forgiveness. Knowledge of the nondual nature of reality ends the suffering bred by the illusion of separateness.

Oneness is all there is—and you are included.

The Vedic seers chant: "Meditate and realize this world is filled with the presence of One Self."[1] "This One Presence is hidden in the heart of all creatures, and yet it encloses the whole universe within itself, pervading everything."[2] "This Cosmic Self has hands and feet everywhere; eyes, heads, and faces everywhere; ears everywhere; dwells in all beings; all embracing."[3]

The Personal and the Universal Self

When the One Self is reflected in your micro-body, the individual life principle called Atman is illumined. When the same Self is reflected in the entirety of the creation, then a Universal Self is illuminated through the collective bodies, collective minds, and collective souls.

The Universal Self, though the same as the personal Self, is known as *Brahman*, rather than Atman.[4] Brahman and Atman are both qualitatively the same and equally amazing, powerful, and intelligent. "Atman" means "that which is boundless." It is the boundless existence of bliss—pure intelligent consciousness operating from within the confines of our individual body. "Brahman" means "boundless consciousness, existence, bliss operating through every body, every mind, and every soul."

"Just as fire, though one, assumes different forms in respect of different shapes, similarly, Brahman, inside all beings, assumes a form and yet remains the same in all forms."

KATHA UPANISHAD, 2.2.9

The English translation of the term "Brahman" is "infinity, ultimate vastness, or bigness, an ever-expanding dimension that nothing can overcome or surpass." Yet, only radical unity exists. Just like the millions of cells, tissues, and organs in our body serve only one person, all the diversity seen in cosmic form serves only One Universal Consciousness (Brahman, Atman).

According to nondual teachings, when we are self-ignorant, the world of experiences arises. But when we are awakened to the presence of greater reality, of Brahman, the world subsides in our mind, and we perceive the pure bliss of Brahman. Thus, the world we see is only an "apparent transformation" of Brahman, not its absolute transformation as there can only be one entity, which is Brahman.

"I am that soul of the universe. The Supreme Brahman—in whom reside all beings. And who resides in all."

AMRITA BINDU UPANISHAD, 22

At the time of liberation, known as "moksha" in Vedic terminology, the human soul gains knowledge of its identity with Atman/Brahman.

"The one who glows in the depths of your eyes—that is Brahman; the death-less, the fearless, that is the Self of yourself and all beings; the Beautiful One, the Luminous One. In all the worlds, forever and ever sovereign!"

CHANDOGYA UPANISHAD, 4.15.1

At this stage, the phenomenal world of separation perceived by the ego recedes to the background, while universal love, greater understanding, inclusive awareness, and symptoms of universal consciousness emerge in the mind.

That is why the *Isha Upanishad* says: "The one who perceives all beings as not distinct from one's own Self at all, and one's own Self as the Self of every being, does not, by that recognition, hate anyone."[5]

The Disappearance of Sorrow

This knowledge frees our minds from the spell of disempowering maya. First, intellectually, then emotionally, we begin to perceive unity over diversity.

A student observes:

> *"These teachings have brought an understanding of how to see my relationships in this world. We get so caught up in our judgments, our likes and dislikes, thinking this is life. No, it is only our small shadowy selves believing this is the real world, but it isn't. What is real is that we are all part of a Oneness, a unity consciousness that has no favorites or judgments."*

These realizations are not merely words, but actual experiences of countless beings all over the world who have been "liberated" from egoic consciousness into discovering a limitlessly powerful and joyful Self. In Sanskrit, such people are referred to as *jivana mukta*, which indicates their "freedom" from conditioned sorrowful existence and release into ever-free, joyful existence.

Watch Out for Spiritual Bypassing

This great Advaita approach, which is the heartbeat of the Upanishads, is unfortunately the philosophy that leads to the most spiritual bypassing. These concepts cannot be appreciated by every mind. It is subtle knowledge, takes years to fully comprehend, and needs systematic exposure to the knowledge.

Many teachers, who may or may not have studied it methodically from authentic sources, offer their own selective interpretations. Some extreme teachers even resort to psychedelics or sex to achieve a state of oneness through chemical or sexual euphoria.

Such teachers universally emphasize "Oneness" emerging from the nondual vision as a one-dimensional panacea to all evils of our duality-ridden world, without preparing the ego-mind to receive and work with this higher paradigm. Pithy statements like, "We're all connected," "There is no separation," and "It's all one big consciousness," make it easy enough for almost anybody to quickly imagine themselves embodying oneness, floating in a sea of nondual consciousness.

On a popular online forum about spiritual matters, a self-confessed "oneness junkie" reports that not only within days but hours of coming across nonduality teachings of Neo-Vedanta teachers, "the whole world took on an ethereal, dreamlike appearance, as all distinctions and dualities melted before my eyes. . . . I have vivid recollections of walking through the halls of my high school near Seattle, Washington, with an inner smile bubbling away as I looked upon everyone and everything as nothing but an illusory display of light and energy. Nothing was real, nothing was important, for all was nothing but a timeless dance of purest Consciousness."[6]

However, the author then goes on to explain how she had allowed her mind to operate from a self-hypnosis, no more than a daze, that left her unequipped to deal with the very real problems of her very real (duality-ridden) world. Her short bubble of universal love and oneness burst, leaving her in an ongoing state of "existential depression . . . aimlessness . . . and esoteric apathy."

What went wrong?

Samsara Purification Must Precede Nondual Teachings

As you can see from previous chapters' emphasis on cultivating discernment, detachment is critical because the main obstacles on the path of nonduality are vasanas, the innate psychological urges or subconscious predispositions that reinforce the egoic individuality (jiva) that is unfulfilled and separate from others.

Until vasanas are seen through and set aside, can the ego really accomplish the leap from duality to nonduality?

According to Arthur Versluis, professor and department chair of religious studies at the College of Arts and Letters at Michigan State University, neo-Advaita is part of a larger religious current that he calls "immediatism," the assertion of immediate spiritual illumination without much if any preparatory practice within a religious tradition.[7] In his book, *American Gurus: From Transcendentalism to New Age Religion*, Versluis describes the emergence of "immediatist gurus": gurus who are not connected to any of the traditional (paths) religions and promise instant enlightenment and liberation. According to Versluis, immediatism is typical for Americans, who want "the fruit of religion, but not its obligations." Versluis points to Ralph Waldo Emerson as its key ancestor, who "emphasized the possibility of immediate, direct spiritual knowledge and power."[8]

Again, when modern teachers promise to teach the path to "instant awakening to Oneness" and completely omit discussions on preparatory practices, do modern seekers have any recourse but to fall victim of confusion?

There was a reason why the ancient seers of Vedic nonduality, who first gave this beautiful teaching to the world, stressed samsara purification and study under a qualified teacher. It is likewise important to develop an eye for critical analysis, rationality, and common sense, especially when it comes to mind-transcending theories. This prevents premature transcendence based on personal insights alone!

But with right preparation through the cognitive disciplines, which we are assiduously exploring in this book, you can hope to experience a state of almost magical Oneness.

It is equally important to learn to *maintain* that state of Oneness and not slip into hatred and disgust or codependency and victimhood when faced with the din and roar of life—relationship conflicts, political chaos, discouraging and disturbing life circumstances, wars and acts of terrorism, horrifying losses and unfair emotional attacks, sexual and financial betrayals, and personal aspirations that conflict with each other.

Inadequate or nonexistent preparation can explain the tendency to use the Oneness teachings to push away issues from the relative realm. It is common to find oneness followers who lose their way, dismissing their or someone's else's suffering as merely the "play of maya," someone else's sorrow as just illusion or a circumstance they should take as a life lesson. "If all is One, then nothing is wrong," said the notorious murderer Charles Manson.[9] The idea of the unity becomes just another way to further bolster the sleepwalking ego.

The next sections explain additional important points about Advaita that most modern teachers do not convey when teaching about nonduality.

We Must Embrace the World, Not Push It Away

Would you be surprised to hear that we must embrace the world, not push it away? The ancient seers explained that at any time, there are three levels of reality: personal, relative, and absolute.

1. *Personal reality* is that which we conjure up in our minds (samsaras) while thinking, imagining, and dreaming (our private subjective world).

2. *Relative reality* is that which we share with each other while awake in this empirical world (objective world). We do not share our world of dreams, unlike the objective world, which we share with other ego-actors.

3. *Absolute reality* is that which is nondual, permanent, and real. Personal reality and relative reality are not the ultimate truth because they come and go (only one exists at a given moment; they do not occur simultaneously). Absolute reality can be known only by a truly awakened seer, one who has gone beyond maya.

Bypassing occurs frequently because modern teachers teach upholding *absolute reality* all the time, while dismissing other states as lower orders of reality. That is why, to the newly converted eyes, the phenomenal world and our worldly roles as moms, dads, bankers, and artists appear pointless, even absurd, and as mere illusions.

But this was never the premise of Vedic nondual teachings. They were not meant to push the world away. They never pooh-pooh the duality-ridden world over attainment of nondual consciousness.

Just as things and events in a dream become meaningless upon waking, when one awakens spiritually, the world and all its objects, pain, and pleasures carry much less "charge" or power over us. The world does not disappear into thin air because it is a mere phantasmal "illusion"; upon awakening, our obsession with it simply recedes to the background and our true Self comes to the foreground.

The world is not the issue here. If you are living in this duality-ridden world, learn to respect it and navigate it with knowledge, say the Vedas; do not simply deny it all as an illusion. It is our unexamined attachments that must be given up. While transacting in the world of duality, remember in your heart and in your meditation that a higher, nondual reality exists beyond what meets the eye. This makes you less invested in the "me and mine" narrative of the ego. This also makes you generally more accommodating to other living beings and their peculiarities.

The nondual verses from the Upanishads engender a greater connection to and identity with the entire universe and its myriad creatures, giving birth to divine love and affection for the common Self pervading everywhere and, ultimately, to the discovery of our own indwelling Self. Nondualism must include dualism. If nondualism doesn't include and validate dualism, then it is an error in our understanding! We must operate wisely within the realm of duality where we are and meditate upon nonduality in our private world of the mind. This is the essential teaching.

The World Is Not an Illusion: Love It, Serve It, Enjoy It

Adi Shankaracharya was a Vedic scholar who lived in India in the eighth century CE. He is often considered the father of nondual teachings because his writings and commentaries are considered the gold standard among nondual lineages from India. He made three statements that are said to summarize the Vedic nondual approach:

1. Consciousness alone is real (*Brahma satyam*).

2. The universe is unreal (*jagan mithya*).

3. Our essential and true Self (Atman) are one with universal Self (Brahman).

Unfortunately, it has become trendy to quote the first two statements of this great scholar and neglect the deeper understanding. When we do that, it appears he is suggesting a duality between the world and consciousness and that the world is an illusion.

However, the scholar never said that the universe is unreal, only that it doesn't have an independent reality. It is *mithya*. The word "mithya" is often wrongly translated as "illusion" by Western teachers. This is not the same as maya, our illusory perception of the world. It simply means "that which has a qualified reality." "Mithya" means "neither true nor false." The world cannot be false because we all clearly see and perceive it. Shankaracharya says that the world is not true either because it is constantly changing and everything that the world has to offer is temporary, transient, and impermanent. But what remains permanent behind these changes is the Universal Self (Brahman).

According to the classical nondual view, this world is
inseparable from consciousness. It is a manifestation of
Divine Consciousness (Brahman).

Therefore, the universe depends on a deeper underlying cause for its existence: it's pervaded with consciousness; it emerges from consciousness and exists in consciousness; and it can't exist without it, quite like our body and mind are not an illusion. They too have a qualified reality since they cannot exist independently. They are dependent upon the presence of Self, or consciousness, *Atman*.

Sadly, the misunderstanding of the concept of mithya as illusion became the crux of Western nonduality. The word "illusion" caught fire in the imaginations of people worldwide. Some even attempt to walk through concrete walls, claiming them to be mere illusion!

Besides, how wonderful to tell yourself that the worldly problems you face right now are mere illusions! It permits us to bypass the world and worldly suffering! If your own suffering, others' suffering, or the suffering of poverty, hunger, sexual abuse, racism, and homophobia is uncomfortable to face, we can dismiss it as an illusion and circumvent the need to do anything about it or even experience vulnerability.

In other words, the misinterpreted version of nondual teachings offers a splendid means to spiritual bypass all the time and even feel contemptuous for those who are invested in the "illusion."

By contrast, look at what the Vedas invite you to do. As preparation to embody nonduality, you are invited to view this whole world as a home of the Universal Self.

Five Veda-Inspired Worldly Relationships

The Vedas ask us to cultivate love and gratitude toward five dimensions of the universe: Mother Earth, parents and ancestors, humanity, divine forces, and gurus. When you do that, you develop an *advaita vison* that perceives unity in diversity. It softens your relationship with the entire world, which you will come to consider your extended spirit family.

Say Thanks to Mother Earth (Mother Nature)

The Vedas say that we, as humans, are deeply indebted to Mother Earth: her soil, rivers, mountains, trees, fruits and vegetables, animals, earthworms, birds, butterflies, honeybees, cows, horses, air, sunshine, and five elements: space, air, fire, water, and earth. She nurtures us like a mother while we are alive, and she willingly accepts our discarded body at death!

What can you do to show your gratitude toward Mother Nature? The Vedas answer: plant a tree, preserve seeds, and think grateful thoughts at the very least. In the modern context, you can:

+ Eat organic and non-GMO foods exclusively.

+ Recycle and compost.

+ Care for dying species (plant or animal) by supporting a reputable sustainable growth initiative.

+ Do your part to clean our polluted air, rivers, and seas.

Say Thanks to Parents and Ancestors

The Vedas ask us to plan to be consciously "present" when our parents are diseased or dying, especially when they are physically, financially, or mentally feeble. They may be cranky, cantankerous, wrinkled, and anger-arousing at times, and yet we are asked to consciously overlook any errors in our upbringing since many parents are unconscious themselves, victims of spiritual ignorance. Not everyone is lucky enough to receive spiritual knowledge in their lifetime. To show your gratitude, you can:

+ Deliberately think grateful thoughts toward your parents, grandparents, and great-grandparents, dead or alive (even if the care or love you received was minimal or lacking).

+ Write and send them a card.

+ Say a prayer for them.

+ Visit them more often.

+ At the minimum, think kind thoughts about them.

Say Thanks to Humanity

Everything we consume today—be it knowledge from published books that make wisdom available to us in our own home, laptops on which we access communities and record and share our thoughts, utensils to cook our food, electricity to run our gadgets, clothes to wear—is due to the accomplishments of human beings, thousands of unknown faces, hearts, and minds, whose hard work, sweat, and sheer industry have made it all possible for us to lead the life we lead. So, we must cultivate gratitude and give back where we can. According to the Vedas, you can:

◆ Think grateful thoughts toward this nameless, faceless humanity that comes to your assistance.

◆ Give a helping hand to any human in need who appears before you—this human may have been involved in the pipeline of your own well-being!

◆ Be generous, be kind, provide charity, and practice nonviolence and compassion. Go out of your way to help distressed human beings—this is an essential aspect of a spiritual life.

The thoughts that connect you to your inherent generosity and compassion open doors to an entirely new portal of conscious existence.

Give Back to Divine Forces

The Vedas ask us to bow inwardly (and outwardly too, if we wish) in recognition of an all-pervading divine principle. This divine principle is the underlying, undeniable intelligence that makes all wisdom from every culture, including the Vedas, available to us through the speech of purified seers. In recognizing a supreme intelligence that weaves our experience in its divine colors, we are acknowledging that our ego is not the beginning and end of existence, but that it is a part of a greater divine Self. We therefore cultivate grateful thoughts toward this divine power in any way available to us. Daily, you can:

◆ Connect to all-pervading Spirit Divine via your mind with meditation, worship, mantra, or chants.

◆ Place a flower or fruit on your altar (at home or in nature) or light a lamp or a candle, and give even simple acknowledgment to the Spirit Divine that dwells everywhere, and within your heart, via your grateful thoughts.

Give Back to Gurus Who Awaken Your Inner Guru

The Vedas guide us to express our humble gratitude to teachers of sacred Vedic knowledge. Thanks to their teachings, we can journey from darkness to light—even just a little bit every day. Without teachers of yoga, Ayurveda, Vedanta, and other wisdom fields, we would continue suffering, never knowing that happiness and immortality are our true nature. In the modern context, you can:

- Thank your teachers in your heart via meditation, mantras, or simple acknowledgment.

- Thank them and support them with your words—write letters or make heartfelt comments on their blogs and social media venues.

- Share with others your personal story of transformation and the role your teacher or guru played.

- Share what you have learned and are learning from your teacher with your circle and beyond.

- Express your gratitude through gifts of service, skill, or donations.

Without the presence of genuine teachers in our lives and their honest preservation and transmission of the timeless wisdom, we would never learn how to turn on the light from within and achieve an inner transformation. This acknowledgement of grateful interdependence by the Vedic sages differs from the individualistic approach to life in modern times.

The Vedic view extols the execution of one's dharmic roles (that we will explore at length in part III of this book), as it automatically fulfills the rights of others. Emphasizing dharma, or value thoughts, fosters a climate of social and spiritual responsibility, something especially necessary today. This contrasts with the current world trend toward entitlement and expectations, which creates a culture of blame, compensation, and irresponsibility.

As best I can, I gratefully serve and acknowledge the five representatives of my nondual essence, my spirit family: Mother Nature, humanity, ancestors, God, and teacher(s) and guru(s), daily. It brings me untold peace and happiness. I serve where I can. I let no opportunity pass of serving, caring, and sharing for the universe and all its creatures—the crux of nondual living for me.

Employ Absolutist Beliefs Judiciously

It is imprudent to impose absolute nonduality-based beliefs, such as universal love, universal acceptance, universal compassion, and universal forgiveness, without discerning whether or not the other party deserves it.

For example, Krishna, the greatest teacher of Vedic nondual wisdom, while teaching his student Arjuna about nonduality, did not advise him to opt out of an imminent battle against insane members of his own family in the name of "Oneness." Instead, Krishna taught Arjuna hard, transactional intelligence to deal appropriately with conflicts in the world marked by duality, evil, and suffering. The right thing for Arjuna to do, according his teacher Krishna, was to fulfill his worldly duty as a soldier for everyone's sake by going to war and trying to win it, for long-term peace on earth.

Lord Krishna teaches Arjuna four ways of conflict resolution:

- *Sama*: Try to sort problems out mutually and amicably first (talk it out). This is a winning approach, and try your best because, after all, we all share the same Self.

- *Dana*: If that fails, try to resolve by offering valuable gifts (for example taking the person out to lunch), or offer incentives to choose harmony, like pointing out the benefits of cooperation versus conflict.

- *Bheda*: If problems continue, separate (stop contact) or weaken the opponent by *distance-creating strategies,* such as not responding to phone calls, asking the offender to move out (or you move out), and so forth.

- *Danda*: Finally, use force, such as a restraining order or physical restraint. Ideally avoid using your own body and speech for violence as much as possible, and depend on "dharmic authorities for dharmic violence," such as the police and the law. When violence is unavoidable, act from inner clarity after due discernment and detachment.

Look to these pragmatic approaches versus premature forgiveness in the name of spirituality.

You will find in Buddhism and Jainism—twin spiritual traditions, both of which also originated in India—a preference toward beautiful but absolute teachings on nonviolence and compassion offered by godly figures like Gautama Buddha and Mahavira directed at monks. This makes sense since monks must choose that absolute level.

But in Hinduism, which is maximally influenced by the Vedas, you will find godly figures, like Rama and Krishna, who impart lessons, not just to monks who live outside the fabric of worldly life, but to householders like you and me. These humanized Hindu gods exemplify leading inspired lives as kings, soldiers, husbands, friends, and parents, and like all worldly folks, they dealt with worldly problems and even wielded weapons and lead dharmic wars, not for the sake of the ego, but to restore light to collective darkness.

This pragmatic approach sounds less elevated perhaps, but it's useful for ordinary humans who are not practicing meditation in isolated communities or caves amid mainly conscious and mindful colleagues, but who are confronted by very real suffering or evil in the world, such as suffering due to wars, murder, rape, terror, or racist attacks wherein innocent children, women, men, or loved ones become victims. Therefore, while upholding the higher values, like nonviolence over violence, rather than asking us to choose only those ideals, no matter what, the Vedas ask us to take a neutral position and choose appropriately in our higher mind, using discernment (viveka).

While nonviolence is a core belief of the Vedas, the Vedas also hold that at rare times, judiciously employed violence (dharmic show of power, force, and might) can be an effective tool to protect our self and others against a threat, abuse, or injustice. There is value in both, provided we approach each situation with discernment, not from delusory samsaras.

That is why I am such a fan of texts like the Bhagavad Gita (the CliffsNotes of all Vedic Upanishads). Lord Krishna teaches right action in a truly pragmatic sense.

While battling the sleepwalking (turned evil) family members, Arjuna was reminded by his teacher Krishna to never forget that he and his enemies in the plane of duality, ultimately, shared the same Self in the plane of absolute nondual reality.

This higher knowledge of simultaneous existence in two planes of experience (outer and inner, dual and nondual, worldly and spiritual) allowed Arjuna a 360-degree vision of his imperatives, both as body and as Self. It prevented Arjuna from going to war for petty, vindictive reasons, or the eye-for-an-eye code of law (like Hammurabi's Code). He did not kill out of hatred. He killed from a greater imperative of universal love, to protect his kingdom from being taken over by unconsciousness. He went to war with inner peace to uphold dharma (righteousness) and restore ethical order in the realm of relative reality—where opposites like good and bad, dark and light, and ultimately conscious and unconscious people who can act with evil intent, do exist. This is an undeniable fact, and Vedic nonduality does not leave us living in some false delusion such as "nothing matters" or "love your enemy."

It is not a choice between war and peace.
We must bring inner peace to our outer wars.

Arjuna did not walk away bitter or arrogant from the kill. With nondual peace in his heart, he did his duty as a soldier on the worldly plane of duality. In the same manner, we must accept duality and its imposition of opposites, while meditating upon nondual consciousness in our hearts. We must not mix up the two.

From the nondual perspective, your betrayers, rejecters, detractors, critics, and challengers are also the same Self, dressed in dark, unrecognizable masks, appearing in different body-suits, only to remind you to switch on your own inner light. But from a duality perspective, you can't simply go kiss them as an outward display of nondual knowingness. You must engage them with alertness and appropriate boundaries in the realm of the relative. You must learn cognitive skills like thought management and the science of ethics.

This will prevent bypassing and trying to walk through relationships either emotionally numb, claiming they are all an illusion after all, or overcompensating with uncalled-for and inappropriate generosity, kindness, and compassion just because you know intellectually that you share a common divine consciousness.

Individuality and Universality

The good news is that exposure to nonduality teachings from the Vedas gives us back our expansive heart.

When we see things as they are (united) versus how they appear to us (separate), we become free from unnecessary suffering. Envy, jealousy, and competitiveness lose their grip on us. We find we are more able to feel appropriate compassion, even for people who we don't know or who have hurt us because our nondual truth lets us breathe into a more inclusive state of mind. As a first step toward expanding my awareness toward nondual consciousness, Baba gave me vivid examples from the Vedic worldview:

"Just like when innumerable rivers from the four directions flow into the common ocean, they all lose their individuality, and the ocean becomes their common truth. In the same manner, various beings let go of their small half-truths when they identify with the common truth of the One Universal Self.

The bees who abound around us work very hard. They collect tiny droplets of nectar from innumerable flowers growing in diverse gardens, forests, and fields. The bees are free to collect nectar from every flower growing around them on Mother Earth that day. So, they roam far and wide and bring back cherished droplets of nectar to the hive. Once in the hive, the mass of droplets becomes one giant drop of honey. The individual droplets lose their distinct identity; they no longer know from which flower and which garden they came. So too do all of us beings when we identify with the Universal Self. It no longer matters who we are and where we came from. Individuality that separates is lost, and universality that unites is perceived. One uniting consciousness pervades everything and is every-thing. It lives inside you as your own Self.

Just like salt, when mixed in a bowl of water, makes the water equally salty at the bottom, in the middle, and on the top, the Self pervades all existence. That Self is the truth of truths. That Self is you."

The best way to reveal the underlying nondual truth in an instant is to observe duality from a detached space. That process of stepping back into a higher, more detached awareness will take you out of any egoic investments in a myth-reality, into a space of greater emotional freedom, out of the clutches of duality, into the ever-present nondual truth of oneness. You will experience a breathing lightness in your heart.

I did not awaken to this radical truth of nonduality overnight. Instead, I slowly and steadily noticed irreversible change in all my egoic beliefs. Through renewed understanding, I became more emotionally connected and present with other people and creatures, with whom I was apparently sharing a common Self.

A Competitive King Who Realized Nonduality

The Vedic tradition tells the story of an ambitious and selfish king who turned into a truly awakened yogi by the name Vishwamitra. He is the seer of the third section of the *Rig-Veda*. Prior to his own spiritual awakening to the truth of advaita (radical oneness), his mind was steeped in duality. Not only did he view himself as a distinct creature, disconnected from everyone else, his estranged and spiritually sleepwalking ego felt competitive, enraged, and justified in his actions to clamor to the top.

Vishwamitra's mind was colored with lust, rage, pride, and jealousy, so much so that he even tried to murder another Vedic sage by the name of Vashishtha simply because the latter was famous for possessing spiritual powers and advantages (such as a wish-fulfilling cow) and was acclaimed as a *Brahmarishi*, "a knower of the truth of Oneness." Vishwamitra did not enjoy being simply a plain old yogi in the eyes of onlookers. He was jealous of Vashishtha—and he wanted the cow too.

To his credit, Vishwamitra quit his kingdom, gave up his material wealth, and tried to make sincere progress in the spiritual direction through extended Vedic practices and meditation. But sadly, whenever he heard about accomplishments of Vashishtha, he burnt up inside his samsaras. From the lofty peaks of ascendance that he attained through meditation, he would plop right back into the muddy pool of desire, self-pity, rage, and jealousy. His ego was so entrenched in the duality of separation and competition that he could not get beyond his own envy to make any genuine progress.

Apparently, our guy Vishwamitra was true seeker after all. He did not give up on himself or stop making efforts to see through his own self-created suffering. Vishwamitra's ego did break free from the prison of his samsara quite a bit. People started praising him for his growing spiritual aura. But just as we get fixated on being validated by a special someone to make us feel our achievements matter, Vishwamita's ego, despite being advanced and appreciated by so many people, now wanted to be recognized by the sage he was so jealous of. So off he went to Vashishtha's house, asking for that recognition. He said, "Everyone says I am a knower of the ultimate truth of Oneness, so I am Brahmarishi now, do you agree?"

Vashishtha quietly shook his head no and walked away.

Vishwamitra was so shocked, and he almost lost it (all over again). But then, by providence, he overheard a conversation between Vashishtha and his wife.

The wife asked: "Why do you not want to tell him that he has realized the highest truth? After all, he does have many miraculous inner powers accumulated through years of dedicated samsara-purifying practices and meditation."

The sage responded: "Because I love him, I will not lie to him, after all he is my own Self. I will never deceive my own Self. If I tell him at this stage of his life that he has realized the ultimate truth of advaita, then it will be a lie. He will think that he has realized the highest, and yet he will not be able to get the results of the highest. Because I love him, because we are one, I choose to tell him the truth. I would rather be misunderstood by him, killed by him, than to mislead him."

Hearing these words of true love that can emerge only from a heart established in absolute nonduality, Vishwamitra's ego transformed in that instant. Vishwamitra bowed to Vashishtha as his teacher, a role model in that moment. His heart began to overflow with divine recognition. He saw his own Self shining in the eye of Vashishtha, his wife, and even the cow that his sleepwalking ego once desired so desperately to possess!

And just like that, the proud king knew the truth of all truths: there is no "other." And he dissolved into infinite oneness. He felt like Self. He heard Self. He saw Self in his so-called enemy. All his vasanas had become quiet. His mind was clean, clear, pure, and shining, lit up like a million suns shining at the same time, thanks to the light of truth of advaita. With tears in his eyes, he spoke to his teacher, "I did not recognize you. I did not recognize me. I forgot we are united in love. I forgot we are One. Thank you for reminding me."

Thereafter, the king became a great Vedic seer, who is known as Brahmarishi Vishwamitra.

There were no more episodes of forgetfulness in his mind's playground. Maya was exposed forever, and the Oneness of Self alone shone in his heart.

Sage Vishwamitra was awake to his nondual nature, and he awakened all of us thereafter, by giving us powerful, life-changing mantras like the Gayatri Mantra (see pages 163–165).

> *"The knower remains awake in what is night for all beings;*
>
> *And when all beings are awake, that is a night for the knower,*
>
> *who truly sees what others cannot see, the truth of One Self."*

BHAGAVAD GITA, 2.69

> *"The Self is blemishless or taintless."*

BRIHADARANYAKA UPANISHAD, 4.4.20

To me, Vishwamitra is a perfect example for us modern-day seekers. While oneness feels like a beautiful concept when we are being led through a guided mediation on unity consciousness, once we get up from the mediation mat and reenter the world, we are right back in the cesspools of duality. Be it at our workplace, where we envy our more successful or better-paid colleagues, or in our bedroom, where we argue with our partner on petty domestic matters, once again, the same old duality-sponsored complaints, gripes, and jealousies come flooding back. While most of us don't harbinger murderous thoughts, rage and envy are things all humans universally possess. We may not murder, but we do dismiss, reject, dominate, stonewall, make invisible, backbite, control, disrespect, and humiliate so-called others. We are often far from knowing that who we are treating so badly is really our own shared Self in different clothes.

Knowing that a confused, egotistical person like Vishwamitra successfully made this journey gives me hope. We are all Vishwamitras who must journey on because if we are sincere, one day we will also encounter a role model like Vashishtha who will not budge from the truth of oneness. Then, even our last delusions that keep us chained to duality will fall away.

There is no shame. There are no missed buses. Even murderous people can be seers, if they truly want. That is why I encourage you to start a journey from inner darkness to light, fiction to truth, and ultimately, from duality to nonduality.

Genuine Awakening to "Oneness" Is Possible

Just like Vishwamitra awakened to truth, despite his delusions, we all can slowly awaken over time with the aid of on-going contemplations and ego-purifying disciplines. And hopefully we will awaken, without any spiritual bypassing, to an authentic experience of unconditional spiritual love. If you too try to sincerely imbibe this knowledge and live by it, a greater nondual consciousness can and will arise in your purified mind, replacing default fears and hatred of duality.

*"The Self, smaller than the smallest, greater than the
greatest, is hidden in the hearts of all creatures. The wise,
with the aid of self-knowledge, behold the Self, majestic and desire-
free and become liberated from all [ego-created] sorrow."*

SHVETASHVATARA UPANISHAD, 3.20

This universe is, after all, a divine setup. One Self appears as many, playing different roles in the theater of existence, ultimately awakening us to the truth of our common divine inner being. But, ask yourself this: Are there many actors or one? Who else is there but you? With this will come the recognition of a world family, a unifying awareness of and a deeper relationship with Mother Nature and all her creatures, and a sentiment of universal friendship and benevolent embrace toward all beings.

*"One who is connected to the Self sees all things equally and perceives
the Self in all living beings and all beings within the Self."*

BHAGAVAD GITA, 6.29

PART III

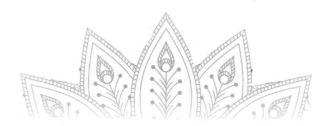

Embrace the Joy of
Your Sovereign Life

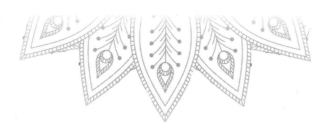

17

Dharma: Cultivating a Life of Meaning

"Dharma ensures material well-being and spiritual progress of humanity."

VALMIKI RAMAYANA, ARANYA KANDA, 8.26

Dharma is one of four *purusharthas*, the life-affirming desires that are the opposite of vasanas. Most of us, if asked about our most important desires or life goals, may rattle off a list of personally relevant goals: getting a promotion at work, starting a family before a certain age, traveling to an exotic location. With time, however, we forget the pleasures we receive from worldly accomplishments. It all fades away, leaving us searching for more meaning. But somehow, we never forget the shine in an old pair of eyes when, unasked, we help walk an old man across the street. The happiness or contentment that comes from such moments lasts and lasts, filling an inner emptiness. This need for greater meaning through conscious and entirely voluntary cultivation of virtue is known as dharma.

"The highest dharma is to wipe out the tears from the eyes of living beings in distress."

VAISESIKA SUTRA, 1.2

The Vedas explain that all the diverse goals of humanity can be categorized under an umbrella of four universal desires, known collectively as purushartha:

Dharma, which is pursuit of virtue

Artha, which is pursuit of survival

Kama, which is pursuit of pleasure

Moksha, which is pursuit of a Higher Truth, of Self, God

I am glad that the Vedas understand we humans come wired with the urge to satisfy these four universal desires. It is easy to see why survival and pleasure would be universal categories. There is no person on Earth who is not driven to materially survive and thrive. The human ego shares these two goals in common with all animals. Our desire for material comfort and security, for play and enjoyment are, within a valid life context, entirely legitimate in the Vedas. Unlike other spiritual traditions, there is no moral judgment of our desires, even those pertaining to accumulating wealth and enjoying sexual and sensorial urges, provided we don't sleepwalk in the process of fulfilling our desires.

Since, artha, or "wealth," can give us only so much security (and our minds can never have enough reassurance anyway) and our senses can enjoy only so much pleasure (kama) before they get bored, it's suggested that we actively pursue the more advanced goals of dharma (mindfulness and virtuosity) and moksha (spiritual sovereignty).

For most of us, the first two goals are instinctually activated. Like all animals, we are conditioned to fulfill them. The latter two desires remain latent until a Vedic master, or the master's teachings and writings, reach us in some way and awaken us to our higher purpose in life. Let us look briefly at each of them.

Artha relates to survival—physical, biological, material, and emotional, the fulfillment of the basic needs of our life: for example, having a job so that we can pay our bills, having a house to live in, having food to eat, and having someone we can relate with emotionally all feel necessary for survival. Artha is especially related to wealth generation. We must not be greedy, but we must make an effort to be abundant, since abundance is our natural vibration.

Kama relates to pleasure, for example going on vacation, buying things that we like for decoration, enjoying sexual intimacy, and so forth. Pleasure may have a limited role in the grander scheme of things, but it plays an important role. We get bored once our tummies are full. We seek play, entertainment, and pleasure of various sorts. And the Vedas say, why not? Don't pretend, in the name of spirituality or God, that you don't care for sensory pleasures; that makes you pretentious and gives rise to yet more delusions. Vedic literature teaches us how to have "out-of-the-box" sex in treatises like the *Kama Sutra*. Vedic teachings on theater (*natya shastra*), dance (*nritya shastra*), sculpture (*shilpa shastra*), and beauty (*soundarya shastra*) celebrate pure pleasure for pleasure's sake!

Dharma relates to virtue, living life with nobility, following a good value system, and conscious living. When we help others, we feel good. This goodness can be a goal.

All humans sooner or later experience an inborn psychological urge to find greater meaning in life by becoming virtuous, giving back, and selflessly serving all beings. This innate impulse for inner expansion—to become aligned with greater, universal ideals, the quest to refine our ego with noble values and live by these values—is dharma. It makes us mindful in interpersonal, societal, moral, religious, and environmental contexts. Does egoism, anger, greediness, unrestrained sexuality, cruelty, and violence deserve residence in our samsara? Or should we carefully cultivate those values that inspire compassion, integrity, kindness, and accountability?

Dharma relates to living a deliberate life with noble values and higher personal standards guiding our deepest beliefs. Dharma is evident from the sense of right and wrong that is the unique heritage of humankind. Inspired by dharma, we humans go beyond our obsessions and expand our consciousness to align with a greater truth operating through us. When we begin thinking dharma thoughts, we become a self-healing, self-soothing, self-uplifting, self-comforting, self-liberating entity, all through the agency of our own mind.

Dharma can be understood as willful self-restraint of our lower nature. It acts as an internal check, a preventive against stupid, freedom-destroying actions. We are invited to grow out of our unexamined passions, impulses, and selfish and egoistic interests to lead a life of more refined consciousness. When we engage in the world of maya, dharma protects us with an armor of values. As my father, Daya Prakash Sinha, a Vedic scholar and renowned Indian playwright on dharmic themes, wrote, "Dharma is sometimes wrongly translated as 'religion.' Dharma has nothing to do with God, faith, hell, heaven, or the other world. Dharma is concerned with this world and only with this world. Dharma is a set of social, ethical, all-time universal code of conduct that is essentially secular; it enables every human to meet their life goals with integrity, peace, and harmony." According to Sage Manu, dharma has the following ten attributes: (1) patience, (2) forgiveness, (3) mental steadfastness or mental strength, (4) non-stealing, (5) cleanliness, (6) restraining of senses, (7) cultivating wisdom, *and* (8) knowledge for (9) truth (10), and non-anger.[1]

Moksha is about suspending all outward seeking for happiness through artha and kama by finding happiness in Self. Though dharma is a great goal, moksha entails going beyond even our dharmic résumé to discover a hidden metaphysical reality. Moksha relates to psychological freedom from the above three goals for exploration of the Self, whose real nature is unalloyed bliss. It is about ending spiritual ignorance that veils and hides this bliss from us.

If you analyze the objects you pursue, be it money and relationship-based security (artha), pleasure (kama), or even virtue (dharma), you will see that you are searching for the sense of freedom you assume you will experience once you have obtained those things; furthermore, your mind will not rest until you have achieved it. Then you will realize that *it is freedom that you value over everything else.*

Realize this: you are seeking only you! Vedic scripture informs us that we are the source of that which we seek, that our very nature is boundless fullness, peace, bliss, and happiness. Once you become convinced beyond a shadow of a doubt that the wholeness of your own essential nature is not be found in the objects of the world, then you will make the search of this inner treasure the primary focus of your life.

Moksha, in the final analysis, is a direct experience, an immediate awareness of ultimate reality and absolute truth. When moksha is achieved, we remember, at last, who we are and reclaim everlasting power, freedom, authority, and autonomy from within.

The Role of the Noble Goal of Dharma

Dharma paves the way for moksha, while artha provides the material support and sustenance along the journey, and kama, the necessary emotional and physical comfort.

Once the two primeval goals of survival and pleasure are met, we humans often begin searching for a deeper value or meaning to our life. Then, we find helping others, even strangers, sometimes at the cost of sacrificing personal pleasure or even risking our survival at times, imparts a greater sense of purpose to our life. Values and principles, ethics and morality support a life of meaning. Meaning in life increases happiness in life, and this happiness is of a more lasting nature, much more happiness than accumulating money or pleasure can ever bring us, in this or the next life. Hence, moksha is the ultimate goal of human life, and in its support, dharma is primary because dharma leads to moksha; artha is secondary, and kama is tertiary in the scheme of intelligent goal-setting behavior.

Dharma must moderate our pursuit of the first two goals. While it is our birthright to enjoy security from money in the bank and pleasures ranging from tasty food to sexual ecstasy, it is also our spiritual business to manage our healthy desires with dharma-born discerning thoughts such as, *How much is enough?* and *What is okay, and what is not okay to indulge in, dharma-wise?* Such human pleasures as singing, dancing, playing, enjoying material wealth, and gratifying sex are valid pursuits, provided we do not hurt or abuse another for them and do not impede our own sattvic-dharmic journey of the soul. Dharma enables us to control our desires and create within our self the capacity to realize eternal reality even while enjoying a rich material life.

Ideally, when our survival goals (artha) are tempered by our values and ethical principles (dharma), then wealth will come to us naturally and with ease, and we will be moved to share it as well as offer it in service of other needy beings. Under the ever-expanding umbrella of dharma, even the smallest of jobs, rendered honestly, will yield honest and sustainable artha that abides and nurtures our material and spiritual existence.

However, sometimes in the name of survival, we humans overconsume, hoard, scavenge, and even steal what isn't ours. Without moderation and a regard to dharmic use of resources, dharma is lost in the ensuing blind consumption, and artha is defiled. Greed is a fundamental cause of loss of dharma. And greed is a consequence of forgetting that we are the limitless Self. Lack of spiritual knowledge makes us blindly material and never satisfied. While economic prosperity is a valuable goal, it should never be our exclusive and dominant goal, without any consideration of the impact on our community and nature.

But there is no escaping the all-knowing, all-pervading gaze of our own Self. Who did we hurt and steal from but our own Self in a different body? That is why the one who defiles artha with non-dharmic actions is a host to morbid fears and even physical diseases from psychological stress and inner conflicts with the Self.

When dharma informs our life, it feels good to be honest and say no to bribes or manipulation, to speak the truth even if it leads to unpleasant consequences, to restrain our own lower nature before pointing a finger at others, to help a person across the street even if it means we are late to work. Thus, dharma is a moment-to-moment choice, exercised not to reap advantage, acceptance, or to get a pass to "heaven." Dharma is chosen again and again by any true seeker, even in difficult circumstances, as it is the natural and rarefied expression of our highest Self, expressed through emotionally mature and self-responsible human-hood.

Dharma also must always be applied in the pursuit of self-knowledge. There is no sleepwalking our way to self-realization. False gurus who discard dharma for rapid notoriety and wealth suffer in the cobwebs of their own minds. On the other hand, Vedic literature abounds with stories about dharmic kings, mothers, sons, doctors, priests, soldiers, farm boys, and even dharmic enemies and dharmic prostitutes.

Unlike security- or pleasure-seeking activities, dharma is not automatic or conditioned behavior. Also understand this: dharma is never externally imposed (like moral policing in some cultures), but rather an internally experienced spiritual urge to align with a greater ethical principle, as the voice of our conscience. When you are ready, you will make a conscious decision to choose dharma over and above survival and pleasure urges, every single time.

Dharma takes us beyond our survival and pleasure goals to express our higher spiritual values, innate human kindness, and sense of social responsibility. A dharmic individual will never knowingly hurt feelings, transgress boundaries, or injure another. One would do to the other only what one wants for oneself. Compassion, kindness, forgiveness, justice, and truthfulness are gems decorating the crown of dharma. Dharma leads to personal and collective stability, maintenance of social moral order, and general welfare of all. Dharma connotes emotional stability and maturity and *adharma* ("absence of dharma") connotes instability.

Peace and harmony in our own mind, the natural environment, the social environment, and the moral environment are the fruits of dharma. In fact, this ideal of dharma is lodged within each human heart, but to discover it, cherish it, value it, and live by its guidance is a factor of unique personal conditions and the divine task of each embodied soul to unearth.

In conclusion, we must be aware that while we do what we can to accomplish security and pleasure in this life, we'll never be fully satisfied or check off every item on our list. It is simply not possible. So, we must also cultivate inner contentment and meditate on the statement, "I am Atman, the Supreme Reality. I am enough unto myself." As you meditate over time, *you will become what you believe.* With this truth as our focus, dharma is possible in the midst of accumulation and acquisitive activities, and even carnal desire and sensorial indulgences can be had within a dharmic framework.

The Desire for Virtue vs. Compulsive Desires

Dharma does not mean renunciation of security and pleasure. It simply means exercising detachment and discernment in the pursuit and enjoyment of the greater good. Without dharma, we can get trapped in seeking security and pleasures our whole life. We are then in bondage of these otherwise legitimate goals. They become compulsions, or vasanas. The mind full of cravings remains restless as the wind. It is dissatisfied with whatever it gets and grows more and more restless by the day. Compulsive desires creep into even the legitimate pursuit of security (artha) and pleasures (kama) and virtue (dharma).

Body vasanas can replace the legitimate goal of kama: we never have enough sex, clothes, or sensory objects to make us happy. World vasanas can replace artha: despite being well-off or even wealthy, we may feel desperate for more money and power, disturb our work-life balance, or even compromise our ethics to earn more, or become our boss's pet to get ahead in our professional life. This leads to ill health and physical and emotional stress. Knowledge vasanas can disturb and dislodge the third goal, of dharma itself. When this happens, our speech may be full of noble-sounding words, like altruism, compassion, community upliftment, environmental protection, the importance of self-care and well-being, or social and gender equality, while our core beliefs remain selfishly conventional or even non-dharmic.

When we are caught up with vasanas, dharma remains a mere illusion. Another mental trap in maya!

Dharma Is Naturally Aligned to Sattva

If the mind receiving knowledge of dharma is in rajasic (selfish) or tamasic (destructive) mode, it cannot retain the knowledge. A sattvic mind alone most appreciates learning about dharma.

Fortunately, when we pursue dharma, the quality of sattva, with its attributes of clarity, balance, purity, serenity, and peace, increases in our mind. And when we cultivate sattva, our thoughts become naturally dharmic—more conscious and evolved. Our inner whispers are always dharmic!

Alternately, people who seem caught up in artha, always working extra hours or working too hard on their relationships by overanalyzing, ruminating, or explaining are operating from rajas, with its attributes of mental overactivity. Those who put pleasure even before security, perhaps by sleeping in or catching a movie while ignoring work deadlines or domestic commitments, may be experiencing increased tamas in the mind, with typical traits of dullness, lethargy, and increased desire for bodily comforts and self-indulgence. By making dharma first, you are saying yes to sattva!

Dharma Is Intrinsic to Your Soul Nature

The Vedas tell us that deep down, all humans are inherently sensitive, kind, and nonviolent. Our goodness, compassion, kindness, and fairness are intrinsic to our true Self. This is a huge declaration, is it not? We are not sinners, but good people. We are simply ignorant of our true bigness! That is why when we expose our ego to dharma teachings, we all begin to melt.

When exposed to higher principles to live by, often even the darkest criminal wants to change for the better. And most of us, if we have not gagged our inner voice by numbing our conscience, fall apart with self-reproach, remorse, guilt, and shame when we know we have violated or hurt another living creature and when we have been unfair, cheated, or lied. We may even lose our sanity or our physical health. Our own greater Self expects better from us!

After all, we relate to each other and even animals and plants through a common cord of consciousness. If, as the Vedas teach us, we have different body-suits but share a common Self, we simply cannot afford to be non-dharmic, can we? It is like going against our own deepest nature.

I breathed a sigh of relief when Baba told me this:

"Shunya, dharma is the voice of the conscience, that part of your ego that still faintly remembers you are part of something bigger, deeply compassionate, interconnected, and divine. From that first impulse when it is revealed in your heart as an inner knowingness of right from wrong, dharma is not the bidding of strict tradition, teacher, god, or the conditioning of society or religion. It is solely and purely the gentle, sovereign voice of your own soul. It is your purest option, your truth-uplifting course of action, your higher mind's decision regarding what is best for you and for everyone you sincerely love."

Therefore, explore dharma as your primary life goal. If you put it before even money-making and pleasure-seeking choices, it will be the start of a more mature, conscious, expanded, and mindful life.

Some of us suppress this inner call to dharma; some ignore, distract, medicate, or even bury it under mindless pursuit of yet more wealth and pleasures; but it is there. We cannot deny it. After all, our ego-mind has two roles. One is to get lost in the world, seeking happiness in wealth and pleasures (I want more, more, more!). But the other hidden, less obvious purpose of our ego is to remember its true, inherently abundant, joyful nature.

And it is this latter, more spiritually aligned part of our mind that makes us want to be good, seek good, and share goodness. Our inherent memory of dharma is an innate understanding of right from wrong. It urges us from within to do the thing that is right for ourselves and the largest number of people. That part of us wants us to choose dharma!

Dharma Is Critical for Psychological Sovereignty

Your own conscience is the highest judge of dharma. Living by dharma values will bestow upon you not only social approval but also a unique sense of self-approval (*atma-tushti*) because my dharma teachings will awaken you to higher personal standards, even as you go through the routines of securing (artha) and enjoying (kama) your life.

Technically, whatever holds, sustains, and allows something to be itself is dharma. For example, the dharma of fire is heat. Without heat, there can be no fire. So, from that perspective we can understand dharma as that which allows us to be who we truly are, not just roles being played out by sleepwalking bodies dressed up in fancy clothes!

Each time dharma is willfully exercised over the ego's self-serving tactics, sovereignty prevails. Only the pursuit of dharma will give lasting freedom—much more freedom than what wealth can buy and more than relationships and sexual or other pleasures can ever bring you. In fact, those bind you through clingy attachments. When you uphold dharma, dharma will uphold your rule over your own life and protect you from psychological missteps leading to emotional bondage. It will give you great inner confidence.

Dharma Is the Teaching of Our Innermost Voice

Baba told me we don't need to know Sanskrit or read scriptures to know right from wrong or ethical from nonethical because most Vedic dharma rules are common sense. They are universal.

The inner Self is the highest teacher of dharma. When we listen to that innermost voice, we know we should perform only those actions that do not arouse any doubt, fear, or shame in our heart. Any action that does is treading on slippery ground and may indicate that we are about to embark upon a non-dharmic course of action. Inner turbulence or discomfort is indicative of being out of alignment with what our spirit wants from us. It suggests we are following the dictate of our ego or senses, ignoring our larger reality, our spirit.

Dharma connects your happiness with everyone's happiness—humans, animals, plants, and even inanimate nature, rivers, and mountains. Dharma teaches us a unique way of being fully human as an instrument of compassion, goodness, and joy in the world, and when you share happiness, you will receive happiness back from the divinely orchestrated universe.

Usually dharmic action is so harmonious with inner Self that it naturally meets social sanction without contrived efforts to win or seek approval. As a mother, my dharma is to care for my son. If I recognize my duty and fulfill it to the best of my capacity, societal sanction is a natural consequence. When harmony and integrity exist within, it is only natural that harmony and integrity also are reflected outside. When I abandon my dharma toward my son, social disapproval is one reality, but my inner agitation and inner pain are even worse. Sometimes the dharma toward my Self can conflict with the dharma required by society, and in that case, I must listen to my heart and carefully evaluate the situation with sincere deliberation.

An important Vedic law book comments in this regard: "If a person in their conscience feels ashamed or guilty to do an act, while doing an act, or after doing an act, it is the clearest indication of tamas quality of action—clearly the act is a transgression of dharma."[2]

The soul will always tell the person who has committed the offense that they have transgressed dharma. Even though that individual may try to pose as a good or even a great person, they will feel ashamed within.

We know what is proper or improper without formal education in dharma. That is why a burglar steals in secret. Is the thief hiding from society? Or God? Maybe. But ultimately, they are hiding from their own conscience. Deep down, we always know what is good versus what is bad. The very fact that we become secretive when we flout dharma is evidence that every human being knows what is wrong. Even a child knows stealing, lying, cheating, deceiving, misrepresenting, and abusing are wrong.

What Happens When Our Ego Forgets Dharma?

But when due to ignorance and delusions our inner light is concealed, our ego-self forgets dharma.

In absence of dharma, the mind, beset with rajas and tamas, begins to behave as a selfish agent, a smooth operator that needs no other guidance or overseer that recognizes no other power, entity, or realm as above, deeper, subtler, or higher than itself. When such a mind acts for the gratification of the mind-based shadow self alone, it is the beginning of great worldly suffering and psychological bondage. Doubt, jealousy, abuse, paranoia, violence, murder, rape, massacre, war, and great emotional instability imprison our happiness. The mind becomes cluttered with negative emotions such as rage, competitiveness, jealousy, hatred, pride, and resentment.

Therefore, when we are without a dharma-based value system and higher ethical beliefs restraining our mind from delusory thoughts (samsara), speech, and actions, we can blatantly lie, cheat, or mock others to get wealth (artha) and pleasures (kama) at any cost! We can even hurt and insult the common Self in other beings—as in those with different-colored skin or with different sexual preferences—and feel no compunction because nothing pinches us from within.

The following is an ultra-simple definition of dharma, universally acceptable and applicable from my lineage: If you do not want anyone to harm you, then embody the dharma of not harming anyone. If you do not want anyone to insult you, embody the dharma of not insulting others. If you want everybody to respect you, you should offer the same respectful behavior to others. If you want everybody to help you and treat you compassionately and fairly, you should help and treat others the same. That is why never do that to another which you regard as injurious to your own Self. This, in brief, is the rule of dharma. Yielding to impulse and acting differently, one becomes guilty of adharma.

I could not always hear the voice of my soul, but now I do, loud and clear, and dharma has become my way of life. It fills me with joy, and with it, I help my students listen to their dharmic whispers too.

Dharma awakening is the first step to our Self-awakening.

Truth begets truth. Love begets Love. Inspired by dharma, human befriends birds and beasts, and they in turn befriend the human. If dharma is the divine law, then truth is dharma's vessel, and right action is its vehicle. Peace and harmony in the natural environment, social environment, and moral environment are the fruits of dharma.

But despite dharma being in our hearts, we seem to have lost touch with it. That is why, even though we know the difference between right and wrong, ethical and not ethical actions, we often transgress dharma anyway. Baba often said:

"The Self itself is the witness of the mind, and the Self is the refuge of the mind. Never despise thy own Self, the supreme witness to the acts of the mind."

Awesome Things Happen When Dharma Is Upheld

Selfishness is your ego's fundamental survival strategy. The most important ego-diffusing and purifying strategy, therefore, is to expose this same ego to selflessness ideals, or dharma. Your sorrow-causing subjective projections, your samsara, will begin dissolving once you dare to operate from dharma rather than from whimsical likes and dislikes—those pesky vasanas!

The seers say, "One who protects dharma, is protected by dharma."[3] Our dharma thoughts elicit divine grace and protection of higher power in the form of good luck, divine grace, and unexpected fortune of all kinds in this or future lifetimes. These are the only side effects of living with dharma values: stability, beauty, and divine grace.

According to the Vedas, when dharma values inform our choices, it ensures a blessed next birth. Good luck, support, fame, and all types of material fulfillment are our reward from the cosmos in this and upcoming lifetimes. Our mind becomes a pure crystal, radiating soul power, divine abundance, and a more awakened state of consciousness that manifests positive experiences. And finally, dharma is the first rung on the ladder toward moksha, or total awakening!

In the next chapter we will explore twenty dharma values that you can embody in your day-to-day life for greater emotional sovereignty.

18

※≫≫≫◆◆◆◆◆※

Yamas and Niyamas:
Nurturing Higher Values

"Even a little bit of Dharma protects one from great fear in the present and future sorrow."

BHAGAVAD GITA, 2.40

If you are a householder seeker like me—meaning you don't live by yourself amid nature, but within a society of people—then you need a personal code of values. This will ensure society does not cause you to fall asleep to your spiritual goal of sovereignty, but that you remain awake, holding on to your dharma. It will help you sidestep automatic behaviors, and instead of habitual, conditioned responses from your samsara, you will choose more skillful responses from a more self-aware, objective or nonreactive, and contemplative state of mind.

Dharma isn't an end game, but rather a way of being in life while embodying higher consciousness, universal ethics, and humane values. Dharma values take us beyond our survival consciousness to express our higher propensities, innate human kindness, and sense of engaged responsibility. When dharma is activated, it leads to an awakening of compassion, altruism, and empathy, toward not only humans but all living creatures. With dharma, one not only supports social justice, equality, basic goodness, and morality, but also becomes an awakened participant in all kinds of relationships.

The dharma values that I share with you in this chapter will help you distinguish between what is universally important and therefore worthy of your attention and what is simply your ego making noises. If we are ignorant of dharma, how can we determine our core values? We will simply copy others. Depending on whom we hang out with, we might inadvertently borrow selfish (rajas) or even harmful (tamas) values. We might also unconsciously pick values randomly from our culture, the media, newspapers, or other external sources.

Dharma as a Set of Universal Humane Values: The Yamas and the Niyamas

"Dharma" has many meanings, including duty, ethical conduct, charity, law, universal love, innate duty of things, compassion, and altruism. The Mahabharata says: "It is most difficult to define dharma. That which helps the upliftment of the planet and the welfare of living beings is surely dharma. The learned sages have declared that that which sustains is dharma."[1]

The values conveyed by the Vedic texts, like the Vedas, Bhagavad Gita, and others, guide us toward proper conduct that ensures we remain sovereign seekers of ultimate liberation, even as we go about our daily lives.

Twenty Dharma Guidelines

Various forms of the ethical guidelines, known as the *yamas* and the *niyamas*, can be found in many Vedic scriptures, including the Bhagavad Gita, *Shandilya Upanishad*, *Varuha Upanishad*, *Yoga Yajnavalkya*, *Hatha Yoga Pradipika*, *Tirumantiram*, various Advaita texts authored by Sage Adi Shankaracharya, and of course the *Yoga Sutras*.

The last text, the *Yoga Sutras* by Sage Patanjali, is the most well-known yoga text in modern times, especially in the West. But, by no means is the teaching of yoga exclusive to this one text or its author. In fact, the ongoing discussion of yoga and specifically the yamas and niyamas forms the backbone of Vedic culture. Here is a verse from the *Katha Upanishad* (800 BCE), which precedes the *Yoga Sutras* (2 BCE–2 CE) by about a thousand years: "Only when mind [*manas*] with thoughts and the five senses stand still, and when buddhi [intellect, power to reason] does not waver, that they call the highest state. That is what one calls yoga."[2]

Therefore, dharmic "observances and restraints" are an essential narrative in a culture that emphasizes yoga as a way of life, not only for ascetics but also worldly folks, or householders.

While Sage Patanjali presents a total of ten rules, I offer twenty, sourced from various ancient texts, including the Bhagavad Gita. I decided to do that for two reasons. First, the teachings by Sage Patanjali of five yamas and five niyamas can be found everywhere, while the rules I am choosing to highlight are relatively lesser known outside Vedic lineages like mine (they are immensely helpful too). For ease of comparison, see the following table.

While a few rules are common in the two lists, most of the dos and don'ts I am highlighting support the spiritual quest of everyday people who are caught up in everyday relationships.

As an illustration, let's take the case of the yama *brahmacharya*, which literally translates as "no sex" in the classical exposition of eight-limbed yoga, the *Yoga Sutras*, which was composed somewhere in between 2 BCE and 2 CE. "No sex" means absolute celibacy because its author, the esteemed Sage Patanjali, was purportedly talking to advanced yogis (monks), who were ideally done with the urge to mate and procreate. However, when this text became universally popular beyond yogic monks, even twenty-year old yoga aficionados started considering the "no sex" mandate and failing at it. It caused confusion among yoga practitioners (along with guilt). Some even went rebelliously to the opposite route, which gave birth to the "sexy" side of yoga.

Neither extreme was required.

From time immemorial, human sexuality has been celebrated in the Vedas. Many of the sages who gave us the holy Vedas were married and sexually active family men with wives or love interests as well as children. (At that time, men and women could choose to be with more than one life partner.) The Hindu gods and goddesses are likewise depicted to be enjoying conjugal bliss with beautiful homes, jewels, and clothes. The Vedas celebrate sexuality and even prescribe it for a balanced life in Vedic medicine (Ayurveda).

The Vedas tell us that we should all strive for four universal goals, the purushartha. One of these goals is kama, which means using our senses to enjoy all kind of sensorial delights—delicious foods, beautiful clothes, enchanting perfumes, scents, flowers, and bedroom delights. Vedic seers even compiled the ultimate compendium on sex, the *Kama Sutra*.

When we don't understand the context in which a certain dharmic recommendation is made, following that dharma suggestion blindly does not aid sovereignty; it can retard it. I suggest we use wisdom and thoughtful discernment to understand our desires (including sexual ones) and take responsibility for fulfilling them in a wise way. Providing a context of wisdom (what, when, where, how much, with whom) was more important to the Vedic seers than any blanket prescription banning sex, marriage, wine, nice foods, music, or dance.

But somewhere along the march of time, we forgot to check in as to who Sage Patanjali was giving his teachings to. Was he teaching to householder yogis enjoying their interpersonal, sexual, and professional relationships and security from material comforts, or to yogis who sought to renounce the world? And what were the insightful Vedas really communicating about the yama of brahmacharya?

Patanjali defines "brahmacharya" as "absolute celibacy." But in an Ayurvedic context, "brahmacharya" means choosing a balanced and healthy expression of sexuality between committed partners. I write in my book *Ayurveda Lifestyle Wisdom*, "An ancient Ayurveda text from the eighth century, the *Ashtanga Hridayam*, puts it this way: 'From a disciplined indulgence in sex through brahmacharya, one gains memory, intelligence, health, nourishment, sharpness of sense organs, reputation, strength, and long life.'"[3]

In fact, the Ayurvedic sages go on to say that if the sexual instinct is forcefully suppressed, mental perversions and countless physical diseases result. Therefore, brahmacharya can mean many things in the Vedas, from no sex (absolute celibacy), to consensual sex, to monogamous sex, to simply leading a life with higher awareness in pursuit of true Self (also known as Brahman). The last example is the way I explain this term and live by this rule in my life.

Celibacy cannot alter the course of human consciousness; it can only influence the curious few. Hence, the Vedas remain pointedly inclusive of sexuality as a legitimate goal of life. That is why I applaud the Vedas and their commonsense approach for common folks like you and me, who would otherwise be set up for failure, guilt, and shame in the path of spirituality. And for all these reasons, I have made the effort to curate a whole new set of yamas and niyamas because it is about time humanity has a new set of dharma values to go by in our worldlier spiritual life, in addition to what is already out there.

PATANJALI'S COLLECTION	MY SELECTIONS
Yamas (Don'ts)	**Yamas (Don'ts)**
1. No violence	1. No violence
2. No lying	2. No lying
3. No stealing	3. No stealing
4. No sex	4. No unconsciousness
5. No possessions	5. No intolerance
	6. No shakiness in the face of challenges
	7. No insensitivity to others' suffering
	8. No deceptiveness toward others
	9. No slothfulness (yes to healthy food and lifestyle)
	10. No impurity (in body, mind, or speech)
Niyamas (Do's)	**Niyamas (Do's)**
1. Cultivate purity	1. Cultivate remorse
2. Cultivate contentment	2. Cultivate contentment
3. Cultivate austerity	3. Cultivate gratitude
4. Cultivate knowledge	4. Cultivate knowledge (seek a teacher)
5. Surrender to higher power	5. Cultivate trust (of teacher, path)
	6. Cultivate devotion (God, guru)
	7. Cultivate a self-mastered mind (in daily life)
	8. Cultivate a higher mind (buddhi) for discernment and detachment
	9. Cultivate steadfastness (of character)
	10. Cultivate desire for moksha (but not in absence of artha, kama, and dharma)

These values exist as a single word each in the Vedic scriptures, but they were modeled for me by my teacher. He lived by them, day after day. And then in my own life and relationships, I worked hard to embody them. Now I impart them to my students. What I teach is my interpretation that I put to work in the laboratory of my own life and relationships. They have yielded me increasing inner peace, joy, and immense satisfaction. I believe they will be of immense value to you too. I am still working on perfecting the yamas and niyamas in my own life, even while I teach them with all my heart. Remember, dharma is an ongoing lifestyle that even teachers refine and then enjoy until the last day of a given lifetime.

The Yamas: Ten Suggested Don'ts

A typical self-ignorant mind with its governing instincts of fear, anger, greed, jealousy, and lust will benefit from a contemplation of yamas, or dharmic "restraints." Without dharmic restraints, a typical mind can quickly collapse in its own negative pool of rajas and tamas and never touch its own hidden potential! As we deliberately think an opposite, constructive (dharmic) thought and restrain a non-dharmic thought, we break the chain of selfish thoughts and actions, and we shed more and more egoistic impurity until we realize our Self.

1. Ahimsa: Don't Be Violent / Practice Nonviolence

Ahimsa is key. It will determine the quality of your consciousness. We should expand our awareness to gradually identify with other members of the planet to such an extent that we should be able to feel others' pain. Only when I begin to feel another's pain will I never hurt another human being. Can those of us who wish to blossom spiritually afford to be violent in the jungles of our egoic existence? Violence indicates slavery to dysfunctional, entitled egos. Nonviolence means restraining the ego's base impulses to become conscious about the impact of our thoughts, speech, or actions on other sentient beings, including plants and animals. The *Yajur-Veda* says: "May all beings look at me with a friendly eye. May I do likewise, and may we all look on each other with the eyes of a friend."[4] Be willing to find nonviolent means to settle disagreements and disputes, and live harmoniously with a spirit of mutual accommodation. However, unlike in Buddhism, which came later, in the Vedas ahimsa is not an absolute value. The Vedas acknowledge that violence may have to be used as a last resort (such as in self-defense) after all nonviolent methods are exhausted. Even then, deliberation should be given before acting with violence to avoid delusory, impulsive behavior rather than the calibrated use of violence for the restoration of justice and truth (dharma).

2. Satya: Don't Lie / Practice Truthfulness

Satya involves refraining from lying, deceiving, manipulating, or revealing confidential information. It means speaking that which is aligned with your thoughts and feelings after due deliberation. Follow this ancient code of communication from the Bhagavad Gita: "Speak only that which is true, kind, helpful, and necessary."[5] Be unbiased, precise, and forthright in your speech. Do not engage in backbiting, slander, spreading rumors, or gossip—make that a personal commitment. Truth in speech strengthens, protects, and illumines you from within. Not every truth need be spoken. If the utterance of a truth causes hurt or violence, desist from giving expression to it. This does not mean you should lie. You can observe silence instead.

3. Asteya: Don't Steal / Practice Non-Stealing

Live from a position of non-selfishness, non-greed, and non-coveting. Due to rajas and tamas in the mind, humans are often reduced to becoming petty thieves in this abundant universe, be it a theft of ideas, words, music, luxury goods, cars, money, lovers, or even the power of others. With dharma, you would rather live without something important to you than stoop to appropriating because only that which comes to you nobly and in due course is acceptable to you. Therefore, you will also never fail to repay a debt, you will control your cravings, and you will live nobly within your means.

4. Brahmacharya: Don't Be Unconscious / Practice Self-Awareness

The Sanskrit word "brahmacharya" means the "path or practices that lead to the ultimate reality of Self." It involves cultivating an entire spiritual lifestyle in quest of the true Self. To be contemplative means to be able to face yourself, love yourself, and take stock of yourself in all its good, crazy, and amazing parts (self-observation). For the one who wants self-knowledge, it is very important to value being with oneself to contemplate in quietude. Cultivate the regular habit of returning to seclusion. Proactively seek out a spiritual teacher who imparts self-knowledge and teaches the art of self-contemplation. Read spiritual texts or books like this one, and practice disciplines like meditation, discernment, and dispassion regularly. At a physical level, this means purifying the biological impulses of food, sleep, and sexuality. This means voluntary sexual restraint (not necessarily celibacy or suppression, which is how Sage Patanjali defines "brahmacharya") and seeking "wholesome" relationships and recreation (not necessarily holy), and always choosing dharma over base instincts. By adopting this value, you are declaring to the world that your spiritual pursuit of your Self is more important than any other goal. While not neglecting material or pleasure goals through relationships of various kinds, you will automatically be focused on cultivating greater self-awareness.

5. Kshanti: Don't Be Intolerant / Be Tolerant

Consciously and magnanimously accommodate those who may hold opinions different from yours. Do not be impatient. Attempt to tolerate as a soul what your ego may label "intolerable." You are more resilient than you think! As best you can, exercise patience with challenging egos. Let others behave according to their own nature. Remember, the greatest souls were once criticized, belittled, or even stoned by sleepwalkers, but they remained focused on their higher path or mission. You are on your own mission. You need not let criticism ruffle your ego feathers. Accommodate and tolerate personality quirks, idiosyncrasies, and generational, cultural, or religious differences with understanding (remember everyone is asleep in maya, after all). Don't preach, judge, quarrel, defend, or argue at the drop of a hat. You need not always have the last word to be right. Don't force your opinions; live them instead. To be accommodating or tolerant, generally lessen your expectations from other egos. Avoid mechanical reactions (of disgust, rage, irritation, repulsion) and make them deliberate instead. Look at the soul behind others' egoic actions, and respond to the soul, not to the action. This softens the impact on your own ego. Then you can feel free to choose your attitude of tolerance and accommodation in thoughts, words, and deeds. No one will be able to disappoint you, only surprise you! Stay calm and focused on your goal of inner sovereignty, regardless of any provocation, by making spiritual tolerance your dharmic practice. Remember, the dharma of tolerance is not resigned sufferance. It is born out of positive acceptance.

6. Titiksha: Don't Mentally Tremble in the Face of Challenges / Practice Forbearance

"Forbearance" means exercising mental resilience in the face of the vagaries of life. This entails cultivating mindful hardiness to persevere through life's difficulties, disappointments, and disasters while resisting the default desire to complain (and build mental negativity) and fix the adverse circumstance right away (which leads to more egoic nonacceptance, fear, and panic). Forbearance comes from willingness to shift our attitude from nonacceptance to acceptance. "Acceptance of what is" and knowledge that "This too shall pass" are the essence of inner resilience, while continuing to practice self-compassion and self-care by seeking and contemplating self-knowledge throughout the challenging period. Knowledge of your higher Self will help you remain connected to your Self and keep your head above the water. You won't get bogged down and enslaved by your embittered and angry samsara or caught up in the "why me" syndrome. Cognitive practices from this book, such as discernment, dispassion, and meditation, will help you see beyond the confusion and hyperreactivity of your samsara. No one can have zero reactions to relationship and other life challenges. Thankfully, that is not an expectation of the realistic Vedas. But by practicing conscious resilience, you can avoid violent, extreme, or delusory reactions and retain your psychological freedom to make smart choices. Gradually, you will overcome fear and inner resistances and cultivate tenacity, endurance, perseverance, willpower, courage, and inner freedom instead.[6]

7. Karuna: Don't Be Insensitive to Others' Suffering / Practice Compassion

Compassion is the root of dharma; bereft of compassion, there is no dharma. The practice of compassion helps us overcome our ego's self-obsession (rajas), indifference, apathy, and even callous, cruel, and insensitive behavior (tamas) toward other creatures and their needs, pain, or suffering. Instead, operate from sattva, where compassion, sympathy, and empathy all are possible. Have compassion for your own learning curves since self-compassion is a step in the right direction toward feeling compassion for others. Criminals and aggressors are clouded by the same strain of self-ignorant delusion that we have had to some degree ourselves. While condemning their crimes, feel compassion for how lost they are and keep the possibility of forgiveness open. With compassion for suffering, we can selflessly assist those who are weak, impoverished, aged, or in pain. We treat all birds, animals, children, and people who have less power than us with kindness. Therefore, compassion can be the cord that connects us to our shared humanity. A Vedic saying goes: "Those who think, *He is mine* or *He is not mine* are petty-minded. Those who are large-hearted regard the world as one family. Compassion comes naturally when we regard the world as 'one family.'"[7]

8. Arjavam: Don't Be Deceptive to Others / Practice Uprightness

Arjavam means cultivating integrity or uprightness in thought, word, and action. Practically speaking, arjavam means being straightforward, honest, sincere, and authentic, not divided due to conflicting motivations. To practice arjavam, you must authentically express what you feel, want, or need, and not work against your own inner knowingness. With integrity in place, we can act in our own evolved self-interest, not just for another's sake. Being straightforward is helpful for your own health and peace of mind. A lack of integrity causes psychosomatic strain and inner guilt and shame. Therefore, try to maintain impeccable honesty and renounce duplicity and deception. Act honorably even when it's difficult. Frankly and openly accept your limitations, slip-ups, and faults without blaming others. The life of an upright person will be beautifully fearless and free from worry.

9. Ahara-Vihara: Don't Be Slothful / Practice Conscious Eating and Lifestyle Habits

The Vedic science of Ayurveda teaches how to have a conscious relationship with food and how to live a life of balance, including good sleep, timely and seasonal meals, healthy exercise and sexual rhythms, and communion with healing nature. Yoga and Vedanta books also emphasize the importance of food and lifestyle in mind management and spirituality. The Upanishads mention how the gross part of the food we consume becomes our body, but its subtle essence becomes the mind. That is why it is important to make sattvic food and lifestyle choices versus dulling and agitating choices. Self-care and cultivation of a positive state of health with bristling vitality and abiding immunity is dharma.

10. Shaucham: Don't Indulge in Impurity / Practice Cleanliness of Body and Mind

Shaucham means both inner cleanliness and outer cleanliness. The latter is a well-known benefit. A clean body, home, and surroundings fill the mind with quantum vibrations and make it more attentive and alert, too. Inner purity in thoughts and emotions, intentions and motives, passions and urges is as important as physical cleanliness. Without establishing inner purity, your samsara can become inundated with negativity, despair, and resentment. Use the spray of self-knowledge to cleanse away the smudges and streaks of envy, annoyance, meanness, self-loathing, unnecessary guilt, and self-condemnation. Practice discernment and dispassion to maintain minimum likes and dislikes. Convert your needs into preferences rather than compulsions or dependencies. (However, always sublimate rather than suppress your desires.) To cleanse your samsara of jealousy, anger, hatred, fear, selfishness, self-criticism, guilt, pride, and possessiveness, choose dharmic thoughts over self-shaming and other-blaming thoughts and resort daily to meditation and witnessing practices. Dharma lies in assiduously cultivating a pure and sparkling body and mind, internally luminous and outwardly shining abodes of your Self.

The Niyamas: Ten Suggested Do's

The ten niyamas, "do's," or the spiritual "observances," will help nurture something more beautiful within us—the superior, soulful sattvic qualities of the mind, hitherto concealed by the rajas and tamas content, elevating our awareness into the higher emotions of selflessness, compassion, universal love, divine creativity, and abiding joy.

With niyamas, you radiate who you truly are—the bold and fearless soul—not the controlling, hoarding, forever-discontent ego! You are Self, not just an individual segregated ego. How will you act? With sensitivity or indifference? With resolve or overwhelm? With trust or suspicion? With gratitude or entitlement?

1. Hri: Cultivate Remorse

Dharma is a great samsara purifier. Only a self-restrained ego can recognize when it has transgressed dharma and caused sorrow to another. Instead of self-condemnation, feel remorse and allow yourself its genuine expression; apologize sincerely. This is dharma. Frankly admit your errors and misperceptions. This always helps carve a way forward. We are all spiritually vulnerable. Dharmic remorse represents a desire to make amends and establish spiritual restitution.

2. Santosha: Cultivate Contentment

Santosha is the happiness that comes from cultivating peace with what's given to us and what's taken away, all as part of a greater flow. Acceptance is our only choice. Can you stop the unexpected rain from pouring? Can you stop the sun from shining? But you can choose to enjoy the sunshine and the unexpected shower, even if it got your coat wet! Everything is a hidden blessing. Live in constant gratitude for what and who you have in your life—your health, family, friends, pets, possessions, and chance to spiritually evolve through life challenges. Don't complain about what you don't possess yet or have lost. Identify with the eternal Self, not the ephemeral possessions and relationships that come and go. Cultivating inner contentment is a sure source of inner peace and happiness.

3. Dana: Cultivate Giving from Gratitude

From birth to this day, you have received gifts, nurturing, skills, and loving gestures from countless people and maybe have even been fortunate to receive the teachings and blessings of a spiritual teacher, or guru. Will you take these gifts for granted, or will you give back with generosity? Giving back opens the heart, diminishes for a moment one's self-absorption, and places value on the well-being of others. In small ways, humbly express your appreciation for someone's presence, actions, or offerings toward your better, more blessed, and enriched life. Impure motivations to give back include giving to receive a favor or to cover your ego's darker side. Giving without expectation of return is the purest giving. It releases our ego from the slavery of self-absorbed entitlement and vasana-tinged greed.

4. Satsanga: Cultivate Self-Knowledge

The Upanishads summon all humanity to undertake a great adventure of raising consciousness so our ignorance- and darkness-filled minds can shine with understanding, purity, luminosity, and universality: "Arise! Awake! Enlighten yourself by resorting to the great teachings and teachers."[8] Hence, dharma lies in not merely pursuing material goals and accomplishments but also making specific time for spiritual studies for evolution of our consciousness. This entails finding a qualified teacher and studying systematically, long-term if possible. Dharma can also be upheld by taking shorter spiritual and self-development classes or online courses, workshops, and retreats, and at the same time taking time out to breathe and meditate while communing with inner and outer divinity. This dharma has three steps: First, attentively hear the teachings or study the original texts under a qualified teacher (take the time it takes and enjoy the journey of self-discovery). Second, contemplate the teachings in the privacy of your own mind. Let them wash over your previous prejudices and misperceptions that blinded you to your own true Self. Third and finally, practice the new teachings in your daily life. The Vedas bless all sincere students and teachers of every path that leads to a higher truth of sovereignty, oneness, love, truth, and compassion.

5. Shraddha: Cultivate Trust in Your Spiritual Path and Teacher

Shraddha means cultivating an unshakeable trust in the Vedic teachings and the teacher who imparts the teachings. By trust, the Vedas do not suggest a blind trust, but an open-mindedness until you have refined your own discernment. Trust in the Vedic context is a noncritical approach, giving the benefit of the doubt to the teacher and the teachings until you more fully understand. Eschew those people and influences who try to destroy your trust with arguments and personal attacks. This discerning trust will strengthen your journey toward your own inner light. It includes cultivating loyalty, not blindness, toward your teacher, path, and lineage (if you are fortunate to have them). Trust is critical. After all, even if you were to complete your degree in computer science or environmental science, you must cultivate "functional trust" in your teachers, the textbooks, and the institution or tradition imparting the knowledge. To fully benefit from my teachings in this book, you will need to have a basic trust in my capacities as an ambassador of Vedic wisdom. Cultivating discernment-based trust versus blind trust imparts confidence, hope, and knowledge. Indulging a habit of perennial distrust, skepticism, cynicism, doubts, fears, or causeless suspicion hurts our spiritual progress and makes our egos unteachable.

6. Ishvara Pranidhanam: Cultivate Devotion Toward Divine Allness

The Vedas declare that "God" is not a person or a specific book alone, but an all-pervading *Divine Allness*—a formless, nameless, universal intelligent principle or presence that we humans can choose to worship in any form or name, if we so desire: Jesus, Krishna, Buddha, Durga, Lakshmi, Mother Mary (all are representatives of Spirit Divine). In fact, this father or mother God is also one with our true Self. Dharma lies in accepting every life experience without resistance, as divinely ordained, and not allowing any experience to generate delusory thoughts. This radical acceptance of whatever life throws at us with equanimity and divine consciousness is dharma. When we look at the world merely with material eyes, we indulge our likes and dislikes and complain in an entitled fashion: "I am going to be picky and complain about what I want but don't have." But if every experience is divine and if this world itself is a manifestation of this Ultimate Reality, then we can move beyond our attachments and aversions to appreciate a transcendental Divine principle at work, shining beyond birth and death, health and ill health, gain and loss, success and failure. The petty arithmetic of our ego, or samsara, dissolves in the face of a higher principle where all experiences lead to Truth and Truth alone. Let the voice of Divinity speak in the sanctuary of your soul!

7. Atmavinigraha: Cultivate a Mastered Mind

Dharma lies in attempting to fully master your mind. This is called *atmavinigraha*. Because of maya, or self-ignorance, we find that the master is the slave of the mind or even afraid of the mind. But the dharmic one calls the shots and not only enjoys the sattvic qualities of the mind but almost plays with the mind like Play-Doh. Yes, you can make the mind do the soul's commands, and your thoughts, speech, and actions will not only benefit you, but will also naturally take into consideration the benefit of the whole planet. When it is mastered using self-knowledge, your mind can only be an agent of goodwill and nobility. Naturally, by this stage, due to purity of the mind, your desires will no longer be colored with illegitimate compulsions (vasanas) or under siege from impulsive likes and dislikes. However, you will be able to attain your legitimate desires with ease and dexterity. The four worthy universal goals (which I described in chapter 17)—wealth, pleasures, dharma, and progress toward moksha—will be achieved steadily by the mind that has been mastered, offering no resistance, only intelligence, alertness, focus, and connection with the soul's power from within. Instead of impulsive thoughts that emerge on their own, conditioned thoughts that emerge due to imitation, scripted belief systems, or deliberative thoughts that emerge when your buddhi (the evaluating function of mind) consciously examines your thoughts (accepting or dismissing them in accordance with your code of dharma values), a fourth way of thinking will spontaneously emerge. Your mind will effortlessly and unfailingly resonate with universal dharma. It is artless thinking, and yet it teaches you, the seeker, the art of living. You will be helped by your own thoughts. Of course, this spontaneous thinking manifests in only those minds that have properly received and assimilated knowledge of dharma and higher Self—without taking shortcuts. A mastered mind becomes your best friend in the final journey to Self, Atman, the inner boundless one.

8. Buddhimatta: Cultivate an Illumined Cognitive Faculty

You are encouraged to live your life from your higher mental faculties and discerned choices (buddhi) versus acting and reacting from the plane of your everyday or lower mind that runs on scripts, patterns, and memory. But even the higher mind needs spiritual instruction, practices, and disciplines, such as discernment and dispassion. These practices cultivate sattva, the quantum quality of the mind, versus dull and agitated shades. A mind infused with sattva can do its job right. The spiritually instructed higher mind will help you understand your true nature beyond the ego's limiting beliefs, listen to your soul's guidance through intuition, commune with God or the Universal Self, and unlock inner worlds where great power, love, and creativity lie.

9. Sthairyam: Cultivate Steadfastness

Sthairyam means "firmness" or "steadiness." This Sanskrit word is derived from the root "stha" meaning "to stand." It indicates constancy in our resolve and behavior. My teacher Baba felt it was a key value for spiritual seekers because without cultivating this value, we never reach our destination. We may get excited about leading our life free from the bondage of our own misperceiving and subjective mind but never reach the goal of full and complete awakening. Without the dharma of steadfastness, many of my students who start out eagerly enough, quit halfway! Their enthusiasm simply fizzles out, and they slump back into their delusory samsaras, back to chasing vasanas! What a loss to Self and humanity! However, many more students—those who paid attention to my dharma teachings and put them into practice—now enjoy sovereign fullness and power. With firmness and inner resolve, they persevered.

Every day they reminded themselves to be steadfast and attended my lectures in a steadfast manner. Steadfastness comes easy when you think of yourself as the amazing, all-powerful, boundless, and beautiful Self, not the slippery ego. It implies a soul-commitment to the completion of one's pursuit (material or spiritual), irrespective of obstacles and challenges you face. Once a worthwhile objective has been set, the steadfast one works toward it with a soul-resolve and ensures that lethargy, family life, professional commitments, or other inner or outer distractions do not come in the way of reaching that goal. To practice steadfastness, consciously engage with the practices, activities, thoughts, meditations, and spiritual affirmations that make you feel grounded and anchored in your spiritual identity and power. When steadfastness is your inner value, you can be resolute and more confident in your intimate-relationship, school, community, and work-based trials alike. You will come through them successfully because the steadfast don't give up before achieving their set goal.

10. Mumukshutvam: Cultivate a Desire for Self-Realization, Moksha

Mumukshutvam means the burning, intensely compelling desire to know our own true Self, which is our inner guru, the God of all gods. This desire shows up only in a self-mastered mind that has received self-knowledge from a qualified source. It is marked by an unquenchable desire for enlightenment, an urgency for awakening to our greater and grandest inner nature. Then, all other material and worldly desires pale beside the desire to know the Self, which is one with the Universal Consciousness, God. Liberation (moksha), with its internal wholeness, fullness, divinity, and perfection, marks the end of external desiring. The more one quests for ultimate freedom by understanding one's true desireless, ever-full, spiritual nature, the more one becomes emotionally free in relationships because then, neither the presence nor absence of objects or people will cause stress. Now we know what we previously did not know about our true nature, that *I am "complete" unto myself.* This dharma value therefore sets apart individuals—those who are hunting for happiness, wholeness, and divinity outside themselves from those who are beginning to explore their inner world and its original infinite treasure of godliness by seeking out correct knowledge and practices to do so. The desire for the Self ends the desire for everything more mundane, or subsumes it. The Vedas are clear: you will manifest what you desire, so desiring to know the invisible but truly abundant and powerful Self is a great desire to actively cultivate. No wonder it is a dharma value unto itself. In many ways, this book is stoking that ultimate desire in you too, and because of that, your whole life is about to change. When you choose to engage only with what is eternal, there is an infinite capacity to connect with abiding inner wholeness. Get ready to receive unending gifts from within.

Benefits of Living by a Dharmic Code of Conduct

Those who live by higher principles begin to connect to an inner soul power. We may choose to live, leave, or change our profession, relationships, and calling, but we will do this from an inner position of personal power and a big okay from our conscience (the voice of our soul).

Living outside the samsara box, with the help of values, is truly liberating and blissful! Let us look at some amazing benefits of adopting values and living by them.

Attachment to Dharma Purifies Samsara

Exposure to dharma can modify the very attachments and aversions that cause delusional sorrow, making them more universally selfless in nature. For example, if we get attached to the values of "speaking truth," "upholding nonviolence," or "practicing kindness in speech" and we become averse to white lies, violence even in our thoughts, and unconscious speech, then we are making the samsara setup work for us rather than against us. This itself is a big dent in samsara, which thrives on desire-based egoic attachments and aversions. Dharmic attachments confound the samsara machinery. Besides, acting from dharma is the quickest route of enhancing the balancing and illuminating quality of sattva in our minds!

Dharma Bestows Self-Approval

In relationships, when we consciously practice restraint, nonviolence, accommodation, or other ego-sublimating values, we enable others to do the same. Living by a dharma code of values bestows upon us not only social approval but also a unique sense of self-approval that our earnest conscience relaxes into.

If you value dharma, practice it in your relationships until it emerges from your thoughts into your behavior. With dharma, you will feel supported from within, strong inwardly and outwardly, and free to navigate through existence as a valuable and self-valuing individual, choosing to coexist with the entire manifested universe, with harmony, peace, and accord.

Dharma Directs the Ego in the Right Direction

Ultimately, dharma is a way of life for those who want to remember that they are not the ego. Dharma is possible in carnal desire. Dharma is possible in accumulation and acquisitive activities. And lastly, there is dharma to be applied in the pursuit of Self. By promoting dharma as the mindful code of conduct for all humanity, the Vedic civilization aspired to and attained the zenith in human experience—physical, sensual, mental, material, social, and spiritual. That is why the Bhagavad Gita says this: "One who is of dharmic mind to the good-hearted, friends, relatives, enemies, the indifferent, the neutral, the hateful, the righteous, and the unrighteous, excels."[9]

Guided Practice: Adopt a Dharma Value

Review the list above. If you want to ensure you are following the don'ts (niyamas) and cultivating positive virtues (yamas), then first make a soul-resolve toward a specific rule (choose one at a time), known as *atma-sankalpa*. Then make attempts to implement that value, even in small ways, through thoughts and actions each day, for several days, until it becomes an unconscious habit.

Here are a few more suggestions to firm a given yama or niyama in your mind:

- If you want to ensure you don't act violently, spend time with nonviolent people. And by that same logic, avoid friends who embody what you don't want to embody (violence, lying, deception, and so forth). Company is key. Try to locate high-minded friends or a spiritual group or tradition where people seem to already possess a certain yama as part of their behavior (or are conscious of it and make efforts to embody it). Spend time with them when possible in conscious dialogue. If you have a teacher who lives by dharma values, then join them frequently on retreats and classes as often as you can. Make it a priority to be around dharmic folks and teachers. When we are surrounded by living role models, yamas grow in us the fastest, as if by osmosis.

- Read books like this one that remind you of your dharmic imperative. Read autobiographies of spiritual teachers, leaders, and seers who have lived their entire lives with one or another dharma value.

- Let the yama you are working be the last thing you think about at night and the first in the morning. Preplan the thought. It takes practice, but it works. When I was working on cultivating devotion (*ishvara pranidhanam*), my last thought of the day was about God as Divine Mother, and that was my first, too, in the morning. If I forgot and my mind started jumping ahead, I gently bought it back to Divine Mother. Now, my thoughts automatically turn to the Divine Truth (which is beyond gender), softening my ego and letting me rest in that higher contemplation. When I wanted to become steadfast (sthairyam) in all areas of my life, I told myself at bedtime, *May my sleep make me steadfast.* Upon waking up I thought, *Ah, another day to practice steadfastness.*

- You can also begin your own yama-niyama journal, and every day write your progress with disabling the niyamas (rejecting urges of acting out from violence, lying, and so on) and enabling the yamas (acting from compassion, gratitude, and so on). Make entries in this journal, not from an attitude of scolding yourself, but for connecting with your innermost voice. The voice of Self is always dharmic, and yamas and niyamas help you to connect with this voice. Our inner guidance is usually drowned in our mental clutter. Accompanying your journal writing with meditation and contemplation on that value will allow this concealed voice to reemerge.

You may not know it right away but adopting at least a few dharma values to begin with will lead you to a more thoughtful, deliberative, spiritually spontaneous, and sovereign way of life.

19

❖❖❖❖❖❖❖❖❖❖❖❖

Swadharma: Embracing
Your Innate Purpose with Integrity

"Truth alone wins;

Never untruth."

MUNDAKA UPANISHAD, 3.1.6

Pure joyful existence, Self, is your true nature. How does it want to express itself through your body, senses, mind, ego, and intellect? What is your dharmic life purpose beyond personal survival? What did you come here to blossom into, and how can you become a gift to the universe? How can you be that which existence celebrates and supports?

The Four Swadharmas

The Vedas describe four root propensities, called *swadharmas*, that will help you boldly embody your worldly dharma. Swadharma is a specific form of dharma, pointing to your inner nature, authentic traits, inclinations, and aptitudes. These four root propensities are the mystic, the guardian, the entrepreneur, and the pleasure-seeker. They each represent a type of personal dharma. "Swa" means "self," and "dharma" in this context means "inherent nature," like heat is the nature of fire. The Bhagavad Gita explains like this: "The wise person must live in accordance with their unique inner calling, or swadharma. Better is one's own duty, though devoid of merit, than the duty of another, well discharged."[1]

Your swadharma reveals what upholds you deep within, and your sense of purpose evolves through this upholding. You may identify with mainly one or possibly two propensities. If your natural propensity is recognized and lived, it can become the basis for a much more deliberate, conscious, and fulfilling life in the worldly sense of choice of profession, vocation, inner seeking, partners, colleagues, priorities, and understanding your experience of the roles you take on.

When you uphold your deepest propensities, you become of incredible value to the cosmos. When you act and respond from knowledge of your swadharma, particularly if you do so while upholding dharmic values, you feel supported from within and more fearless to be who you are. You can use this knowledge to say yes or no in relationships and maintain beautiful, values-based boundaries. It makes you more authentic in all your interactions, more able to face challenges. Let us briefly explore each propensity now.

The Seeker of Higher Truth / Mystic Propensity

You are a born mystic if from childhood you have been wanting to know Self, God, or truth; if this desire has gone beyond a passing or occasional wish in your mind and translated into a full-fledged lifestyle where you read spiritual books, seek out spiritual teachers, attend spiritual classes, or even have a deepening relationship with a living guru (or are yourself a guru); and if the goal of acquiring self-knowledge and living in inner joy is your top priority. Mystics may or may not be religious in an institutional sense (though it's highly probable that they are), but every being with a mystic propensity is "spiritual." They feel an undeniable inner call to know what lies beyond what meets the ordinary eyes. Sadly, without knowledge like the Vedas, which sets us free to boldly be who we are, many of us, especially if born into nonspiritual families or anti-God or overly science- and technology-driven societies, bury this propensity or fail to identify it. They may even become depressed. From a Vedic life-goals perspective, people with the mystic propensity are most attracted to pursuing the goal of moksha.

The Seeker of Higher Values / Guardian Propensity

Are you a guardian by nature? Guardians are always driven by a cause that is bigger than their personal agendas. Do you possess opinions and ideas with which you want to protect the unprotected and make our Earth a better, safer, and happier place to live? Then do that, say the Vedas. Accept yourself as you are—no apologies. Guardians are sometimes misunderstood or labeled as "protestors" or "rebels." With knowledge, we can now define and accept ourselves, saying: "I'm a holy warrior, a guardian of truth and dharma. And because of who I am, I make this world a better place." Don't give up your inner voice just because your spouse, partner, family of origin, friends, or state of polity in your society rewards the meek. Maybe to challenge the status quo (while upholding universal values) is your job. Thanks to this propensity, the world has been blessed by the likes of Gandhi, Nelson Mandela, Martin Luther King Jr., and the countless unknown everyday guardians who make our schools, families, neighborhoods, and global communities safer and more radiant with shared power. From a Vedic life-goals perspective, people with the guardian propensity are most attracted to pursuing the goal of dharma.

The Seeker of Wealth / Entrepreneur Propensity

Are you someone who dreams of wealth? The Vedas say that is great. Accept yourself as an instrument of the divine intelligence that shall use your original propensities to create wealth on our planet, and you can nonapologetically, boldly, and enthusiastically enjoy it, share it, and circulate it by creating jobs, service, and so forth. Your bliss may express itself more fully in creative wealth generation, and your inner growth may be hidden right there too. You must not spend time trying to be a guardian or a mystic since that won't be authentic to you. Of course, even as a wealth-seeker, you will, if you are smart, continue to uphold the universal values we have already discussed. Wealth-seekers can benefit from spiritual education and meditation. This can only enhance their wealth-generating propensity. But they must not confuse propensities and least of all plan spiritual careers. Similarly, we don't want mystics running businesses, as their inherent disinterest in money will be counterproductive. Guardians also are best placed inside social-cause-driven outfits where they can keep harking humanity to greater social order. From a Vedic life-goals perspective, people with the entrepreneur propensity are most attracted to pursuing the goal of artha.

The Seeker of Pleasure / Flowing Propensity

When you are happy assisting others, if you can make a decent and ethical living, enjoy a family or social life and the little pleasures that a stable life can unfold (for example gardening, home-decorating, entertaining, hosting friends and family), then you may be enjoying an inward propensity for flowing along with life as it comes and drawing pleasure where you can. In fact, most of humanity has the flowing pleasure propensity—80 percent of us. Pleasure propensity? Is that a sin? No. The Vedas say enjoy it—you have every right. Maybe you have done the other things that require sacrificing pleasure in some other lifetimes or will be called to do so in future ones. This lifetime, in this story, if you are ready to lead a life of ethically earned joys and pleasures, such as earning money to buy a home, luxuries, clothes, vacations, and so on, then you are welcome to do that. Thus, the pleasure-seeking (pain-shunning) propensity is also a propensity recognized by the Vedas. From a Vedic life-goals perspective, people with the pleasure propensity are most attracted to pursuing the goal of kama, which can be pursued alongside dharma and moksha. If you are a pleasure-seeker, go for it, but be careful of body and world vasanas.

Empowered by Authenticity

Swadharma is not your highest nature, but it is a deep memory of the part of your ego that is closer to the Self. When you embody your swadharma, you will be living a bit closer to your Self. You can negotiate more freely for your needs and values in relationships and feel less intimidated, vulnerable, or imprisoned by your own masks. We feel unfulfilled in our relationships when we do not know about and own our swadharma. We pretend to be who we are not and suffocate under our own masks. I urge you to contemplate: What do I represent; what do I stand up for?

Vedic knowledge empowers us to live a more self-determined, naturally authentic life. The law of swadharma mandates that you first use knowledge to recognize, then value, and finally live your true calling without apology. When you do that, your inner contentment will not go away. Your wholeness will accompany you all the time. You will inspire others too!

Pure existence has room for everyone and every kind of propensity. We must believe in ourselves and honor our deepest desires. The desire to cultivate a tiny garden in our home and delight in it is as valuable as the wish to change the history of racism and apartheid on our planet. Who decides what is less or more important? It is One Self flowing in so many ways and pleasuring itself in myriad ways.

In the Upanishads, the qualities of *satyam* ("pure continuous existence"), *chaitanyam* ("consciousness or awareness"), and *ananda* ("infinite bliss") describe our true Self. Two additional qualities are *bhati*, meaning "light," and *priyam*, meaning "love or pleasure." That is why everything in the universe, whose underlying reality is Self, is shining as if with its own inner light, and we are all attracting each other because we are suffused with "loving pleasure" (priyam). Isn't that beautiful?

A problem arises when we don't know or can't accept our inner swadharma of pleasure-seeking or somehow think this propensity is less valuable, less appreciated, or outright sinful. Then we hide behind a mask and begin pretending to be who we are not. This leads to tremendous sorrow. I have met people (many are students) who were not content with their life as homemakers or parents, or are in the retail, tourism, insurance, medical, or beauty industry, for example. They instead wanted to become spiritual teachers overnight (imitating the mystic propensity), start nonprofits with fiery social-transformation agendas (imitating the guardian propensity), or start business ventures, taking a lot of financial risk (imitating the wealth propensity), and naturally it all fell flat. Sooner or later, each of them felt overwhelmed from within, causing great regret and sorrow in the aftermath. Perhaps they could have cultivated their "garden of pleasures" by staying in their old homes raising children with gratitude and poise, holding jobs, drawing salaries, and leading lives with simple pleasures such as PTA bake sales, neighborhood barbeques, and weekend movie marathons. I also have students who have a mystic propensity but are afraid to own it due to fear of rejection from their partner, spouse, parents, or culture or of the loss of worldly identity. I tell them that they can have everything and more, provided they embrace who they are and begin viewing all their relationships with more discerned detachment.

The teacher Krishna says in the Bhagavad Gita: "The wise person must live in accordance with their unique swadharma or inner nature. All beings follow their inner nature. What good can repression do? . . . It is better to do your own duty badly than to perfectly do another's; you are safe from harm when you do what you should be doing. No one should relinquish one's swadharma-based work, even if it is flawed."[2]

No propensity is fixed. We may be born with certain inclinations, even a mix of them, but they may change with time. This is not a sudden process, but gradual and realistic. When we are exposed to a spiritual master with self-knowledge, our inner mystic may start emerging. Dharma must be lived by everyone, not just the guardians (who have the inclination to protect it).

Over this lifetime or several, our inner propensities rotate from pleasure to wealth generation to dharma until, in a critical lifetime, the mystic propensity inspires us to reach the climax of our existence by seeking moksha, the ultimate freedom.

Swadharma in Relationships

As human beings, our authenticity is predicated on us recognizing our inherent value as Self rather than seeking external validation for our false "being-ness" and "doing-ness." Ultimately, only you can approve of you. Your own self-approval through upholding your inner nature makes you more authentic and capable of bringing forth your inner gifts to serve others. As Fred Rogers once said, "One of the greatest gifts you can give anybody is the gift of your honest self." This is dharma. One of my students has this to say about recognizing swadharma in relationship:

> *"I have a well-defined mystic propensity. My husband is a pleasure-seeker. We are poles apart. While earlier I would hide my inner spiritual quest and contend with watching movies every evening after work and on weekends, after learning about swadharma, I began to say no. I also had a private mystic propensity to take care of; I did that with greater enthusiasm by making time for it. Since I clarified my strengths and weaknesses, I stopped bending myself out of shape to be something I'm not! As I accepted who I am more, my partner also accepted me as I am. He had to. Two decades later, we are still together. Even today, my partner and I live in the same house but do completely different things. That's okay; we are better friends than ever now. I had to risk conflict. But what I did not risk losing was my own swadharma."*

Dharma demands that we voice our propensities and values with more clarity—when to give in, collaborate, or sacrifice—and know where to draw the line firmly, not quit on ourselves and our swadharma! The Hindu epic Mahabharata says: "The tiger dies without the forest, and similarly the forest is cut down without the tiger. The tiger should protect the forest, and the forest should defend the tiger."[3]

Therefore, Dharma does not teach sacrificing our swadharma (propensities) or purusharthas (goals) for others. In fact, it is essential to remain true to our relationship with them and only then relate with people.

We are all worthy and deserving of sovereignty in our worldly life. Despite our emotional delusions, instability of mind, and ignorant ego suffocating inside its myriad masks, our true nature is unconditional freedom, oneness, power, light, and grace.

The Importance of Integrity and Letting Go of Masks

Remember, this universe is a divine setup. Separately and collectively, we are each playing different roles to awaken ourselves and each other to the truth of our forgotten nature.

Attachments are attachments—they blind us
and enslave us to our expectations.

We humans often put ourselves in situations that are emotionally, verbally, even physically and sexually dangerous, all for the sake of our relationships, hoping they will fulfill us once and for all. Our enslaved mind endorses us in leading risky lives of lies and deception of ourselves and others, simply to have a relationship at any cost and avoid being alone. We become isolated, egoic islands—each unfulfilled and lacking love. Then we become conceited, fake, non-upright, and often untruthful—obsessed with meeting our needs and our needs alone. We all have something lacking in this state naturally, and only spiritual knowledge can fill those gaps.

Because liberty, not bondage, is your natural state, fortunately, your conscience may question you. You may feel regret: *Oh, how did I land here?* However, once we begin imbibing dharma values and start acting from dharma, things begin changing for the better, even inside the most difficult relationships and challenging life circumstances. We develop new emotional competence to deal with complex issues and make more self-respecting, self-affirming, self-valuing decisions that free us from the bondage-causing delusions of our own mind.

Dharma Is Not Martyrdom
but Profound Self-Acceptance

Upholding dharma values teaches us not to hide and pretend or keep up appearances or a false persona. "Let's be real" is the essential invitation of dharma, especially when it comes to relationships. With dharma, there is always time to come back and take off the clothes of affectation we were wearing. After all, what can be more bondage-creating and more joy-killing than not being who you are?

Our relationships begin improving when we start taking off the ego's masks. To be who you truly are is dharma. Yes, voluntarily, literally peel your personality masks off, one after another.

We all take on masks—of pride, vanity, arrogance, falsehoods, egotism, malice, hard-heartedness, cruelty, feebleness, weakness, martyrdom—because from the time we are born, we are often greeted by sleepwalkers, each flashing an egoic mask or persona. We don't know who we are and what we stand for, so we hide behind our masks in relationships. Before long, we become warped by self-deception and manipulation (non-dharma).

That is why I recommend, for success in relationships, dropping masks first and foremost and beginning from ground zero. Build renewed clarity by adopting and implementing dharma values, explored in previous chapters, from the ground up. In this chapter, let us revisit the important value of arjavam, or "integrity."

Be Straight Like an Arrow in
Following Your Swadharma

The dharma value of arjavam means cultivating consistency in thought, word, and action.[4] It can be summed up as uprightness or straightforwardness. *Be straight as an arrow* in your dealings by paying attention to your thoughts, feelings, and desires because they matter. You matter, and you deserve to spend time exploring your own inner landscape, so your alignment comes from greater self-familiarity and an intentional cultivation of self-alignment.

Adopting the core value of arjavam, or straightforwardness, will make you direct in your communication. As you speak, so you think, and so you feel deep inside you. You won't have suppressed, ignored, or hidden agendas, and you will be open and candid with discerned clarity. There will be a beautiful consistency between your thoughts, words, and actions, keeping your samsara free, with an uncluttered mind, to uphold the value of truth.

Our ego-self can say, "I hate Coca-Cola!" But privately, we may like it. It is better to say, "I like it; I am trying to wean myself off it." We all have an egoic personality, a theatrical actor self, acting out in deceptive ways merely to earn more approval, likes, and admiration. We must make the effort to bridge the gap between our posture and our truth.

When straightforwardness takes priority, our conduct is pleasant, nonviolent, truthful, and assertive versus passive, aggressive, or passive-aggressive. Instead of dropping hints, skirting around issues, or hiding behind the unspoken, we put our spoken and unspoken cards on the table, honestly and openly. This opens the field for sattva and dharma to prevail.

In the beginning, greed, selfishness, excessive and unchecked ambition, and power play stand in the way of our consistency in thought, action, and deed. That is why, without this sattvic value guiding us, humanity often lies to attain material fulfillment: a job, lover, good grade, or illegal permit. However, in the long term, a lack of integrity rocks your samsara with delusions.

Let us not hide and pretend, keep up appearances, or maintain a false persona. Vedic texts remind us that humans are "the only animals on the planet that pretend to be what they are not" and that we can drop masks, first and foremost, by adopting the value of arjavam, or uprightness. Here is one of my students' journeys with adopting the value of arjavam in parenting:

"I get a lot of practice in straightforwardness as a parent, not only in the way I speak to my children, but also in how I uphold my dharma as a mother in the outside world. I used this once when a close relative and authority figure allowed my kids to do something that was not safe and that they should easily have known was against our family rules.

A surge of anger overtook my heart and mind when I heard about what had happened. I sat with that emotion, allowed my anger to wash through me, allowed my mind to fantasize the things I could say to shame and blame this person into submission, and let those angry words wash away too. I was left with the truth that as a mother I could not hide from my duty to protect my children from hazardous risks, and I had to correct this. Later, during the key conversation with this person, my heart was fluttering, my palms were a little sweaty, and fear was coursing through me. Yet I tapped into the courage to press on because I was aligned in my heart, mind, and soul that letting this adharma stand unaddressed was not an option.

I was able to calmly tell them how I felt and explain that I needed this close relative's teamwork and support to keep these children that we all love safe. I noticed a change in this person afterward. I felt a deeper kind of respect from them going forward. This is a person who in the past had taken similar conversations from others very personally and carried them around as wounds. This seemingly sensitive conversation in which I spoke from the heart and owned my power in a straightforward manner strengthened both of us."

Thus, the life of a dharmic person is worry-free, fearless, bold, inwardly esteemed, and therefore inwardly soaring. It comes from a fierce commitment to your own wholeness and truth—never compromising it. It leads to the critical habit of pausing to discern what you really live for, what you value in this moment. Upholding dharma leads to improved self-esteem, personal power, and self-confidence every single time.

Shed Your Unconscious Egoic Barriers to Dharma

One reason we wear masks is conceit. That is why consciously practicing the dharma of non-conceit, called *amaanitvam*, becomes important. This is significant because, otherwise, our own conceit and false pride can get in the way of practicing the dharma of straightforwardness (arjavam). Conceit can also keep us stuck defending roles and responsibilities of a swadharma type that was never ours to begin with. Conceit feeds the ego and prevents awakening. My teacher always said to me, "Shunya, be proud, not vain."

If false pride and self-admiration are present in our ego, they not only conceal our swadharma but prevent us from finding an authoritative source of knowledge. We become unteachable. Our ego refuses to acknowledge it has lessons to learn or homework to do or that it needs to find a worthy teacher. This is the biggest tragedy because without a true teacher guiding us into growing into who we really are deep down, we may never embark on the journey toward embodying swadharma. Thanks to egotism and false pride, we will remain stuck upholding unsuitable roles and wearing multiple masks for others' sakes.

Conceit has additional side effects. In any field of life, be it fiction writing, scientific research, art, or music, when we possess conceit, we cannot tolerate people who are gifted and so cannot benefit from their presence, insights, collaborations, and teachings. That is why in the Vedic tradition, besides cultivating straightforwardness, to be without conceit is a number-one requirement for seekers of sovereignty.

It is worth contemplating the difference between healthy pride and unhealthy pride. Healthy pride arises from upholding dharma. It arises from completing given tasks well, upholding responsibility well, behaving ethically, achieving something worthwhile, and not transgressing boundaries. This yields healthy self-worth and self-confidence. Healthy pride is generated from being a socially valued person. It encourages future behavior that conforms to higher standards of worth or merit. Feelings of pride for meeting or exceeding morally relevant standards (and for inhibiting impulses to behave immorally) may serve important motivational functions, rewarding and reinforcing one's commitment to autonomy, community, and divinity. Morally arisen pride imparts self-worth, self-confidence, and self-esteem.

Healthy, constructive pride—such as taking pride in our work or responsibility—is different from unhealthy pride, which is conceit. Conceit is not related to actual achievements, but an imagined sense of superiority and self-importance and a tendency toward self-admiration. It stems from covering a feeling of basic inadequacy, generating a need to constantly reassure the ego and to desire reassurance from others. The ego often feels ignored and invisible. Excessive self-estimation and self-deference, leading to an expectation of being constantly praised, pandered to emotionally, given importance, or even glorified, is plain conceit.

We must use our higher mind to question the ego. For example, we should ask: Is this complaint realistic or overblown? Is it someone else's fault (say, your significant other's) or your own emotional wounds born of egotism? (Those can only be healed by self-knowledge that reveals the illusions around such so-called wounds.)

The problem with conceit is that to maintain it, one is always comparing oneself to others and wanting to come out above. One turns a blind eye to their own weaknesses and imperfections and is quick to judge and condemn others. It's hard to apologize (How can we accept fault?), hard to compliment anyone (How can we recognize someone else?), hard to accept criticism, and hard to give positive strokes (but we want the strokes ourselves).

I am not talking about people diagnosed as narcissists. Conceit is not always grandiose; it affects humanity universally in subtle ways, perhaps by overly depending on our loved ones to acknowledge us so we can have a good day or else we feel moody, invisible, and hurt. Yes, I am talking about all of us. All humans, estranged from our own totality of Self, suffer from shaky self-esteem deep down, and our covert or overt need for positive strokes, reassurances, validation, and approval arises universally. The ship of esteem sinks the moment we feel ignored, rejected, or not given the importance we think we deserve!

If false pride or conceit remains unchecked, it starts showing up in our behavior. We become artificial, vain, superficial, pretentious, hypocritical, and outright fake. This is called *dambhitvam*. It makes us false. While we are all organically different or special, when we try to portray that we are different via our clothes, postures, facial expressions, or habits—name-dropping, exaggerating professional experiences, or bragging about wealth—it is pretentiousness. It makes us false. This strengthens the estrangement of our ego from its natural state of dharma and takes us even further away from the straightforward path of swadharma.

Dharma Lies in Willfully Cultivating Non-Conceit

If you truly want to be sovereign, stop looking to others to make you happy through praise or approval, and stop trying to fit in shoes that don't belong to you. Embrace your own swadharma, as it is, in a straightforward manner, without false pride or pretention.

For example, I quit trying to be a perfect homemaker a long time ago. While I am sincere and conscientious as a wife, mom, aunt, and daughter-in-law, my obvious tendency toward the mystical swadharma made me accept my so-called shortcomings on the domestic front without defensiveness or offensiveness. It is what it is.

And it is okay to not be perfect. There is no need to excel in all swadharmas at the same time. Once we accept ourselves as we are, we return to authentic ground. We do this by accepting our limitations and not needing to be anything more in this moment. To make our mind a fertile ground, where plants of true dharma can grow into beautiful fruit-giving trees of self-worth and self-respect, we must face our own false pride—a mask covering our egoic limitations. Pierce your dependency-causing illusions with the spear of knowledge. Cultivate genuine self-worth by cultivating knowledge of swadharma within.

When the dharma value of modesty, the opposite of conceit, is our primary motivator, we become self-accepting, self-healing, self-soothing, self-uplifting, and self-comforting beings. We become truly admirable and pleased with how our lives are unfolding, instead of being a burden on this planet, defensive about our shortcomings, sensitive to criticism, afraid of being exposed, and begging to be admired and constantly stroked. When we accept our swadharma, we become an asset for all because we experience more stillness in our heart through the act of spiritual self-acceptance. *I am enough as I am! (Even if I can't bake a perfect apple pie or do laundry on time!)* We can consciously choose to make our ego prideless or humble and realistic through honest self-assessment and by valuing of "non-pride."

This is how we cultivate humility, amaanitvam, "freedom from self-conceit." Once we accept ourselves as we are, we return to the authentic ground of swadharma. This return to "pride ground zero" is a relief for true seekers of harmonious relationships and self-knowledge.

Unpretentiousness, genuineness, authenticity, and ingeniousness are traits that describe the value of non-pride. Let us be content with who we are, what we know, what we don't know, what we feel excited about, and what turns us off. This is the path to embodying authenticity through swadharma.

Be Who You Are

Another way to avoid the external expression of conceit and pretentiousness and follow our swadharma with ease is by adopting the core value of naturalness known as *adambhitvam.*

Nature is simple. It is nonpretentious. A daffodil plant is not trying to grow roses; an apple tree is not trying to grow a mango. Each blade of grass is content being its authentic grass-self, shining with inner simplicity. Swadharma aligns with authenticity, not hypocrisy.

The dharma of simplicity does not mean austerity in lifestyle, severity in dress, or bluntness in behavior. It simply means refusing to be superficial, coming back to who you are deep inside you, again and again . . . being your soulful, heartful, mindful natural Self. It means speaking and living your humble truth. It means not letting your outer appearances sabotage your swadharma. The value of simplicity is a strong support for being spiritually straightforward (arjavam).

Value of Truth for Final Freedom

Truthfulness is your true inner nature. When we live a lie or speak deliberate lies, we know it deep inside us, even if we are never caught. When we follow a life path that is against our swadharma, we judge ourselves as a person who cannot do what they must do to uphold truth, and we dislike ourselves, deep down, even if we publicly profess otherwise. We become internally split, and then tranquility of mind is impossible. Lying to ourselves and others creates deep inner psychological conflict. We know when we lie, and we don't like it, even if we outwardly defend our lying.

There is nothing like falsehood to activate a delusory non-tranquil samsara python. Speak your truth in all your relationships and walk away free. Embracing truth is really an invitation to disarm your egoic personality from the armor of false pride and pretentiousness. Truth reflects your innocence and soul purity. Truth is your true nature. There is no getting away from your love of truth, since every cell of your being instinctively values and thrives on it. No wonder you demand truth from your lovers, children, politicians, and friends. Consequently, if you want to be tranquil and at one with your sovereign truth, start expressing your truth gently, pleasantly, but consistently, and enjoy your inner garden of freedom.

For the sake of your higher truth, you must deliberately unsettle what you have settled into for the sake of the world or your worldly relationships, be it a role, a script, an image, or even a career path. Actively dismantle expectations; make sure your life is not all about meeting other people's expectations. Regain your right to determine your own swadharma, not to hurt others, but so you are always in alignment with the highest dharma and not the falsehoods you have come to identify with over the course of time.

As for people who attempt to hold you down in a fixed role for the sake of their insecure samsara, ignore them; forgive their ignorance in maya.

Integrity: The Best Antidote to Spiritual Bypassing

Embodying dharmic values like straightforwardness, non-conceit, non-pretentiousness, truth, and simplicity have one more benefit. They collectively prevent spiritual bypassing.

As an ordained *acharya* ("spiritual preceptor") of my lineage, I try to model the path of non-pretentious, real-life spiritual teachings in here-and-now circumstances. I do not try to prove my holiness, but rather embrace my inherent, undeniable inner battles with my own darkness too. I talk about my own relationship struggles openly and my not-so-perfect past, when I struggled with demons in my samsara. That is why, though I graduated from my spiritual studies with my guru Baba at age twenty-four, I took the time it took and did not take on my first spiritual student until age forty.

What was I doing up till then? I was certainly not leading people on journeys I myself had barely started. I was honestly employing the wisdom I learned from my teacher in my real-life laboratory of relationships, discerning and detaching, and trying to explore what it feels like to be in my swadharma, to embody arjavam. I was learning to hold on to something authentic inside me even when the price I would pay would be great.

When I could come clear of my own samsara cobwebs—and stay clear—I knew I was ready to be a teacher, not one day sooner.

You, too, can awaken to your innate propensity and
inner flow without ever needing to pretend to be who
you are not! Embrace your swadharma!

20

◈◈◈◈◈◈◈◈◈◈◈◈

Atmashakti: Bringing Soul Power to Relationships

"Never do that to another which you regard as injurious to your own self. This, in brief, is the rule of dharma. Yielding to impulse and acting from ego, one becomes guilty of adharma."

MAHABHARATA. 18.113.8

In a village in ancient India lived a snake that was a bit bad-tempered. He would bite for no reason. Once, a saint was passing by and gave some discourses. The snake's mind was highly moved, so he decided to change his nature and not bite people anymore. He decided to practice unconditional ahmisa, nonviolence.

The next time the saint went by the same village, he found the snake in a precarious physical condition; small children had thrown stones at him, and people and even other animals, like the monkeys, had trampled all over him.

"What happened to you?" the saint asked the snake.

"After your discourse, I decided to not bite anyone," replied the snake.

"That's nice that you've decided to stop biting people for no reason, but did I tell you to stop hissing and keeping others from biting you? Why did you choose to become so powerless that you could not even defend yourself?" the saint questioned.

This story beautifully illustrates how we must have our personal power in place, always. That is how we can assert healthy boundaries in relationships; we do not to have be offensive, but we can have boundaries in self-defense against the sleepwalkers whom we are bound to meet sooner or later.

To live in accordance with our unique nature, we need personal power. We must develop familiarity with our power, learn to live from our power, and ultimately act from this power. It is ours, and we must accept it and embrace it. That is why I call true power *atmashakti*, which is a word derived from two Sanskrit words: "atma" ("self") and "shakti" ("power").

The snake who forgot to hiss in self-defense forgot his atmashakti in trying to be overly "nice." But atmashakti is beyond good and bad. It is our unquestionable power of Self to lead our life with physical and emotional safety, to act as sovereign of our inner realm.

Every violation of our personal boundary is asking us to clarify our relationship with our own personal power. If you are aware of your atmashakti, then people around you will sense your power too and automatically come to respect your boundaries. They will stop seeing you as less important than themselves, disrespecting you, or threatening you.

Soul power, or atmashakti, is like that. It is invisible, but it can be sensed from miles away. When you see a lightning storm, do you dare go into it? No. You admire it from a distance. In the same way, when you are established in your atmashakti, people will sense that you have power. You don't have to be angry or loud or hold up your fist. You could be relaxed and silent, and still be the most powerful person in the room.

Atmashakti makes you powerful whether you have a college degree or not, the right career or not, a lover, partner, or spouse or not! I ask you to act powerfully whether you are young and strong or now dealing with wrinkles and disease by becoming familiar with atmashakti.

You can use your advanced mind to draw upon its great spiritual strength, knowledge, skills, and creativity. And you can wield this power in ethical ways, not biting others, but still able to hiss in self-defense.

Atmashakti Is Always a Dharmic Power

When our ego is sleepwalking in rajas and tamas, it births an unconscious egoic power that can hurt others and make you suffer the consequences. This is *ahamshakti* ("aham" means "ego").

But when the same ego is awake to its true nature, colored by sattva and anchored in dharma, it gives expression to atmashakti, a blessed power that the purified ego channels from the Self. Atmashakti invariably protects you and uplifts others. *You always have a choice.*

Upward-rising
Atmashakti
(Soul Power)

Downward-dragging
Ahamshakti
(Ego Power)

	ATMASHAKTI	AHAMSHAKTI
Whole vs. Part	Soul power is always whole and enables an expansive perspective of what's possible.	Non-dharmic egoic-power is self-deceptive and limited in conceiving options.
Abundance vs. Scarcity	Soul power supports the mind to first seek out mindfulness (dharma) and freedom (moksha) and does not neglect material acquisition (artha) and pleasures and enjoyment (kama) either. It is a balanced quest.	Egoic power supports a mind focused excessively on money and pleasures while neglecting higher ideals (dharma) and even becomes enslaved by not valuing spiritual goals (moksha). This is an unbalanced and self-destructive quest.
Known vs. Confirmed	Soul power is known from inner eyes.	Egoic power needs outer confirmation/approval to be activated.
Strong vs. Weak	Soul power will ensure you stand your ground with firmness and equanimity even if challenged; will still feel internally validated; knows when and how to find help and asks for it.	Egoic power breaks down; mind falls apart or ensures a stress-attack when challenged; will try to be a perfectionist and not ask for help.
Original vs. Copied	Soul power is original, inspired from the infinitely creative limitless Self; it enables writing one's own script, creative solutions, inspirations and imagination.	Ego uses its power to imitate; follows scripts given by others; stays stuck.
Infinite vs. Limited	Soul power in the mind is infinite. It keeps increasing despite responsibilities and challenges, due to positive, constructive, win-win thoughts.	Egoic power cannot meet challenges with ease; enables limiting thoughts in the mind that shame and blame self-and/or others.

Figure 20.1: Ego Power vs. Soul Power

	ATMASHAKTI	AHAMSHAKTI
Flexible vs. Rigid	Soul power makes the mind flexible—not trying to prove a point. A person driven by Soul power may win or lose; asks for help when needed; admits mistakes when made without guilt or shame for self and others; takes charge, not control; is willing to consider others' needs and values.	A mind fueled by egoic power chooses rigid standards that punish self and others; takes control, not charge; ignores others' needs and imposes their own needs.
Accommodative vs. Punitive	Soul power accommodates ignorance of others; sees sin, not sinner; allows personal and others' learning curves and mistakes with sense of dignity. This power includes compassion.	Ego connects power with punitive ability, remains judgmental and critical, condemns own self for silliest of mistakes. There is no redemption or room to make mistakes.
Sharing vs. Hoarding	A person with Soul power shares knowledge, money, decision-making.	Ego hoards power, knowledge, money, decision-making power.
Expressed vs. Suppressed	Soul power enables speaking up in the face of injustice, can give a clear yes or no, enjoys healthy boundaries.	Egoic power makes the mind vulnerable to injustice; is easily bullied, agitated, disturbed, or enslaved by others; remains mute in face of fear or injustice or overreacts. Unable to say no or honor yes; gives unclear responses.
Surrendered vs. Controlling	A Self-driven ego surrenders outcomes to a higher power, trusts universal intelligence beyond personal ego, lives more and more in the now, feels tranquil, turns inward to find God as parent and friend.	The default ego uses its power to control outcomes; can't let go, trust, or relax; fluctuates between past regrets and future worry; feels stressed out; experiences existential aloneness and orphaning.
Straightforward vs. Manipulative	Soul power enables one to speak the truth fearlessly; expresses vulnerability. No compulsion to be or become anything—will blossom into what feels natural and organic.	Truth is hard when all one has is ego power. One expresses defensiveness; compulsion to be or become someone or something that feels unnatural and forced.
Flowing Love vs. Flowing Fear	A person in touch with Soul power enjoys inner contentment and peace; experiences gratitude; silently emanates acceptance, peace, gratitude, and love. The positive Soul power makes one's life beautiful and in sync with the inner Self.	An ego-driven person attracts mental negativity; experiences lots of emotional challenges; finds people to be hurtful and bothersome; experiences mostly fear, anger, even rage; silently emanates hatred and resentment. The power is completely negative.

Figure 20.1: Ego Power vs. Soul Power *(continued)*

Atmashakti Powers Dharmic Relationships

True power emerges from within us when we sincerely try to live ethically. Dharma ethics teach us how to value all beings and creatures, even inanimate plants and mountains, but not before first valuing ourselves as embodied spirits. Therefore, soul power is first and foremost about self-respect and self-value.

Offering your blind respect or allegiance to the undeserving just because they enjoy a prestigious position in society, have a lot of money, or are older than you is not dharma. This is what the ego does. People with soul power bow only to those who earn their respect. Power is not higher than dharma. In fact, dharma qualifies what kind of power you possess—soulful or egoic.

Vedic wisdom is practical; it offers realistic versus sentimental or absolute spiritual teachings. It does not make sweeping statements like "Love everyone, even if they are non-dharmic!" The Vedas recognize that we are both body and spirit, and while our Self is one with all beings, our body and mind must dwell in a world where goodness and evil coexist. Dharma lies in making the correct choice between the two. That is why soul power is always accompanied by a discerning mind.

In the Bhagavad Gita, Krishna instructs Arjuna that he must not quit an imminent battle simply because he cannot bear to see his grandfather and teacher killed. They deserve no special handling, even if older and beloved by him, since for whatever reason they chose to support a despotic contender to the throne. The choices they made despite being presented with facts make them liable to face the consequences.

Upholding dharma through exercising your soul power will not erase sorrow or transform the egoic personalities you are challenged by overnight. But it does lead to a profound inner resolution to live consciously, from here onward. The relationship challenges will feel lighter. With knowledge of greater spiritual remembrance, the issues won't bleed in our hearts or make us unconscious.

A happy ending is not always possible. But dharma is always possible.

When dharma informs our mind, we take responsibility. Instead of shaming ourselves relentlessly, we make positive changes by putting our soul power toward constructive inner growth and cultivating emotional resilience. We accept where we must change and accept what we cannot change. Using our higher mind and its faculties of discernment and detachment, we know what to do, and when. Instead of blaming others, we attempt to understand that people are born with different strengths and challenges, and everyone is struggling in maya, the spell that makes us ignorant of spiritual reality. Even if we must fire someone, break up with another, or even punish or admonish others, we can do this from soul power, with honesty, respect, and integrity. You may win a person's cooperation, or you may lose that person, but either way, when you act from soul power, not the ego's shenanigans, you will gain your own self-approval every time.

I cannot promise you will win another person's attention, affection, respect, or love in all your relationships. But I can promise that with dharma by your side and by acting from soul power (never egoic power), you won't lose your own self-respect.

Dharma gives us an option to have higher personal standards. That is why when you are operating from soul power, you will not compromise your standards simply for the sake of holding on to a relationship. You will no longer choose another over yourself and simply throw yourself away. At the same time, you will not selfishly cherish only yourself and walk all over the feelings of another in indifferent disdain.

Dharma demands you slow down and become conscious of how you use your power. It asks you find deeper, win-win solutions rather than superficial ones, categorizing people into who is powerful and who is powerless, who started it, and who is whose victim. When a greater truth of Self is known, the ego loses power. The power equations fall away, exposing our inherent soul equality, vulnerability, and spiritual potential. We relate to the cord of our shared humanity and our common godly Self, which is the source of our collective spiritual power.

Establish Soul Power–Based Boundaries

Any kind of relationship violation—physical, sexual, emotional, or verbal—is teaching us that we need better emotional boundaries, known as *maryada*. Boundaries are about personal power—the need to revamp it, reassert it, or revoke it. Most of us assert egoic power. Then, the upkeep of boundaries takes work. They can cause emotional strain. However, when we assert boundaries with soul power, the hard work can become soft work.

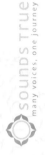

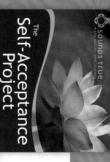
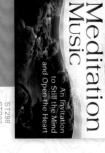

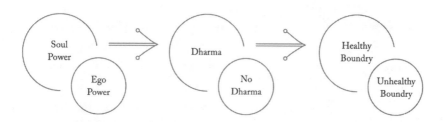

Figure 20.2: Always Choose Dharma

Egoic power can never give us a healthy boundary. Having a soulful bound-ary in place means you know what your reality is (Who are you: Self or ego?) and what your values are. It means you will consistently uphold your dharma, even in the face of other people denying your right to be you or questioning your choices.

Either unite with another in dharma or separate from another in dharma. Don't simply act and react from an out-of-control ego. Boundaries should not make us belligerent, bitter, hypersensitive people ready to fly off the handle if someone so much as approaches us. They should simply make us alert so we become aware of our own atmashakti. And when we are aware of our own soul power, then others who are challenging our boundaries somehow sense it too. But if we are unaware, then there are good chances that we can scream and shout in self-defense, and yet our boundaries will be encroached.

Egoic pleasing, begging, entreating, yelling, screaming, threatening, or any such iteration of ego will only lead to loss of true power. Eschew such uncon-scious behaviors like the plague. Watch your mind and choose dharma thoughts over self-shaming and other-blaming thoughts. Establish new healthy bound-aries, outer and inner, aligned this way through dharmic vigilance. Leave or stay in a relationship with awareness of right from wrong, rather than leaving or staying while defending positions of your separate, battling egos.

Boundaries are beautiful in that they allow us to truly own who we are, including our dharma-driven soul power, and accept who others are without trying to change them in any way (or unnecessarily making them powerless to feel powerful).

Slowly, with soul power and dharma by your side, you can become quietly pleased with yourself. You will realize that for successful relationships you don't need to please, pacify, or pimp your egoic power. You can simply be yourself, self-possessed and within your own self-defined boundaries, enjoying your atmashakti . . . as you are, possessing compassion for your learning self and sincerely trying your best to live by soul power, peacefully, gratefully, and joyfully. You accept you are not perfect this very moment (who is?), but at least you are experimenting with beautiful, dharma-aligned soul power in your imperfect samsara! Isn't that something worth patting yourself on the back for?

The Power Talk vs. the Power Walk

When should you stop talking from power and start acting from soul power instead? What if you uphold dharma and speak your truth to negotiate your core needs, but the person you are in a relationship with simply doesn't want to hear you? Or rejects you in some other way?

If they just don't want to hear you, then you must no longer communicate your truth. You must act on your truth, with all your soul power backing your truth. And to do that, you must gauge whether you have sufficiently contemplated upon your core values or not. And, ask yourself: *Do I have enough courage to express them? Do I have enough conviction not to drop them? Do I have enough soul power to make them a priority?*

> *Perhaps your difficult relationships are asking you to explore*
> *and live the truest and highest version of who you are.*
> *Never let the cost of intimacy be self-betrayal.*

Refuse to take on any shame that may be shoved toward you by any sleep-walker. Remind yourself: "I am spiritually shameless."

Because of your own clarity about your core values—for example, *I will live and speak truth, and I won't let anyone's poor behavior rob me of my right to align with truth*—any rejection based on your values will be a minor event in your life, rather than a major event.

You can go beyond dire scenarios in relationships, where we are victims of a bad world made of bad people, or we're bad, and everyone else is good. These are delusions that will no longer blind you or trap you in an egoic power wrestle. You may find that your atmashakti is even more strengthened by rejection—your truth shall set you free. You may become even more tranquil and powerful in the face of challenges. All darkness leads to light, especially when we use Vedic knowledge as our matchstick. You will be guided from within.

You can stop any conditioned or scripted pleasing behaviors by repeatedly reminding yourself that all beings deserve more from you than false niceness. They deserve dharma and truth, soulfully owned and assertively lived with atmashakti—even if it means walking away with your head held high.

When your partner is operating from egoic power, you can change the stakes by choosing soul power that is inherently connected to dharma and moksha. Simply refuse to play delusory power games. The one who explores *dharmic soul power* in relationships listens to the voice of the spirit within and thereby has no more accidents, passivity, manipulations, or power games. Many people will not understand you, but that is not a reflection on you.

Often, we respond with pleasing behavior, yet the more we please, the more we are rejected. That is how egoic power works. The one being pleased becomes pumped with false power. This may make them even more distant. The one who pleases loses power, as the very act of pleasing goes against the soul's nature. What can we do?

Being steadfast in one's own inner truth of Self will set you free from the need for external validation. Don't waste time ensuring others "get" you! Simply ensure that *you* get you and move forward with inner freedom and soul power intact.

Upholding Dharma in Relationships

Relationships by their very nature are ever changing; this is to be expected. Living beings give us pleasure and sorrow. If we rub each other the wrong way, it will only lead to unhappiness. Instead, we should understand what to fight for and where we should become accommodating—this discernment itself is upholding dharma.

Dharma dictates that we all deserve respectful, honoring relationships; for that, we must be ready for compromise and non-compromise, giving and receiving, sacrificing and withholding as guided by moment-to-moment discernment but not a maya-born ego script like "I am a giving person, and I give to the deserving and un-deserving both!"

At times we may need to respectfully draw lines between right and wrong, discern whether we are giving away too much of ourselves or too little, or ponder upon what our dharma is toward others and what our dharma is toward our self. Will we walk away, stay and work on it some more, or file for divorce? We must listen to our legitimate anger and other dark emotions. They convey a wealth of information.

Lending your power to rajasic and tamasic characters is not dharma; it is false compassion that arises from lack of discernment. Instead, reinforce your ethical boundaries and proactively affirm your new dharma lifestyle with expectation of reciprocity. Direct your compassion and flow of soul power toward *deserving* beings. Openly accept and celebrate yourself in the face of rejecters and detractors.

Demonstrate through actions that you are willing to watch out for egoic power. Prioritize maintaining your samsara hygiene.

Sadly, sleepwalking individuals who do not proactively embody dharma and atmashakti are bound to fail each other sooner or later. Therefore, do not control what relationships look like externally—simply ensure you are aligned with your dharmic values and soul power (they always go together).

Making one dharmic choice after another is what began my transformation into who I am today—no longer a resistant, angry, or guilty person, but one at peace with her life, enjoying her atmashakti.

Today, I can stay spiritually awake for all of us. I can be with other sleepwalking egos without my ego falling back asleep. We can, if we wish, be supremely self-disciplined in the use of power, prioritizing our sovereignty through emotional maturity and spiritual awakening.

Guided Practice: Soul-Powered Thoughts for the End of a Relationship

If a relationship is causing us suffering of body or mind, it is often a message to wake up, spiritually speaking. When dealing with a relationship crisis, either believe in a power outside you or believe in a power inside you.

Believing in power inside means believing in your infinite potential, freedom, and fullness. This is how you became truly, soulfully powerful—worry-free, and joyful, despite any rejection. You can establish yourself in your soul power by making new inner agreements that support dharmic boundaries in relationships, beyond samsara attachments. Try surrendering to your inner source of power, the Self, and see what happens next.

I am enough unto myself because power lies inside me. Even if my most precious relationship ends, it will not diminish my power, by even one-millionth of a percent.

Let me not search for power outside of myself in relationships. Let me henceforth relate from soul power, rather than seek it from others. No one can take anything from me in any real sense. I am forever powerful. Power is my true nature.

I am enough unto myself because the love I seek to experience is not merely contained inside you (or anyone else).

We often become powerless when it comes to love. But contemplate on this: love is everywhere, in every particle of this universe, in every heart. It is a matter of perception. When I perceive this infinite, ever-present, pure love as my own true nature and in every being, it reveals itself everywhere. I experience it inside me, for me. This self-love makes me even more powerful, in an abiding sense.

I am enough unto myself because I am already the love I seek. Knowing that I do not need anyone to complete, approve, or even love me, I do not need to depend emotionally upon _____ (name the person) to be who I am in all my fullness.

Because I do not seek love, fulfillment, or approval outside of myself in relationships, I can be radically powerful, honest, and authentic in all my communications in all my relationships. I can role-model dharmic authenticity.

I am enough unto myself; therefore, I am consciously letting go of seeking love, approval, or support outside of myself so I can now focus on discovering it inside. It never lay outside me anyway.

I love you, but I don't need you.

I love your company. But if you leave, I will enjoy mine.

Your judgments of me are entirely your own. They don't destabilize my inner knowingness of my truth.

Thank you, but I don't want the burden of having to complete, fulfill, or love you. You can complete, fulfill, and love you. I don't need you to complete me either. I am complete without you. I am the sovereign Self.

I don't need to project anything different for you than what or who I am right now, in this moment.

I am ready to take off my mask first to spark the truth that dwells behind the mask of others too. My rawness in who I am, as I am, is sheer power sourced from my naked Self.

When I start pleasing and rejecting, essentially manipulating others to seek love, attention, approval, power, or respect, I become bound or enslaved and made powerless by what I seek. By stopping this incessant, mindless, all-consuming seeking and manipulating, begging, and cajoling (conscious or unconscious), I set myself free. I simply like to be me in relationships and welcome others also to be themselves, rather than versions of themselves that please, seduce, or reassure me. This is my ode to my Self. This freedom is an expression of my soul power.

Despite the differences between us, let us find a place where can meet beyond the story (at a soul level).

True love is all that remains when our egoic power games, seeking, grabbing, possessing, and manipulating behaviors subside.

When I wait for _____ (name the person) to complete, love, and make me whole, I begin leading a hand-me-down, powerless life.

I no longer beg, plead, threaten, manipulate, fight, or numb myself with addictions for crumbs of love, attention, and approval.

I am the cake. I am enjoying my own sweetness.

Your relationships can be renewed by your own radical self-acceptance and willingness to embody true dharmic soul power, self-respect, and divine love. Your self- and other-honoring process will impact others too at some level since we are all connected, and differences, distances, and separation are a mirage. Others will begin viewing you with new eyes and wonder if they, too, should change something.

Let Go of Shame and Sin Mentality

If right now you have a dark samsara, crawling with egoic power that binds you, often making you irrational and non-dharmic, and suffocating you with a loss of freedom, it is not personal. None of this is anyone's fault. Maya, which casts a hypnotic spell on our minds, strikes universally and almost "bewitches" our minds. It is a setup, and we must not get caught up in power games.

You can feel remorse and desire to break free from old patterns, but do not feel shame or think you are a sinner if you have hurt someone else through use of non-dharmic ego power (emotional or physical violence) or got hurt yourself. *You did not know what you did not know.* It was simply a case of spiritual self-ignorance, not evilness. Besides, the Vedas say this: You can never be a sinner. You are simply a student of life. You are a divine being who has temporarily forgotten your power. That is why an ancient text says: "Bright is the Self, indivisible, untouched by sin, wise, immanent, and transcendent."[1]

In great compassion, the teacher Krishna says this in the Bhagavad Gita: "Even if you are the most sinful of all sinners, you shall cross over all sins accumulated in your samsara by the raft of self-knowledge."[2]

Yes, in the Vedic universe, there is no sinner, no sin, so no reason for shame … only ignorance of who we are and how to act and react from learned and practiced wisdom. Bewilderment, agitation, and sorrow are our ego's lot. Hence, as I continue to say, relax, and continue to proactively seek self-knowledge, which includes the knowledge of wielding atmashakti versus ahamshakti.

After checking that you are aligned with your soul's—not your ego's—mandate, you will powerfully express your true voice, your deepest values, and soul desires. You will express your core beliefs fearlessly as Self and make your spiritual evolution, truth, and freedom your priority, even as you conduct your worldly roles with dharmic power and self-assurance. The world will not be able to shame you, nor will you need to blame the world. Understanding and acting from soul power versus egoic power is a kind of liberation.

21

◆≫≫≫◆◆≪≪≪◆

Vaaktapas: Employing Ancient
Communication Protocols

*"Nonviolent speech, which is truthful, pleasant, and beneficial, and used to
utter the Vedic truth, is called austerity of speech."*

BHAGAVAD GITA, 17.15

Five thousand years ago, in the Bhagavad Gita, Lord Krishna gave humanity its
first lesson in conscious communication known as *vaaktapas*. The Sanskrit word
vaak means "speech" or "communication," and *tapas* means "discipline" taken on
voluntarily.

Lord Krishna said let us all embody:

nonviolent speech (*anudvega karam vaak*)

truthful speech (*satyam vaak*)

pleasant speech (*priyam vaak*)

beneficial speech (*hitam vaak*)

All four points work together to describe dharmic communication, which is
assertive and clear, but also compassionate, constructive, and truthful.

Embody Nonviolent Speech

Violence emerges in our speech when we feel powerless, helpless, and separate.
We lash out to regain some sense of power. Underlying our violent speech is an

illusion of nonfulfillment or a vasana to control a personal loss and an attempt to temporarily reclaim egoic power. The ego's illusions are fueled by self-ignorance. Violent speech belongs to an ego that believes it can author life as it wants, control outcomes, and even inflict violence and not feel the pain (or burn) itself. This is the ultimate spiritual illusion of separateness, when the truth is that all beings share the radical One Self, despite separate bodies.

Make it your conscious discipline to communicate with constructive, compassionate, and never hurtful speech, even when offering a critique or registering a legitimate complaint. We think that demanding, intimidating, threatening, accusing, criticizing, reproaching, sarcasm, put-downs, making others invisible, labeling, judging, mocking, shaming, blaming, comparing speech with accompanying facial expressions, expletives, and even physical aggression like slamming fists, is justified at times and that it makes us more authoritative. But it does not. It hurts and wounds hearts. It puts us in bondage of our own shortsightedness. Pay attention to your content, pitch, and tone and offer the same conscious speech to friends and foes alike.

Embody Truth in Your Speech

Once you dare to bring the value of truth (satyam) into your speech, you won't unfairly insult, judge, blame, and least of all shame others with your speech. Likewise, when you value truth, will you conceal your real feelings and emotions and disown them? Will you paste a smile on your face and say, "I'm okay" when you are not okay? Speaking truth is a reward unto itself. It is the basis of dharma in relationships.

So, go back to who you were as a child, a truth teller, a truth celebrator, a truthful expression of Self. Express your observations, needs, desires, requests, opinions, and boundaries truthfully. You can ask yourself these questions:

Are my words emerging from my ego?

Is my false speech engaging and abetting false speech in others?

Or, is my speech emerging from a deeper place of vulnerability and openness within me, where lies my truth, my wholeness, my entirety . . . where I faintly recollect our shared inner Self?

Reminding ourselves that it is only One Self staring at us from different pairs of eyes can amplify the truth within us. How can we lie, cheat, and deceive our own Self in different bodies with our words, and for how long, without getting caught up in samsara delusions?

Let us make our speech deliberately truthful. We can begin our spiritual journey with our speech. Is there a difference between a white lie and a black lie? So-called white lies only strengthen the ego's illusion of powerlessness and need to manipulate to get ahead with vasana fulfillment. Truth in speech strengthens, protects, and illumines us from within. In my opinion, truly nonviolent speech is truthful speech. There can be no greater violence than infecting other humans' samsara with our delusory lies and false promises. Silence is better than lying. If it is not safe or if it's inconvenient to speak the truth, simply say, "I do not have a comment at this time."

Dharma is not asking you to embody higher consciousness only for the benefit of others. First and foremost, consciousness helps *you*. Thanks to consciousness, I don't give up or stop making an effort, until I and those I am closely engaged with in domestic or professional situations (my partner, son, students, and so forth) are on the same page. I don't stop till I feel content that I have communicated my *whole truth*, not merely a part of it, and did not conceal, mask, or repackage it as something else, simply to make them feel better; nor hid behind my own false beliefs that tell me I don't deserve to be heard.

Let us also make our speech deliberately dharmic. To do that, let's avoid egoic haste in speaking. Buy time. Say, "I will get back to you when I know what I need to know from within me first; let me think it over!" The Vedic tradition recommends mindful silence over mindless lying.

Besides, speaking lies to deliberately misrepresent is not a natural state of the Self. It is a learned behavior of our poor struggling ego, a false coping mechanism in the absence of right knowledge of dharma. Deep down, innocence, truth, fairness, goodness, and compassion are our true dharmic nature. Truth in our speech is an expression of our true being, and that is why when you try to be more genuine in your speech, you will feel good, confident, and aligned deep inside yourself. When you start upholding truth in your life, you will more easily see through anyone wearing a mask of deception and lies.

I have found that when I use dharmic speech protocols, somehow my truth, even if stark or intense, becomes more palatable, and people thank me for sharing.

They feel empowered with the way I own my reality and express it gently but firmly through my choices of deliberate thoughts and words, no matter what the consequences.

Therefore, make dharmic communication your prime value in relationships. Convey what you are thinking and feeling rather than what you think your significant others want to hear. This is upholding the value of arjavam. Soon others will begin respecting you, as truth is always aligned with soul power. Truth will set you free to create and recreate your life, as you wish.

Embody Pleasantness in Your Speech

Baba said we should speak as though every word is being recorded and echoed throughout lifetimes. What do you want your soul recording to sound like? If you find your tone is shrill or aggressive, understand and readjust to what you wish to communicate from your heart—the voice inspired by your true Self is always pleasant. We can examine the tone of our voice, the underlying attitude, volume, and pitch each time we speak. Can we make eye contact that is reassuring and reaffirming of our common spirit truth (Atman)? Can we choose to take a deep breath before speaking, if necessary, and bring intentionality into our speech?

After all, the word for pleasant communication is "priyam," meaning "that which is happiness-imparting, pleasant, or dear to the heart." Can our communication be such that it supports heart-to-heart connection and makes us gladly conscious, both when speaking and hearing such communication? Even if we agree to disagree, can each person walk away fortified emotionally by the communication versus misunderstood or wounded? Perhaps when we bring in our vulnerability, honesty, empathy, care, compassion, and even some mutual fun and humor, thanks to our shared human experience, our communication will become more heartfelt.

These aspects of speech are connected to the aspects of truth and nonviolence. If truth is conveyed nonviolently, it must be pleasant or agreeable because this communication fosters greater connection between the two communicating egos. Here are six suggestions to embody pleasantness of speech that I teach my students:

Breathe evenly. Throughout communication, check to see that you are not breathing rapidly or have not stopped breathing altogether due to gathering inner tension. You can even place your hand on your belly to observe if it is gently undulating or not. (Practice deep belly breathing versus shallow lung breathing). At the least, take a breath at the end of every sentence. In the Vedas, breath and mind are deeply connected. The more slowly you breathe, the calmer your mind becomes. Breath is also prana, or "life-force." When you keep breathing, your mind is filled with prana. Breathing allows you to conduct a much more positive and pleasant communication even if you must convey hard things, like laying someone off or breaking up.

Speak calmly. Raised voices signify challenge or conflict. They invariably negatively affect the listener's ego since they stimulate the button of emotional danger. Keep your voice calm or serene (but firm). Breathing slowly and easily will help you modulate your voice and keep it soft. Remain conscious of your facial expression and hand gestures. Above all, gift calmness by listening patiently. Identify with the struggles and pain of the other person too, who is another struggling human like you. In other words, listen with empathy.

Speak unhurriedly. Pace yourself. Speak slowly. Avoid run-on sentences. The gap between words is important. It can convey something deeper—your inner silence, soul presence, and caring facial expression.

Be concise. Long sentences encourage your mind to drift and lose focus. They also cause your communication to lose power. So choose shorter statements. Importantly, balance your speaking time with hearing time—otherwise you lose connection with the listener and your runaway speech sabotages the very purpose of your communication.

Pause often. Vedic communication is not just about the art of speaking but the art of listening. Pauses also allow you to remain conscious and allow others to process what you have said. Pause to check in with your higher Self and stay close to the end goal of communication.

Lock eyes. It is important to look at the person you are communicating with. Then use your eyes to convey unspoken emotions like understanding, empathy, respect, interest, curiosity, appreciation, support, sympathy, and emotional safety through the communication that makes all humans equally vulnerable, whether they say so or not.

The greatest leaders of Planet Earth—Gandhi, Mandela, Martin Luther King Jr., César Chávez, John Lennon, the Dalai Lama, Bob Marley, Henry David Thoreau—have delivered truth, hard and real, cutting through the dense ignorance of billions of humans; yet, it was a pleasant experience for the speaker and a memorable one for the listeners.

No one knows for sure the origin of these words, but they fit beautifully:

Before you speak, let your words pass through three gates:

At the first gate, ask yourself, "Is it true?"

At the second gate ask, "Is it necessary?"

At the third gate ask, "Is it kind?"[1]

Embody Beneficial Compassion in Your Speech

An awareness of the intention behind our speech is also important. Is it coming from ego or soul? Insensitivity or compassion? We should not speak just for the sake of speaking. Along with making it nonviolent, truthful, and pleasant sounding, let us also look at our speech's impact on the listener.

Ultimately, what is the agenda of my communication? Is this mere venting of my unfulfilled desires? Do I think this communication will help both the listener and the speaker? Or is my speech merely satisfying my desire to run my mouth? What is the hidden intention behind the speech—ego aggrandizement, venting, lamenting, self-pitying, gossiping, judging, flattery, dominance, control? Is my speech truly aligned with my deepest spiritual intention and the furthering of understanding and dharma (win-win, ethical harmony)?

When you begin discerning the impact of your truthful speech on others, beneficial or not, you are telling your ego that it is not the sole player, that it is a team player. That is why, even if you have all the wisdom, insights, and suggestions in the world, do not offer them, unless you are asked or invited. It is important that your partner is ready to receive what you have to offer. Perhaps for a change, your peaceful silence will be more beneficial to that person than your words. You must be willing to accept that and discern, case by case.

This dharmic self-restraint will go a long way in facilitating effective communication in relationships.

My student Elliott R. writes:

"As I settle down and focus on the four qualities of speech, I see that the other person and I both emanate from the same source (Self). Impatience fades, and we are in a field of mutuality. I listen to and appreciate what the other is offering and what they must say. I let go of my 'agenda' and am not urgent to move on or to accomplish a result. I communicate clearly and directly and am in the present. The exchange is peaceful, truthful, pleasant, and mutually beneficial. With speech discipline, communication becomes communion. The four qualities pave the way for community to blossom—from the inside out."

Keep flowing your deeper awareness of your true Self versus your ego in speech. To do this, you must remember that your current personality with its speech pattern involves two parts: one is your identity, the Self, and the other is your egoic identity. You are a cosmic actor obliged to act on a virtual stage. From now on, why not speak the lines from your true Self and let go of costumes, makeup, and the shadow didactics of the changing, suffering ego?

Positive Speech Begets Positive Experiences

I often remind my students that each thought they allow to dwell in their mind has consequences; thought by thought, they create their own destiny.

Watch your thoughts, for they become words.

Watch your words, for they become actions.

Watch your actions, for they become habits.

Watch your habits, for they become character.

Watch your character, for it becomes your destiny.[2]

We may not realize it when unconscious negative thoughts and feelings colonize our mind and then become stronger and stronger until they crystallize into words and begin to influence our language. For example, if you mentally berate someone in your thoughts as a loser, one day, inadvertently, you may call that person a loser out loud.

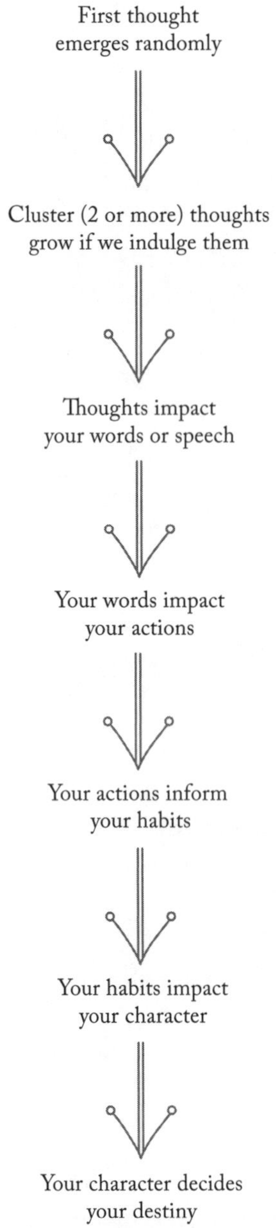

First thought
emerges randomly

Cluster (2 or more) thoughts
grow if we indulge them

Thoughts impact
your words or speech

Your words impact
your actions

Your actions inform
your habits

Your habits impact
your character

Your character decides
your destiny

Figure 21.1: Thoughts Impact Your Destiny

The word "loser" that emerges from your mouth is not a random word. It is riding the force of thousands of similar thoughts that called this person a loser (and more) in the safe confines of your mind. Your speech is the gross manifestation of thought buildup. If you find you are mad and screaming and shouting, again it is most probably a buildup—over minutes, days, or even years—of frustrated thoughts preceding their expression in words.

By using your higher mind to ensure the perpetuation mainly of clean and pure sattvic and ultimately ethical or dharmic thoughts in your lower mind, you can take control of your speech effectively. It will become quite intentional and deliberate as a result. You will never be caught off guard with an "Oops!" or embarrassed moment.

This is important because your thoughts and speech determine your destiny! This is how it works, and the seers say: "You are what your deep, driving desire is. As your desire is, so is your will. As your will is, so is your deed. As your deed is, so is your destiny."[3]

Your thoughts become words. Your words later become condensed into deeds or action; therefore, action is the grossest product of the subtlest thought.

By using free will from your illumined intellect, you can not only direct and control your thoughts and speech but also your actions. The type of actions we take defines our character in society, which ultimately determines our destiny. Through thought control, you become the writer of your life script, the builder of your destiny.

When dharma contemplations begin to routinely inform your thoughts, your speech will undergo radical changes. You will increasingly let go of your speech masks and embody your soul power and soul authenticity. Your speech will become naturally truthful, compassionate, and humane.

Therefore, assiduously practice thought observation. Actively watch your mind and its contents to avoid coming under the spell of selfish-rajas and reckless-tamas thoughts. Make your thoughts, speech, and actions worthy of your soul instead. Continued exposure to self-knowledge will help you develop higher standards.

Embody Inner Silence to Support Conscious Speech

Besides mindful speech and thought observation, one of the best ways to access a more sovereign mind in day-to-day life is to embody mindful silence for a few moments every day.

The egotistical approach to regaining our power is to go up against the world and somehow prove we still have it. We may make a lot of noise, but often we chase a fool's paradise since we have little control over external conditions or, for that matter, over our own senses, thoughts, feelings, and perceptions. We often become more disempowered than empowered. The spiritual approach is to work on our internal conditions. While external events deplete us, our internal life can more than make up for it. If we want, we can be abundantly powerful and autonomous, even in the most challenging situations.

I instruct my students to reclaim soul power from within:

Embody silence within and without—

Allowing what is. Surrendering to what is emerging—wanted or unwanted.

Not controlling what is.

Returning to silence after speech, action, and every thought.

Resting in silence, not ever needing guidance.

*Even as fire without fuel finds peace in its resting place,
when thoughts become silent, the soul finds strength and
peace in its own source.*

*A quiet mind overcomes both good and evil thoughts, and in the
silence, the ego is one with Self; then one feels the joy of eternity.*

*When the mind is silent, beyond trying to fix weaknesses of mind
or even concentrate the mind, it can enter a world far beyond
the mind: the highest, which is the domain of Self.*

*In this silence, the polarities merge into Oneness. Fear and
sorrow, too, end in this silence. In this silence, birth and death
become resolved into one existence.*

Silence, called *maunam*, is the faculty of activating soul power, inner freedom, restfulness, and intuitive wisdom. In the fertile silence, we can connect with a greater truth. This practice begins by autosuggestion, rather than shutting off the mode of speech: "Let me embody my inner silence now."

Baba reminded me:

*"Shunya, there is an infinitely powerful presence abiding within you.
It dwells beyond your thoughts and beyond your speech, but it can be
accessed in your silence. In fact, it will self-reveal itself to you in silence
and make itself silently known to you. It is the supreme unknown that
lies beyond even our subtlest thoughts. Let your mind rest in that silence
occasionally . . . enjoy the inward revealing of your soul power."*

Guided Practice: The Practice of Silence

Try spending time daily in solitude. Simply closing your eyes removes 80 percent of stimulation to your brain. Sit by yourself in a terrace or backyard. You can also take a quiet walk alone, without your cell phone or headphones. Then, become aware of the inner silence—a subjective inner state.

The inner silence is of a different, subjective quality that pervades the universe from inside us. It will slowly start emerging from your entire being. You can soak it in like a healing balm. As water relaxes when it meets water, fire with fire, and air with air, so also your mind becomes comforted when it meets its source, the Self, and rests in a spiritual, silent serenade.

Sometimes, despite choosing silence, thought waves may increase. Know that this is a ploy of your conditioned ego, forcing you to speak, even if to tell others, "I am silent today." When you activate the faculty of silence, you need not constantly assert this thought even to yourself: *I won't talk.* Silence is not necessarily the opposite of talking. This kind of enforced silence that we employ in cold war speaks more potently than words.

I am talking about a peaceful inner state, a silence that is an expression of your soul's inner power that does not need to exert itself—*it simply is.* If you must think anything, think repeatedly, *I am the Self. Silence is my inner nature. Power is my natural expression.*

Seeking solitude is helpful. It means deliberately removing yourself from the collective and being willing to be alone for an extended or set period without giving this time spent apart from the world familiar maya labels of lonesomeness, aloneness, sadness, and so on. If anything, you can label it a spiritual sadhana (spiritual discipline).

The benefits of each encounter with silence in solitude include emergence of inner clarity, inner capacities, and a very clear experience of an unshakeable inner power. We feel more internally powerful to handle challenges with a calmer state of mind.

As we become adept at activating and deactivating our faculty of silence, we can deploy it any time, even amid day-to-day life, in a grocery aisle, on a noisy train, on a bus ride, or in a movie theater.

The Difference Between Inner and Outer Silence

We don't necessarily need outer silence to activate inner silence because silence is the essence of our true being. Outer silence is dependent upon the absence of external sounds. Recall the case of the man who wanted outer silence and became enraged when he felt his classmates were too noisy for him to meditate and pursue spiritual contemplation. He felt spiritually cheated and annoyed. He was powerless over his obsession with something he could not control. But outer silence does not quiet the mind. Our friend in chapter 4 could have made the personally empowering choice to descend into deeper depths of consciousness and activate the faculty of inner silence that does not compete with speech, activity, or other cognitive brain functions. If anything, inner silence complements them because it leads to a greater inner connection.

Another benefit of getting in touch with inner silence is that we become naturally empathetic listeners. We gift soul presence to others by mindfully listening to their woes while resting in our inner healing silence. Sometimes our silent yet deep listening is more healing to others than anything we might say. Our silence indirectly activates others' inner silence to be with whatever difficulty they are undergoing. In that sense, the power of silence is more powerful than the power of speech. And our speech becomes divine when balanced with inward silence.

There are mundane but important social benefits for silence. Embodying inner silence frees us from power-depleting habits of gossip, negative self-talk, exaggeration, unnecessary arguments, disempowering chitchat, and power-grabbing habits of constantly interrupting others as they speak. We no longer indulge in monologues or forcefully dump our opinions on others. These forms of speech are a waste of energy and fuel emotional unrest. In all such cases, mindfully embodying silence is like allowing the mother to hold a restless baby until it stops squirming and experiences inner ease. Then, our divine speech becomes established in its natural godly partner, which is silence.

My long-time spiritual student Arjuna shared some of his contemplations on the sadhana of silence:

"I am learning that silence is not about 'waiting my turn' or 'shutting my mouth.' Rather, it is a practice of turning inward to have a profound experience of the true Self. I am learning that compulsive talking, storytelling, gossiping, and the 'conversation' is all outer-directed, caught in the push-pull of attachment and aversion: 'I like this, I don't like that,' 'I want this, I don't want that.' Each day, I see more clearly that outer speech (the way we talk with one another) is mostly run by social convention and polite niceties.

Silence, as Acharya Shunya says, has led me to discover 'the great friend in my own Self.' Silence is the womb of stillness. It gives birth to what we really need to say or do. In silence, my mind is quieting down. As I leave the chatter, as I let go of the opposites, I come closer to the one truth. Life is becoming much sweeter."

With practice, when our silence complements our mindful speech, our inner tranquility increases greatly. Your words will carry spiritual weight, and your silence will be transformative. Your Self will shine forth from your words and your silence alike.

22

Samatvam: Cultivating Equanimity by Accepting What Is Arising

"Water flows continuously into the ocean, but the ocean is never disturbed:
in the same manner, desire is continuously flowing into the mind of the seer,
But the seer's Self is not disturbed."

BHAGAVAD GITA, 2.70

Once, a king revered a yogi who lived in the forest just outside the kingdom. Every day the yogi came to the palace after dawn and gave his student, the king, a wild fruit, such as a fig or an apple. The king politely accepted the fruit, but given he had a royal feast waiting for him, he never ate it. In deference to the yogi, he did not throw out the fruit but stored it a special room—all of it accumulated there over the years, rotting.

One day, a monkey got hold of one of the pieces of fruit and eagerly ripped it apart. Out fell a shining diamond onto the floor.

The king was shocked. It became clear that he had rejected the yogi's gift, thinking it was a mere wild fruit, but all along, there was a diamond hidden in each fruit. How generous of the yogi! He ran to the yogi's abode and begged his forgiveness.

The yogi said with kind eyes, "But all human beings do the same thing. In every experience, a gem is hidden for you, a gift from the Supreme Reality, but you don't wait to find it."

Every experience of your Self is a gift from the universe. How can it be anything but a gift? But you only see the outer "wild" form and miss the message hidden inside the experience!

That is right: divorce, childbirth, the death of a loved one, and even betrayal, humiliation, and terminal disease are wild fruits with hidden gems.

But we refuse to read the message. We can't be bothered with the wild fruit—we only want the exotic, pretty ones. We have our artillery of likes and dislikes ready to reject these fruits that we did not order. This sense of "control" that our ego entertains is a delusion. Ultimately, you must wake up and eat the fruit that came to you by divine orchestration. This is the path to total equanimity.

The Connection Between Equanimity and Dharma

The Sanskrit word for emotional equanimity, or inner tranquility, is *samatvam*. Believe it or not, it is a choice. Choosing tranquility means consciously choosing to operate from dharma, in all kinds of human encounters. It means wanting to become more spiritually awake, rather than simply reacting and acting mechanically from knee-jerk thoughts and feelings arising in a cluttered mind. By cultivating an attitude of friendship toward those who are happy, compassion toward those in distress, joy toward those who are dharmic, and detachment toward those who are nonvirtuous, equanimity and tranquility arise in the mind.

Therefore, inner equanimity is a key value on which rest all other values, like truthfulness, humbleness, and compassion. After all, only a tranquil mind (one reposing in the knowledge of the Self always) chooses dharma. An immature, reactive, impulsive mind that is acting out, numb, or hell-bent on having a tantrum can hardly uphold dharma, can it?

This is important because without tranquility, which represents sattva, the illumined quality, in the mind, we can use none of our tools when we are faced with difficulties. Our mind gets taken over by the suffering mind, comprised of agitating rajas, dulling tamas, and delusory attachments! We get trapped in our own overactive imagination that is not anchored in reality.

When the mind is disturbed, we also lose the power to discern and detach wisely. Then, all our decisions go wrong. We lose the capacity to learn from our experiences because we are reacting, even hyperventilating in a full-on suffering-samsara mode. Samsara spells pure powerlessness.

God, Self, and the Universe Are Expressions of One Indivisible Consciousness

Perhaps when you understand that the entire manifested universe is the expression of your own true (manifested) Self and that what we call "God" or "Goddess" is none other than your Self, then you might be more comfortable with whatever is arising in this universe.

The Bhagavad Gita makes this observation: "That person who venerates Higher Power, with the knowledge that this Supreme Power is situated in all living beings (as Self), abides in Divine Consciousness in all circumstances."[1]

When you understand this amazing truth, then whatever you encounter in this creation becomes meaningful—no thing or occurrence is random. Thanks to this understanding of God, not as a special person with miraculous powers or a super-being living in the clouds (accessible only after death and only if we are good) or high up in some mountains, but as a super-intelligent, all-pervading principle or presence, then we can greet God everywhere.

You don't need to die and go to heaven to "meet God." You can meet God every day, everywhere, in every eye because this universe is an expression of the same omniscient presence. And why go far? You can greet the same omnipotent presence at work and in your own heart, and in fact, reposing as your dazzling and divine Self!

I appreciate the endless opportunities to experience divinity as an all-pervading intelligent presence with every sunrise and every sunset. Thanks to this beautiful, divinity-suffused vision the seers from the mystical Upanishads have shown me, even the inanimate rivers and mountains feel sacred, every pebble suffused with the light of the Divine Self. The Vedas reverberate with this holy vision that encompasses wholeness: "O Divine Presence, you are in the tender grass on the seashore, as well as in the foaming waves. You are on the sand banks as well as in the midst of the current. You are in the little pebbles as well as in the expanse of the ocean. You are in the lonely places as well as to be found in the crowded places . . . salutations to thee."[2]

Once you begin to appreciate this entire universe as the theater in which the divine truth is emerging everywhere, visibly and invisibly, in the living and through the nonliving, then you will find divinity radiating in every eye, both the good-hearted ones and dark-hearted ones. Both the sorrow-imparting life challenges and joy-giving circumstances will unpack for you the same essence of the one universal truth of divine, transcendent consciousness.

Equanimity in the Face of Sorrow

"For one who has mastered their mind, and who is tranquil, the supreme Self is self-evident. [The knower of Self] remains the same in heat and cold, pleasure and pain, joy and sorrow, as well as in honor and infamy."

BHAGAVAD GITA, 6.7

If not even a speck of dust or a blade of grass is out of place or unnecessary, then how can a sorrowful circumstance, no matter how dire, be frivolous or purposeless?

Each difficult situation is an integral part of an elaborately intelligent cosmos representative of our Universal Self, or God, with meaning and intentionality. It may be that the message or purpose is hidden in the sorrow. Whether we recognize this purpose or reason now or later, without a doubt, every difficult situation is meaningful and purposeful.

There are too many factors, including shared human consciousness and its collective ignorance (maya), that make circumstances outside the area of our influence unpredictable and outside our control. Whatever is meant to happen happens according to a greater cosmic will. We often distract ourselves by nursing our likes and attachments in our samsara and then rant, rave, and fall apart when things don't go our way. We create mindless futuristic sorrow by resisting, making the sorrow "go away" or manipulating things to make them go "our way."

Whether we experience the inevitable in a mature way, versus in a childish way (protesting and screaming), or in a numbed way (medicating or distracting ourselves), we have no true out except through enlightened knowledge. We must wake up and recognize that nothing is random and that perhaps this bitter sorrow, loss, betrayal, disease, or loneliness is exactly what our ego needs on our path to awakening to its highest potential.

Wisdom lies in controlling what you can control, which is your response to the situation, not the situation itself. Wisdom means trusting a greater intelligence beyond your ego's arithmetic of what it wants and does not want and aligning your will with cosmic will.

You are a boundless being—you are more powerful than you know, even if your ego has forgotten it temporarily. Deep down, you have the intellectual strength to overcome, transform, or peacefully accept any situation or challenge, no matter how painful.

Baba once said,

"If pain has come to you in a divine universe, then you, the divine one, have what it takes to face and grow from it."

If you're in the center of a difficulty, then you're in the center of the resolution also. You alone can find that solution by exposing your mind to enlightened wisdom.

Reality does not create stress, pain, or frustration. Your perception and interpretation of reality does. Not accepting reality is exhausting.

This is not to say that you should not act to improve a situation or protect yourself from harm. As a teacher, I never advocate fatalism or becoming a doormat to abusive or difficult people or circumstances, meekly accepting good or bad. But I do ask my students to spiritually grow up, be realistic about their expectations, and refrain from unhealthy grief, rage, and shame every time an unwanted situation or circumstance raises its unpleasant head.

Perhaps my own story will help illustrate this.

My Inner Guru Has a Stiff Neck!

Some years ago, an inflammatory genetic condition was activated after a nasty accident. As a result, my neck no longer moves with ease. It is almost immobile now. I must move my entire body to address people on either side of me. In the past, I was in excruciating physical pain, and I could not even type an email, let alone an entire manuscript (as I did for this and my former book). Thankfully, my practice of Ayurveda and yoga took away the pain, but the stiffness persists.

Given that I am a public speaker, this could be potentially embarrassing, but this situation became an opportunity to explore some questions: "What truly matters?" and "Who am I, if I am not my 'perfect' outward body?" This neck situation brought me new depths of empathy for people with disabilities, physical challenges, scars, disfigurement, social rejection, and trauma. Others may gape at us as if we are an anomaly when we are simply Self in a different body-suit.

By applying a greater wisdom, my so-called physical challenge or disfigurement has revealed to me the beauty of my soul. It has ultimately given more than it's taken from me. I have imbibed lessons in cultivating tranquility, deepest self-acceptance, and unshakeable equanimity that I would never have known and "lived" at this deeply vulnerable level.

Today, I teach worldwide with my neck as it is. I am unstoppable. Without enlightened wisdom of my true Self and a divine order, without the practice of equanimity, I would have simply curled up in sorrow and retired from the public life forever, feeling like a personal failure (when it comes to health) and crushed and cursed by "God."

I am confident now that every difficulty has a hidden blessing. The blessing is that I will emerge tranquil, steadfast, and more sovereign than before. And in this inner equanimity, slowly, my neck will heal too, even if it takes more time than usual.

Finding the Inner Monk in Karmic Solitude

"I am people-less," was another favorite sad lament in my life, once upon a time.

Repeatedly, I would find myself physically alone, either through deaths of my loved ones or through sheer lack of opportunity to connect with like-minded people (besides my students, who are not peers) at an intellectual or heartfelt level. My husband has long work hours, and also, in the early years of our relationship, we could not really connect. Even now, while we are beautifully harmonious together, we are not great talkers. Our son works abroad. The rare times I would encounter a potential friend with whom I could really have a conversation, they moved away, and some have died.

I used to wonder, *Am I socially unlucky?* The loneliness made me sad. But today, I can tell you, I am not sad, nor am I lonely. That sorrow was the perception of my attached samsara causing yet more grief. But this suffering only exists in our individual minds. We can magnify it to any extent we want. Accepting the reality, as in a flat resignation, is not the goal either. On the contrary, once we inquire and gain clarity on the hidden good in the so-called sorrow, we become better equipped, despite the sorrow, to make decisions that work for us.

Upon reflection I discovered that a supremely intelligent universe has provided me with the perfect external setup to discover my inner monk within a householder situation. I had all the freedom to mindfully cultivate solitude to self-explore, meditate, contemplate, write, reflect, embrace inner silence, and become who I am today. The Supreme Intelligence was saying to me through huge billboards: "Got solitude? Got quietude? Got self-reflection?" My specific and somewhat sparse social situation in this lifetime has helped me befriend my inner goddess.

Now, when I meet with the many people that my role as a spiritual preceptor demands, I come from an inner fullness. I am happy when we interact, and I am happy when I am alone. Students crowd me for my attention, and I can gift them the inner powers that I have cultivated in my alone time. And when I am alone—time I actively seek and protect now—I enter a mystical realm, whose doors open with my acceptance of my life situation as is and finding fullness in what looks like emptiness.

Today, I am a friend to the world. A Divine Intelligence that accompanies my true Self saw to that. I cooperated with my faith in a divine evolution. Nothing is ever random, and what looks like punishment is just the outer covering of a hidden, shining gem! The road God wants us to travel may not be our preferred road. Yet, our ease and flow may lie there, on that road less traveled.

Only Radical Acceptance of What Is
Leads to Emotional Equanimity

The spiritual practice of cultivating emotional tranquility includes *acceptance of what is* in your day-to-day life. Acceptance nips the bloom of the suffering mind in the bud. Agitation (rajas) and stuckness (tamas) don't arise as much or are quickly arrested. Peacefulness, clarity, balance, and joy (sattva) become steadfast.

Your mind will become purer, calmer, more accepting, flowing, trusting, happier, relaxed, and cheerful, radiating a more spiritually aligned state overall.

Let me share my student's observations in this regard:

> *"I went for an interview recently, and I was very nervous to the point that I felt my brain freeze up. I had to give a fifty-minute lecture, and I couldn't even get myself to practice once! This lecture was in front of professors whom I held in very high regard, and I felt paralyzed because I was convinced they would think I was a fool as soon as I opened my mouth. I wanted to run away. But I decided in that moment to test my dharma. I decided to forgive myself for not having practiced. I also realized that I no longer wished to be bound by my (false) myth-esteem, which was holding my mind captive (to somehow earn the approval of these professors). If they think I am incompetent, so be it! My true Self is beyond rejection.*
>
> *So, I said to myself, 'I am here, and I am going to do my best. If I fail, I will fail gloriously!' I could have run away or feigned an illness, but I couldn't get myself to do that. I realized I had to face this situation, honor my commitment, do the best I could, and let my connection to my inner truth lead me. The beauty of the whole process was that once I started upholding dharma, even this outwardly apparent disaster played out beautifully. I was able to witness dharma in action. I spoke my calm truth, so all my answers felt perfect. While moments ago I was experiencing a flurry of emotions—shame, anger, guilt, and inadequacy—the moment I connected with my inner Self, which is beyond outer approval or disapproval, I was able to be an observer, a sakshi. As a witness, I could observe these emotions as unnecessary, rather than being caught up in them. Being grounded in dharma, I was steady as a rock. My dharma spine was strengthened because I was able to transcend this samsara storm and remain steady in my inner tranquility."*

The Bhagavad Gita talks about the greed of wanting life situations to go exactly as we want, known as *spriha*. We humans, alone among animals, have this existential greed—the greed for existence to give us the cookies we want, when we want them, and as much as we want! Once we've enjoyed cookies of happiness, success, approval, or admiration, we become cookie addicts. We want more and more.

But is that even a realistic attitude, given we live in a duality-filled world marked by impermanence, and every experience is always cut short by its exact opposite?

Look how this universe teaches you what to expect from it during your human voyage. The day is always followed by night, light by darkness, spring by winter, youth by aging, birth by death, and death by birth. In the same way, a greater cosmic intelligence sends happiness and sorrow to visit you. Just as you don't go into confrontation mode when it rains or the sun shines, nor do you try to control the weather. Let the rain of sorrow too fall upon your being. When you become wet in it, that alone will lead you to find the open sky within your heart.

Indeed, our equanimity lies in greeting this cloudburst, not entreating it to leave or running away from it.

This Wave Too Shall Pass If You Simply Observe

Can you let the volatile waves in the ocean of existence rise and fall? The ocean always washes ashore pairs of opposites: fame and anonymity, victory and defeat, loss and gain, likable and unlikable, comfortable and uncomfortable, beautiful and ugly, acceptance and rejection—each a teaching of sorrow and joy. Instead of trying to control the opposites to make them vanish or to get more of them, can you be like a lighthouse rising above the crashing waves of duality, steadfast, unmoved, and unshakable?

This, too, is another wave . . . it, too, shall pass.

Give the wanted and unwanted circumstances only so much importance, and remain steadfast in remembrance of a higher spiritual truth, accepting all the opposites with a cultivated spiritual practice of willingness and acceptance.

How to Practice Acceptance and Willingness

The seven-step cycle below can help you identify, understand, and step out of repetitive cycles of resistance when faced with an unwanted circumstance and bring in greater acceptance and willingness.

Our first attitudinal response to unwanted situations and outcomes is generally inner resistance. We simply don't want to face difficult situations, and we go into a "why me" mode. So, we must confront two issues simultaneously.

One is the outer difficult situation. The other is the inner emotional resistance. We spend all our energy questioning the emergence of challenges (resistance); wallowing in rajas-emotions of blame, resentment, and rage; and resisting tamas-emotions of self-pity, sorrow, and shame.

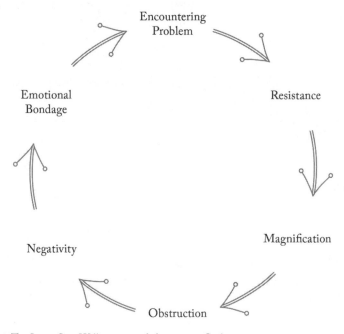

Figure 22.1: The Seven-Step Willingness-and-Acceptance Cycle

Resistance leads to inner magnification. We lose perspective, and things appear bigger, nastier, or grimmer than they may be, and perceived consequences are magnified in our mind. Emotionally overcome with likes and dislikes, attachments, and aversions pertaining to the problem, our rational thinking is concealed. None of it is real. It is all imagined.

Problem-Solving Skills Meet Obstruction

Magnification of negative gloom-and-doom–type emotions obstruct your intellect's natural problem-solving skills. The higher mind cannot use its own intelligence, skills, and past experiences or recall what it has read or admired in others regarding handling difficult situations. It cannot access its own creativity, ingenuity, or, least of all, acceptance or any thought of God or Self. It is simply overcome by the tidal wave of despair and frustration. Negativity takes over your daily life.

Watch out for complete emotional negativity in the form of hopelessness. We feel joyless, despondent, and depressed. We are terrified, stressed, and anxious. We see ourselves as victims of God, fate, humanity, and bad relationships, and we still never pause to inquire if our state of mind has anything remotely to do with our unchecked negativity.

Bondage: Loss of Emotional Sovereignty

Sustained emotional stress or psychological negativity leads to maladaptive behavior and hides the hidden gem of wisdom that may await you in your acceptance of the situation, no matter how grim it may be. We get caught up in pathological greed (for things to be or go exactly how we want them to go). Then, not being able to fill our cosmic holes with our cosmic greed, we experience uncontrollable grief, gut-wrenching fear of future problems, and finally anger. Any soul insights coming our way naturally are drowned in the deluge of negative delusory emotions that now besiege our mind. We are doomed to experience nonstop emotional pain of our own creation just because we could not accept . . . what had come our way.

Oftentimes, we lose our energy, money, and peace of mind in the process. We are simply projecting our undigested emotions all over the planet, not accepting the difficulty we face as an opportunity for inner growth.

Pausing to discern between what is real and what is simply projected reality is like switching on a lone bulb in the dark of night. Redemption can only come when we discern how our mind has become a prisoner of its own resistances. Then we can detach the emotional slugs and debug our samsara. Only then can we choose to cultivate acceptance and willingness over default resistance.

Every problem has a solution. When hunger is the problem, you must eat food. When isolation is the problem, you must make friends. When resistance is the problem, you must cultivate willingness and acceptance through exercise of viveka. Wisdom lies in controlling what we can control, which is our *response* to the experience or situation and not the situation itself.

Whenever I am faced with choiceless sorrow in my life, I have trained myself to breathe deeply every time I feel the urgency to fix things, push them away in resistance, or drown in emotional negativity.

I deliberately slow down by embracing quietude and a meditative-contemplative mode. I ask myself: *What am I being asked to see in this great sorrow that has colored my being with emotional pain? Let me wait to receive the answer within my heart from my Self seated within.*

This is the practice of willingness that follows acceptance—the willingness to have revealed in due time in our own heart, what we must see. This revelation of a deeper insight occurs not through our compulsive and angst-ridden egoic math of "It must be this way," or "It must be that way." It is a deeper insight that arises in the form of pure emotions that accompany insights and clarity when we become relatively still inside with practiced acceptance and willingness with greater spiritual poise.

The decision to not simply act and react from knee-jerk feelings and impulses in the lower mind but to simply observe the situation pulls us into a more transcendent (nondual) state of awareness.

The observing deactivates or weakens the hasty impulses. We become less emotionally reactive; we have purview of greater self-knowledge from within, as the higher mind is activated.

When we practice acceptance and willingness using our discriminatory faculty, despite problems that may feel urgent, the delusory thoughts and negative feelings subside or recede into the background and our greater soul-knowingness arises into the foreground

Any time you deliberately step back to observe your "reactive mind-field," it can no longer exercise the same kind of power over you. Only as a neutral observer of your own mind, can you dissolve the illicit edifice of your own resistances, fueled by irrational attachments and aversions, leaving you free to respond emotionally in a more brilliant, creative, and original manner.

Therefore, we must expand our own understanding; we must wake up and recognize that nothing is random, not even the so-called unwanted life situations, and that perhaps this bitter experience (loss, betrayal, disease, loneliness, or similar) is exactly what our ego needs on our path to awakening to its potential. This recognition will make you inwardly tranquil.

Next time this happens, you can kick the resistance cycle by simply facing the unfortunate circumstance and roaring with all your sovereign power. Tell yourself repeatedly, "If I have a problem, I will find the answer too."

Be a Peaceful Warrior in the Battle Grounds of Life

The holiest Vedic scriptures, the Bhagavad Gita, was delivered on a battleground, when the war was about to begin. The teacher, Krishna, wanted his student, Arjuna, to go to war against an enemy of society and sanity, neither as a victim nor as an aggressor, but as a divine being, as Self. He wanted his student's passion to be accompanied by inner equanimity, his mind in his full command.

Here is how the Krishna defines mental equanimity to Arjuna: "Having made pleasure and pain, gain and loss, victory and defeat the same (samatvam), engage in battle [of your life] for the sake of the battle; you shall not incur sin."[3]

The background of a battle is an appropriate allegory, reminding us not to hesitate before the battlegrounds we face in our life. Today we are more familiar with relationship battlegrounds, far-removed from the dust of hoofs and the beat of shod feet.

Our relationship battles may be in corporate meeting rooms, in the stock exchanges of the world, in the hallways of Capitol Hill, in congresses and parliaments, in towns small and large, or in national or global courts of justice that we humans have instituted for conducting our relational, egoic battles. Indeed, our life bristles with professional, political, and personal relationship battles.

That is why it is essential to cultivate equanimity, making ourselves tranquil warriors for the battles we regular folks face every day at work, at home, and on our commute. Are you ready for the battle for inner equanimity? That is the emblematic question. Not taking a side is not an option, since diffidence is akin to acting, albeit passive action. The Bhagavad Gita has compared human existence to a great battle of ideas (*dharma yuddha*) that begins from the first movement of conception, where sperms battle for supremacy, onward. No wonder Krishna says: "Filled with egoism, if you think, *I will not fight*, vain is this your resolve [for] nature will compel you [to fight for your existence]."[4]

The laboratory of spiritual growth is life itself, where battles may be fought outside you, but with a contemplative, discriminant, and detached mind within you, you can be a peaceful warrior. For the battles of life, more important than a temple, a church, or a mosque is a tranquil mind trained to remain inwardly empowered by the Self.

That is why the Bhagavad Gita says: "Therefore, always, remember the Self, and fight [your daily battles] with mind and intellect fixed or absorbed in Self; you shall doubtless come back to Self alone."[5]

All our life experiences, even the sorrowful ones, can teach us something. But without tranquility, we cannot see what we must see. Only by valuing inner equanimity can you learn to face the transient sorrows and joys coming at you with some cultivated neutrality. Birth, death, youth, old age, hope, and disappointment are coming your way. Are you ready to face the opposites? If you value tranquility and want to make it your prime inner value or guidance system, you must go beyond the word and understand my invitation to live with emotional maturity. By valuing tranquility, you will transcend your own ego and implement the practices I impart in this book.

Equanimity Is Your Best Aid in Relationship Struggles

When a pond is cloudy, we cannot see what lies on its bed. But when the water is tranquil, the mud settles down, and we can see all the way to the rocky bottom. Just like that, when our mind becomes tranquil, we can see all our samsara and take stock of our every feeling and thought.

The Bhagavad Gita says: "In tranquility, the destruction of all miseries takes place. Verily, the self-knowledge of this serene-minded [person] becomes firm."[6]

But, if we don't value cultivating equanimity, even a minor challenge inside a relationship or an old painful memory resurfacing will be enough to set us off in another samsara-suffering storm! The mind is then easy prey to an unending litany of self-created sorrow. Old traumas become fresh traumas every living moment.

Therefore, the only solution is to process pain on two planes at once: you must inquire into the pain by fully being with it (no bypassing) and be in the state of practiced equanimity at the same time. You will feel the full depth and fierce intensity of the pain (or memory), and at the same time, you will transcend it by being able to observe it, from an autosuggested and consciously chosen tranquil state of mind.

For most of us, the mind is an expanse of victimhood where somebody or other—spouse, boyfriend, girlfriend, other woman, other man, mother-in-law, great-aunt, mom, dad, step-mom, step-dad—is out to get us. If it is not a person or group of persons that we know intimately, then the seasons, planets, government, politicians, terrorists, weather, and aliens can do the job.

The victim script is a tamasic state of mind. "Tamas" literally means "darkness," and it represents a state of mind that is thoroughly drenched in self-forgetfulness (blind to the inner light).

Here, we "believe" we are cosmically disempowered. The world or even God or destiny or the higher principle (whatever be the name) wants us to remain so, and we have no right to choose otherwise. Negativity, disappointments, suspicion, and self-doubt are permanent residents of our mind, coloring our everyday self-experience as deeply impotent. We expect failure in all areas of our life: professional, personal, health, and of course, relationships!

Our true Self, which is neither a victim nor an aggressor but always powerfully tranquil, is right here within us; however, under the influence of maya, we fail to see or acknowledge its existence and instead hold steadfast to our version of the story. As long as we keep swinging between victim and aggressor consciousness, we are unable to transcend either. We will keep slipping into one or the other mode of consciousness again and again. Sometimes, our entire life is spent in the clutches of maya, and even on our death bed, we die as the angry unrepentant aggressor, or we die of the unredeemed victim's grief.

When we consciously accept all parts of ourselves, darkness as well as light, we begin to experience a new raw soul-power to simply be ourselves and let others be themselves—to live and let live—by neither becoming a power monger (rajas) nor victim (tamas), shaped and morphed by another person's power. We become someone willing to authentically uphold our sovereignty through spiritually available inner knowledge, practices, and disciplines that make us equanimous (sattva). Can sorrow exist forever without pulling in its opposite, joy? Can powerlessness rule your mind for long, when radical freedom is your real nature? In radical wholeness, which is Self, can darkness exist long, without pulling in light?

"The one whose wisdom is steadfast is sovereign;
This one knows bliss in the Atman and wants nothing else.

Residual desires may cross the heart,

But the awakened one renounces these vasanas too, through wisdom.

I call such a person sovereign."

BHAGAVAD GITA, 2.55

"Not shaken by adversity; nor yearning after happiness:

Free from fear, free from anger; free from the attachments risen to desire,

Such a person is sovereign."

BHAGAVAD GITA, 2.56

"The one who is not limited by body consciousness

May be lucky and does not rejoice; may be unlucky and does not lament

Such a person is sovereign."

BHAGAVAD GITA, 2.57

23

❦

Moksha: Making Awakening
Your Supreme Goal

*"The awakened being, freed from self-ignorance, enjoys uninterrupted,
infinite 'direct contact' with the internally seated divine Self."*

BHAGAVAD GITA, 6.28

Have you ever lost something and then found it?

The happiness of lost and found property is something special. When you buy something precious for the first time, you experience happiness. If you lose it and then find it however, the happiness is greater than when you first acquired it.

That is how it will feel when you achieve true and final awakening: moksha! After searching out there somewhere in the world and web of relationships for inner freedom, autonomy, power, joy, and happiness, you will find those qualities inside you, shining in your purified mind as blessings from your Self.

Yes, in moksha you are liberated from the shackles of your own mind, even past actions and regrets. Your mind is illumined with your spiritual light. While dharma represents waking up "inside" maya by embodying noble traits and the pure ego's values, moksha represents waking up "from" maya—that is, remembering who we are in the first place. Without dharma in our hearts, one cannot even begin to value inner quietude, a pure diet, spiritual self-discipline, and what it takes to awaken to our Self.

The ones who dare to embody dharma shine with the purity of dharma, say the seers. No wonder embodying dharma has been marked as a very important goal in the Vedas, a critical preliminary step that lays the groundwork for achieving ultimate liberation from our imprisoning samsara. Therefore, moksha marks the consummation of the process of moral, emotional, intellectual, and spiritual self-development through exploring, accepting, and embodying dharma in daily life as a dharmic banker, dharmic belly dancer, dharmic baker, dharmic parent—a dharmic human being.

Defining Moksha: The Word and the Types

"Moksha" is a Sanskrit word derived from the root word *muchyate,* which means "free or released" (from the bondage of samsara). It is also called *mukti,* or freedom.

Moksha can be understood in two ways. In one sense, moksha is the destruction of bondage through elimination of the delusional, hypnotic belief systems that keep us spiritually limited and caught up in egoic engagements—the destruction of samsara. This is awakening to our true expansive identity beyond our limited ego.

And then moksha is also said to be a state of unalloyed bliss or eternal happiness. Moksha is declared to be the experience of *param-samatvam,* or the ultimate tranquility, abiding peace, and unalloyed bliss of Self.

In fact, moksha has a variety of meanings:

* Freedom from bondage to anything we want to do or not want to do, feel or not feel.

* Freedom from the chain of birth and death because when we are one with our Self, we will have choice.

* Freedom from suffering caused by one's own emotional misperceptions and delusions.

* Freedom from the chain of ignorant actions that are said to oblige us to take repeated births and undergo repeated deaths.

* Freedom from unexamined attachment to the objects of desires.

* Discriminative knowledge that the self is totally different from the not-Self, so it is the dawn of self-knowledge (*Who am I?*).

* "Freedom, liberation, release from bondage," and in this sense, moksha makes us truly sovereign.

Enlightening, liberating self-knowledge is key for achieving moksha. That is why the Bhagavad Gita says: "To those whose ignorance is destroyed by the knowledge of the Self, like the sun this knowledge reveals the supreme Self, Atman."[1]

Moksha Is a Here-and-Now Awakening

Some people are nervous about the idea of awakening, or moksha. They fear a loss of identity. But the awakening I am talking about is a totally here-and-now phenomenon in the context of your daily life as an awakened mom, dad, employee, son, daughter, spouse, and so forth—you don't have to die to achieve familiarity with your Self.

The Bhagavad Gita sheds light on awakening as freedom from samsara: "With the senses, mind, intellect ever controlled, having freedom as one's supreme goal, free from desire, fear, and anger, the seeker is liberated forever."[2]

Traditionally, pursuing the goal of moksha meant seeking out a Vedic teacher for a long-term systematic study of Vedic scriptures. With ongoing exposure to these scriptures, it is said that lifetimes of self-ignorance may be burned away.

In a nontraditional sense, pursuing moksha can mean living in the world with emotional maturity, inner contentment, and authenticity, not bothering excessively with the world and its scripts. It is my belief that inside each one of us quietly sits a recluse, waiting for its turn. To walk the journey toward permanent awakening, the recluse must appear, sooner or later. Otherwise the crowds, noise, pomp, and show of the world will forever keep us distracted and occupied in the business of everyday living.

When moksha is our goal, our inner recluse makes it a priority to study and practice with qualified teachers, read dharmic books (like this one, perhaps repeatedly), and practice witnessing and meditation frequently—not just to relax or destress before going back into the world for round two of the vasana chase, but to finally touch and reclaim the greater metaphysical reality within.

Moksha is every human's birthright and ultimate spiritual goal, not just the aspiration of a rare awakened individual whom everyone else looks up to or even envies (while loathing themselves deep inside). The Vedas hold achieving enlightenment or awakening as a universal goal of human existence. It is not magic or a super-state, as it is often made out to be. It is simply resting in our true, unalloyed divine nature. It is the natural expression of our evolving human consciousness. We will all encounter our hidden divinity sooner or later, the Vedas promise, and we must all make the effort because powerlessness, bondage, and hypnotic sleepwalking are no way to live!

Moksha Takes Place in the Ordinary World

"Knowledge is enveloped by ignorance, thereby beings are deluded."

BHAGAVAD GITA, 5.15

Trust me, moksha is not achieved from abandoning the world: it is achieved by living in it with inner freedom. Some teachers, both Indian and Western, wrongly interpret moksha as abandonment of the material world. Abandonment matters only to those who are bound and attached to begin with.

In its true essence, moksha is the freedom Nelson Mandela experienced in the confines of prison and is how Helen Keller chose to live freely and follow her original inner calling despite lack of sight. To the undiscriminating eye, they were bound and imprisoned in unfortunate or trying circumstances. However, these brave souls understood that no body, sense, or set of four walls could confine them.

Most of us are miserable because we are under the illusion that we are bound by finite objects like four walls. But how can the soul, which is infinite, be bound? How can that which is free of time and space be entrapped by it? Shattering this illusion is what moksha is all about.

Moksha is not about abandoning your confines; it is about living within the confines of the knowledge that you, the Atman, are free. This is how all great beings have first seen a new way and then shown it to the rest of humanity—by soaring in free skies within!

Moksha Is Connected to the End of Worldly Distress

The connection of moksha with the end of emotional distress and delusions can be seen in the word itself, which is comprised of two words: *moha* and *kshaya*.

"Moha" means "mind-based emotional thought disturbances, projections, and delusions that cause sorrow"; "kshaya" means "the end of those mental knots."

Moksha in this context entails the change of our deepest held false beliefs such as:

My happiness is dependent on accomplishing the goals of physical and emotional survival (artha), pleasure (kama), and higher duty (dharma). This is not true. Even if the other goals don't work out, your Self can be a source of fulfillment for you.

I am limited in how much happiness I can manifest for myself (perhaps none). This is not true. Unlimited, infinite cosmic consciousness is the center of your being.

I am powerless to do anything about a difficult or challenging situation, so I will either be a victim (never have enough happiness) or become an aggressor (snatch happiness). This is not true. At any time, infinite choices to respond, from our discerned will and not from our default reactive samsara, are open to us.

Therefore, the classical Vedic tradition advocates cleansing the mind with the cloth of self-knowledge, much like a dirty mirror is cleaned to faithfully reflect reality. No wonder, moksha means "the end of sorrow-causing mirages," illusions such as, *I need others to accept me before I can accept, like, and love myself.* It is the ultimate freedom to live boldly, with full personal autonomy, and operate from one's own radically empowered nature. Even though your divine Self was always there, shining brightly, you can now become directly cognizant of it. Your ego at last comes home to its source—the bliss, vastness, and freedom of Self.

Moksha Is Inclusive: It's Your Turn Next!

Have you heard about instant-awakening stories such as, "I was depressed until one day, *Swooooosh!* I just awakened to the highest truth, and now I know all there is to know." Such people are saying that they were randomly chosen by the universe and bequeathed an awakening to their sleepwalking mind. This hardly imparts any hope to the rest of us!

Instant awakening is a false promise of some modern Advaita teachers. They say we are already enlightened; therefore, no practices are needed to uncover our inner wisdom. As was stated in a recent article on Neo-Advaita and mindfulness, "The trouble with this viewpoint is that it's more of a philosophy than a practical application. You can think you're free and let go of all ideas of non-freedom all you want, but at the end of the day, you may still not feel very free."[3]

Classical Vedic tradition agrees that the Self is enlightened or all-knowing. But as one scholar puts it, "We have blinders on and cannot see our own enlightenment, and practices (which there are many types of) will remove the blinders and allow our inherent liberation to naturally shine forth."[4]

The Vedic tradition is unequivocally united on this fact: genuine awakening can be earned by anybody willing to do the inner work of purifying and illuminating the ego (samsara), with self-knowledge. There are no awakening "haves" and "have nots."

Moksha Is Permanent: Awakening Does Not Fluctuate

Once the knots that conceal your inner truth are removed with inner work, then your experience of Self will not come and go—it will abide.

"Perceiving the Self in the self [ego], the knots of the heart are untied, all doubts dispelled and vasanas exhausted."

MUNDAKA UPANISHAD, 2.2.8

The freedom that comes from knowledge of the Self is permanent. It is permanent because it already is. All we need to do is test it out. Our Self represents pure freedom and is not dependent on any specific state of mind or our life circumstance. What I am saying is 100 percent supported by this revelatory verse from the Bhagavad Gita:

"Awakening to the ever-full Self takes place both here and hereafter for the self-restrained ones who are free from desire [vasana] and anger and self-pity, whose minds are restrained, and who have known the true Self within [Atman]."[5]

Therefore, whatever was disowned due to ignorance must be permanently reclaimed through knowledge. This is moksha. It means our mind is never again locked in illusory bondages due to misperceptions. Moksha is freedom to remember a greater truth and operate from your true Self, in day-to-day life.

The Neo-Vedantists advise their followers to expect that the awakened state will "come and go." They say it should not matter much if it is not permanent since you are not the ego after all. But what is the point of awakening if we are still haunted by our virtual ghosts? This is not a sovereign state at all. It is simply another egoic bubble that the mind enjoys and then drops when faced with the first adversity.

Once you have achieved that light of all lights, its radiance should not come and go like a blinking bulb. It abides because it is a state of the enkindled soul, the true radiant Self.

The Bhagavad Gita declares this: "The person of steady wisdom [who has achieved awakening] does not ever fall back from it, back into delusion. Even at the moment of death, they remain alive in that awakened state: the immortal Self and the mortal self are one, for the seer of the Self."[6]

The Bhagavad Gita explains the connection of moksha with an irreversible state of inner freedom so poetically in these verses: "True moksha is characterized by your ability to see your Self with your pure mind [that you have efforted to purify or enlighten with the light of self-knowledge]. Only then will this mind relish and rejoice in the Self. In that joyous state, your mind will experience boundless spiritual bliss. And, established in your sovereign mind, you will never again depart from this greatest truth of your Self. Being so situated, you will not be shaken even amid greatest difficulty. This indeed is actual freedom. This is true sovereignty."[7]

Therefore, awakening, or moksha, is not a destination in consciousness to "reach," or a short-lived experience of inner freedom we suddenly arrive upon one day when our awareness is feeling expansive that then reverts to bondage, limitations, and sorrow when our consciousness is once again filled with routine worldly concerns.

Adopt Conscious Disciplines to Prevent Moksha Bypassing

"If you think you are enlightened, go spend a week with your family."

RAM DASS[8]

When small chains in your samsara start snapping apart because of contemplations and meditations on Self, you will feel empowered. This happens to everyone. I will offer some examples of "moksha moments" that my students have experienced later in this chapter. However, to make true progress, you must watch out at this stage for prematurely imagining yourself permanently awakened, especially if you don't have a living teacher to guide.

A tiny time-bound experience of moksha that comes and goes is not the same as the abiding freedom of moksha.

All responsible spiritual teachers give this counsel, and all genuine seekers appreciate it. After all, there is such a thing as spiritual vasana (shastra vasana), which makes us unconscious in the realm of mysticism and turns the spiritual search itself to the desires of the ego.

But despite such forewarning, because of feeling temporarily inwardly empowered, many seekers imagine they have become "enlightened," or at least made tremendous progress, when really they are just starting out. This "premature transcendence" disrupts their growth efforts.

Some delusory ones even step into the role of an enlightened teacher and give out half-baked truths. Many such self-declared messiahs with charismatic personalities command a cult-like following. This does not make them enlightened or sovereign in any true sense. It is these teachers who have given the word "guru" such a bad reputation.

Sadly, the so-called awakening claimed by countless spiritual teachers, alive or now dead, who have been caught with their halos (pants) down, is the hypnotic vasana-conditioned mind acting out its self-appointed spiritual credentials. It is not awakening at all, but deluded spiritual sleepwalking.

As we've discussed, traditional nondual wisdom from India emphasizes instructing the ego in a formalized process that can take years. In the absence of some kind of systematic ego-purifying practices, some well-known teachers have admitted that their "awakening" has not resulted in an end to their suffering. Some have suggested that suffering may increase upon awakening or that the state of being awakened is exhausting.

To this, I respectfully say that until you learn to edit and audit your own behaviors and improve your lot by going to work on your own ego, you will remain caught in a prison of your own false notions, and your suffering will continue unabated. Further, no spiritual shortcuts or even holy rituals will help you break free from your delusions. Fortunately, the classical Vedic process of awakening comes with measures to prevent bypassing and self-deception. The ancient texts are clear when they say:

"Truth seems to arise only from inquiry and the reflections upon trustworthy guidance by an awakened teacher ... not by holy baths [in the sacred rivers], giving elaborate gifts [to pundits], or by accomplishing breath control [like an exercise]."[9]

Due to a long tradition of Vedic *guru-shishya parampara* (the transmission of sacred knowledge from teacher to student), sincere seekers of true Self have a blueprint to follow. It prepares us to internalize these teachings, taking the time it takes, and without bypassing our egoic challenges. This discipline is voluntarily taken up by seekers to qualify their minds to receive self-knowledge (atma vidya) from a qualified guru. The good news, dear reader, is that you have already absorbed much of this practice, as it is the secret basis for this entire book. This blueprint is the series of core mental and spiritual self-discipline practices called *sadhana chatushtayam.*

Guided Practice: Sadhana Chatushtayam—Classical Fourfold Discipline to Purify the Ego and Prevent Spiritual Bypassing

The opening verses of *Prashna Upanishad* describe spiritual seekers who arrive at a Vedic school (*gurukulam*), seeking knowledge about Atman (Ultimate Reality, Self). They ask Sage Pippalada to impart this knowledge. The teacher does not start providing answers immediately, but demands that they first spend time—almost a whole year—with him, dharmically upholding cognitive disciplines, collectively called sadhana.

"To the seekers the sage said:

First dwell around me for a year with tapas [perseverance], with brahmacharya [dharma], with sraddha [trust],

Then ask what questions you will,

If I know, I will tell you all."

PRASHNA UPANISHAD, 1.2

This is significant. The sage's emphasis upon taking up sadhanas that includes tapas, brahmacharya, and shraddha shows the importance of preparing the mind for highest knowledge by all seekers. Second, look at the humbleness of the ancient Vedic teacher. The implicit admission by the teacher with "if I know" brings a healthy sense of skepticism and humility into the process of teaching and learning.

"Sadhana" is any dedicated spiritual discipline consistently maintained over time. "Chatushtayam" refers to a fourfold path ("chatu" means "four" in Sanskrit), which is explained below. This unique, cognitive practice helps to clarify the mind and make it more open to spiritual breakthroughs and spontaneous awakening of spiritual consciousness.

Remember, this is a voluntary discipline.

1. Viveka: The Sadhana of Discernment

As we have learned, "viveka" means "discernment." In this practice, you use Vedic self-knowledge to look at your own mind and discern whether what you are thinking is coming from your shadow self or from an authentic place within you. When we don't pause to examine the reality or nonreality of our own thoughts, often the shadow is driving our car, and we start bypassing reality. Say you hear about your uncle's death, and you don't shed tears because you imagine that enlightened people don't cry for a Self that does not die. You will discern this is a suppression of emotions due to the false belief that enlightened folks are above emotions, and then, you will allow your legitimate grief to take over. But you will not be lost in it too long because you will also have greater wisdom of eternalness of Self. How to hone our discrimination of our motivations, thoughts, and feelings was discussed in detail in parts I and II of this book. So in a way, this entire book is helping you perfect viveka, thereby preventing spiritual bypassing.

2. Vairagyam: The Sadhana of Stepping Away from What Is Not Real

Healthy discernment is always followed by healthy vairagyam, or detachment. This simply means stepping away from whatever was falsely coloring your mind. You will realize that freedom lies in being authentic (feeling grief after the death of a loved one) and not fake (false nondual chin-up). (I talk about this practice in depth in chapter 12.)

3. Shadsampat: Cultivating Six Awakening Propensities, or Inner Virtues

This sadhana can be broken down into six sub-steps:

a.) Shama. This entails management of your mind and its content—thoughts, feelings, motivations, and emotions. We don't simply think positive thoughts to the exclusion of what is negative in our mind. We take a survey of our mind's entire contents through a more neutral, observer consciousness. Then, without suppressing the negative, we move the content toward embodying what is more positive and ultimately what is more "real." This is not a bypass of anxiety, depression, or rage. It is taking a deep and ongoing stock of our mind and then changing its content to a more preferred state "by conscious choice and conscious effort." This entire book is helping you with shama, or mind management.

b.) Dama. *Dama* is the conscious choice to direct our senses toward whatever experiences (food, music, company) will help us be more real, authentic, and self-aware, versus delusional, numb, or living a false reality. Therefore, when we follow these Vedic guidelines and prefer cultivating the vibration of sattva (that illumines the mind) versus rajas (that distracts it) and tamas (that makes it dull), we automatically disconnect awakening from mind-altering substances or even false friends. We automatically choose to cultivate more solitude, healthy relationships, and a lifestyle of pure foods and pure recreation. (See chapter 11 on sensory disciplines taken up by responsible seekers, voluntarily.)

c.) Uparama. *Uparama* means stabilizing in your swadharma. If you are practicing the above three sadhanas that impact intellect, mind, and senses respectively, you are in good shape to begin living your daily life with swadharma (see chapter 19). A seeker with a core propensity of pleasure who allows themselves pleasures (such as ice cream and sex, for example) is more authentic than when that same seeker denies them. They begin lying to themselves and to others. This causes spiritual bypassing. The shadow will rebel. Also, if we are bypassing, we start neglecting and refusing our swadharma because we falsely feel that the Self is beyond all worldly chores and duties, and therefore, we are free to shrug off our worldly responsibilities. Rather, performing our worldly roles and duties is the exact place to keep observing whether or not we are truly awakened and able to perform swadharma without "samsaric explosions," without the spiritual bypass of not upholding our swadharma because we prefer to sit in the bubble of bliss we have created to keep us from our worldly responsibilities.

d.) Titiksha. This word means "endurance." It entails practicing steadfastness in all your above sadhanas when you are challenged. Challenges will come in the form of different enticements to look, feel, and behave more spiritually advanced than you are, to the point of forgiving too quickly or not allowing yourself to feel your needs and desires. But you will want to hold on to what is authentic and real for you in this moment too. Don't let any teacher or teaching that promises instant awakening take you away from the very real awakening that you are slowly and steadily orchestrating using the wisdom tools. There is no bypassing the ego, and it must stay in your soul's wisdom school long enough to not die or disappear, but to truly transform and become filled with light. When you practice conscious endurance, despite life's ups and downs, pushes and pulls, you will remain dedicated to authenticity and cultivate a samsara-free mind. (See chapters 19 and 22, which discuss cultivating authenticity, steadfastness, and equanimity despite trials and tribulations.)

e.) Shraddha. "Shraddha" means "trust." This entails cultivating trust in the words of the teacher and the path you are journeying. Most teachers and most traditions demand absolute faith. The Vedas suggest only reposing functional faith at the beginning and retaining some healthy skepticism until our own mind reaches this advanced stage of trust. By now, using discernment, you will be able to tell whether your current teacher and the tradition are truth tellers or are simply seducing you further into your shadow (to be who you are not). If you are with a truth teller, then congratulations. Bow inwardly to the Self of this teacher. You may end your teacher and tradition search at this stage and repose with confidence in your chosen teacher and tradition going forward. You are safe against bypassing teachers and traditions that encourage sleepwalking. (See chapter 8 on real versus nonreal teachers.)

f.) Samatvam. At this stage, you are almost shadow-free. Or you are fully aware of what's left of your shadow, and you guide it with the knowledge tools you gained through the previous sadhanas. You still have an ego, but its head is above the maya waters. Your ego is working with you, and you enjoy the teachings of your chosen teacher and the light of masters from your path. No part of your personality is faking it; you are who you are, free of vasana scripts. You may still have inner work to do, but you are embracing your darkness with all the light you have—you are not simply stuffing away your darkness in corners you can't see. You want true abiding awakening (moksha) and a genuine encounter with inner divinity. In this sadhana, you consciously live by dharma (yamas and niyamas) and abide in a focused and easeful sattvic mind state for continued periods of time. You must build this balanced mind into a steady, nonflickering flame of devotion to guru, loyalty to path, meditation, and contemplation on the nondual teachings from the path (see chapter 10). You are a perfect spiritual seeker at this stage, primed for success. Do your work.

4. Mumukshutvam: The Sadhana of Desiring Moksha

When the preceding sadhanas are in place, your life as you know it will be totally transformed. In relationships, even at work, you will be a whole new, much more serene and powerful person. This sadhana involves looking beyond a successful worldly life to seek what lies within you—the majestic Self. At this stage, the sadhana is to remain steeped in consciousness of the nondual Self and desire union with it. Everywhere you try to see beyond the body to the Self! (See chapter 16.) All desires will pale in comparison to the desire to realize the Self through achieving moksha! And because we become what we believe (or think about constantly), very soon your mind becomes the meeting ground to meet your own Self. You are waiting for moksha.

In this regard my teacher Baba said:

"Don't chase the Self like a physical object. Through sadhanas, you have prepared your mind, like you prepare your living room to receive a special guest, and the nonphysical guest will simply show up one day, just like that! You won't be able to see it, as it is not an object graspable by your senses, but you will know it, as it can be intimately known by the prepared and purified mind, ego, and intellect."

I hope you appreciate as much as I do the thoroughly systematic, realistic, and inclusive awakening journey laid out by the Vedic seers. They don't skip any steps, and they prevent spiritual bypassing astutely because they are aware that the human mind can be quite imaginative, even in spiritual arenas.

Signs of Awakening

I appreciate the slow and steady nature of achieving the goal of moksha in the Vedic tradition, with no pressure for overnight spiritual perfection (or else people like me would never have made it!). It takes the time it takes before this intellectually received knowledge of our own potential becomes a seeker's living and permanent reality.

The first sign of the dawning of awakening is when you handle conflicts, losses, and challenges with more sattva, dharma, and mental tranquility. The mental samsara does not dissolve instantaneously, but rather gradually, through repeated application of spiritual wisdom and practices in daily life.

First, you will see a reduction in frequency, then in length, and then intensity of episodes of powerlessness, delusions, and self-created sorrow. You will also find an undeniable increase in personal power, inner ease, choice, emotional tranquility, and natural alignment with dharma.

Moksha feels like it should be a special moment in time, but Self is always shining behind our mind, is it not? Your sleepwalking mind simply catches up with its own divine light. This is what happens when the veil of maya is thinned by constant contemplation upon awakening self-knowledge and when this knowledge is applied in daily life.

Enjoy Moksha Moments before Final Moksha!

Until full and final moksha arrives, you can enjoy tastes of moksha or "mini awakened moments." These are like spiritual "aha" moments—deep, even if fleeting, reconnections with your spiritually available inner freedom, perhaps several times a day.

A student had this to say about choosing moksha moments in daily life choices.

"It is difficult to awaken in a world full of sleepwalkers or the semiconscious: the darkness and deception become glaringly obvious and disparate. I liken this to being in a setting with people who are drinking alcohol and you are not. You see the rajas and/or tamas taking over and how, often, their behaviors are caricatures of healthy human engagement. I have had moments where I want to relax into the 'drink' of the cluttered mind, to retreat to 'bed,' to the seeming ease of the 'make-do self' sleepwalking through life. This way of living seems safe and secure because it is known and nearly perfected. I witness how I fall back into the entrenched patterns of the small self—the storylines of victimhood and separation. It is so easy to do, like how a record will skip to the well-worn groove of your favorite song. However, these so-called 'comfortable' default behaviors are not our actual nature. They are learned behaviors nurtured by family and culture, deepened by trauma, and reinforced by limited knowledge.

This is where the teachings of my guru Acharya Shunya come in: the true knowledge of the highest Self, our sovereign truth, begins to illumine the sorrow-causing thoughts and imagined separateness. When I remember that I am the boundless, ever-free Atman and I engage the world with observer consciousness, I witness the trickery of the small self.

While it is challenging to rise out of this mental groove, one that is reinforced all around us in culture, I have had moksha moments where I stand fully in my higher Self. These moments are coming more frequently and starting to break apart the gossamer net woven by vasanas. Yes, it is difficult; yes, it is possible to continue this path."

Let me give a few more real-world examples of moksha moments below:

Lauren's awakened moment in the dentist office.

"I have heard my teacher expound that our likes and dislikes or attachments and aversions are the main sources of suffering in samsara. I had an experience today that brought those lessons home in a new way. I felt fear coming up while waiting for my daughter's dentist appointment to get a chipped tooth fixed. When I examined that fear, it seemed it came from a strong attachment to my daughter never feeling pain or trauma, to her always behaving the way I want her to when I want her to . . . and an equally strong aversion to her suffering or feeling scared, to her not freaking out and causing a scene in the dentist chair. All of these pushing and pulling thoughts were bouncing on a cushion of avidya—the basic ignorant identification of the mind with the body rather than Self, the Atman.

Before I had this knowledge, I would have probably tried to talk myself down from the worry within the samsara paradigm ('Everything will be fine; this is a good dentist; even if she suffers, it is for her own health'.) Being able to stop and observe the roots of fear shooting up, seeing the excessive attachments and aversions brought to light, and noticing how delusional they were (all based on myth-beliefs in my samsara, not on truth), allowed me to then observe how all of that is an overgrown extension of one fundamental misidentification—the ego with the body rather than spirit. It was a classic moksha moment for sure!"

Kristin's awakened moment amid fiscal challenges.

"I had an experience this week that sprang out of nowhere. It was information that directly impacts my family's financial stability. I was really amazed at how quickly I was able to detach from all the logistics of everything and the fear of the unknown. My first response was, 'Wow, I am really seeing the benefits of cultivating self-knowledge and how helpful it is when we are faced with difficulties!'

Between focusing on what is permanent (I am okay inside me, my happiness is up to me) and what is impermanent (things keep changing outside me, so the happiness from them can come and go), I noticed an inner voice, and that inner voice kept talking with me, soothing me, guiding me, and it kept saying, 'Moksha, moksha—trust that the Self that dwells inside me and everywhere and in every being is perfection despite the easy and harder experiences of life.' I know that whatever happens from this point onward will only increase my trust in the Self.

I was sharing with my husband that I had no idea where I would be without these teachings, as in the past I would not recover for weeks and feel a victim. But I was okay. And I could help him be okay too. I think I was enjoying not one but a series of moksha moments despite some challenges externally!"

Prasanna Steve's awakened moment despite a friend's death.

"I had a very good friend pass away suddenly, someone I talked to quite a few times a week. My response was all the natural emotions, but what I didn't have this time was the thought, 'Why did this happen?' I was not railing against the inevitable. I didn't need any of these thoughts where I fight what is before me. The 'why did it happen' thought didn't serve any purpose; whatever happened, happened, and so there was very little disturbance for me in that sense. So, because of that inner acceptance of things as they were, I was able to enjoy a freeing moksha moment!

I was able to fulfill my dharmic duty as a friend by helping his younger brother, who was quite upset and needed someone to talk to. But because there was no such upset on my part, I also had all the normal responses that I should have, just without all this wasted emotion, such as it should've been different, it should not have happened then, or how could it have happened so suddenly (as was my tendency in the past). I felt free, okay, at peace despite my real loss too."

In the above real-life situations, Lauren could see through her own fears because she could apply knowledge of Self over her panicking mind and recognize that her daughter is not the body but the Self, and thereby dissolve her samsara in that moment.

Kristin refused to be bitten by the snake of world vasana, which tells us that fiscal concerns should be our number-one concern (money makes the world go around), and continued to trust something more eternal (nitya) inside her, her true eternally fulfilled Self, despite the outer challenge.

Prasanna Steve refused to be swept away by a very real loss and stayed steadfast on his dharma of helping the bereaved family members, while also not bypassing his grief either, but experiencing the blessings of "pure sorrow" versus sorrow deluded with should'ves and could'ves (likes and dislikes about the choiceless situation at hand).

All three demonstrated a sovereign way of experiencing fear, sorrow, and loss in a balanced way, a way with a greater understanding and tranquility (samatvam) while at same letting the emotions emerge or tears flow if that is what needed to happen (no spiritual bypassing). My teachings on what is permanent (Self) and what is impermanent (waves in the mind) had become a part of my students' systems.

The Vedas say, "What you think you will become" (*yad bhavam tad bhavati*). When you think, *I am agitated, I can't cope, I am upset*, you are bound by such thoughts in perceived limitations. After all, you are the supreme power at your core, so you can decide how you want to feel, and you will feel accordingly. From here on out, when experiencing a challenge, crisis, or loss, you can *choose the dharma of cultivating tranquility through self-knowledge* and audit and edit your thoughts, like Lauren, Kristin, and Prasanna Steve chose to do. They chose knowledge-enabled and soul strength–activating thoughts instead.

Have you seen how gracefully a swan lives in water, its feathers never quite wet? Similarly, just as a swan lives in water but keeps its feathers dry, the one who has self-knowledge and puts it to use in daily life lives in this world full of maya, but is untouched by its illusions and false appearances. The knower dwells in the universe but remains untouched and unpolluted by maya's seductions and mirages (vasanas). Such a one is called a *hamsa*, the spiritual swan—truly a sovereign one.

We can be inspired by the swan and emulate hamsa-like ideals in our personal lives.

The hamsa does not fear pain, nor longs for pleasure.

The hamsa is not attached to the pleasant, nor fears the unpleasant.

The hamsa does not hate, nor rejoice. Firmly fixed in knowledge, the Self is content, well-established within. Such a one alone is called the sovereign one, a knower, whose consciousness is permeated with the perfect bliss. That Atman I am, is known. The goal of Self is achieved.

Remember:

No matter what happens, you are enough because you are Self.

Instead of reacting, you will respond.

Instead of seeking, you will manifest.

Instead of wanting, you will receive.

Instead of complaining, you will be amused.

Instead of agitation, you will enjoy inner peace, wholeness, and fullness, which is your natural state.

Once we know the Self, we don't need to give up those objects that previously fulfilled our legitimate worldly needs. We simply know their real value.

Fortunately, one part of you is already awake. It is the truth in you, which is forever free of maya, beyond maya, which in our self-ignorance we tend to forget. As you internalize awakening Vedic self-knowledge, potent memories of who you are will be stirred in your now pure mind and liberate you from the fog of illusion.

The true Self knows it always reigns supreme.

24

Atmabodha: Knowing the Sovereign Self

"As water becomes one with water, fire with fire, and air with air, so the mind becomes one with the infinite's mind and thus attains infinite freedom."

MAITRI UPANISHAD, 6.19–23

Just as heavy dark clouds can come between us and the light of the sun, an over-expressed, dull, agitated, and self-ignorant mind blocks your sovereign Self from its true and pure expression.

When you use the winds of Vedic wisdom to blow away your clouds of self-ignorance, your pure and enlightened mind becomes the vast, limitless, unobstructed blue sky in which your Self shines like the eternal sun, warming you with rays of happiness, power, wholeness, fullness, and freedom for all eternity. You will realize that the sun had never stopped shining, even for a single moment, even while hidden behind the clouds.

Once you experience *atmabodha*, "knowledge of your true Self," you are no longer carried away by external circumstances and other people's opinions, beliefs, and lifestyles; you do not do things just because others are doing them.

Your inner guru awakens and may begin awakening others too. When you begin navigating your current life with timeless wisdom, that same mind that was once so lost in the dark corridors of maya now becomes the receptacle of truth, wisdom, and light. The qualities of agitating rajas and clouding tamas recede permanently, and illuminous sattva alone shines like a crown jewel in your sovereign mind. The darker emotions, like anger, grief, dismay, and overwhelm are replaced by understanding, born from deep wisdom and self-knowledge.

In moksha, just as a handful of salt mixes completely in the ocean, just as a spark is enveloped in a massive fire, just as a drop of rain becomes one with the tumbling river, so does your estranged and embattled ego, the little self, disappear into your grand and magnificent big Self that is expansive, abundant, and ever free.

In this stage, the suffering mind disappears, and a pure mind that can see truth, the past, and the future while remaining established in the present takes over. You live the way you wish, whether as a monk in awe-inspiring solitude or with full-throttle engagement in society as a dynamic, joyful, spiritually awakened householder, artist, banker, lawyer, spiritual teacher, or parent who never forgets the truth of divine inner fullness. You know you are overflowing. *I am enough, and that is why I am forever free and joyful!*

This enough-ness, fullness, and freedom are not mere intellectual words. They become your living reality. You feel pleased, as if bliss is exploding within you, for no apparent reason. Your earthly relationships become wonderful tool—free, light, and playful, yet heartfelt, sincere, and flowing. Some sleepwalkers may still not get you, but they can't ever get to you.

You soar beyond the attacks of others. Everybody is not awake, after all! But where once your ignorant ego, if criticized, would either lose power or seek revenge out of false power, now you simply live your power through remaining indifferent to both criticism and praise; you understand that both are mere thought waves passing through the not-yet-awakened person's mind. You fear no criticism. You crave no compliments, you experience fearlessness, boldness, and compassion instead because all egoic-samsara delusions have ended forever.

Spontaneously, heartfully, gladly, and god-fully, you teach others how a great soul lives in a body, navigating worldly relationships with those who are still sleepwalking in a more self-valuing, self-respecting, and self-celebratory manner with greater compassion and understanding for all creatures of this universe.

While enjoying your relationships and gifting them your tranquil presence and elevated state of mind, you continue to experience emotional, intellectual, and spiritual autonomy. Before you even speak, you inspire. When you are silent, the discerning ones feel love, respect, and devotion for you because you are in touch with your Self in both speech and in silence.

Claim Your Sovereign Destiny

O fellow human, awaken from your mental slumber, where you have accepted sorrow-giving mental bondages, limitations, and restraints as your destiny! Awaken and recognize your potential to be joyful, resourceful, abundant, and limitlessly expansive! Now is your time to come unstuck and soar in inner skies of limitless freedom, to be or become what you want.

I urge you to explore new pathways where none existed yesterday. Then you will make personally uplifting and planet-benefitting choices you never thought you could make. You will constantly surprise yourself and especially those who may have written you off because your pure ego will become a gateway to your true Self. You will become, for the rest of us, a light shiner, a truth teller, a darkness conqueror, and a peace ambassador.

Remember: You Are Sovereign, Always

In the most ancient of all Vedic scriptures, the *Rig-Veda*, a woman seer by the name of Vagambhrini declared her thoughts upon achieving moksha in a hymn known as "Atma-Stuti"—a hymn in celebration of the Self.

This great woman disbanded the imprisoning bonds of samsara bondages in her mind ten thousand years ago. She recognized her true identity. At the moment she encountered her own unimaginable, limitless spiritual power and psychic immensity, she declared her sovereign truth to the universe. Her inner freedom reverberates through this book.

I conclude these teachings on the bliss and freedom of the Self with her emotionally exhilarating, consciousness-elevating, gloriously unapologetic, and awesomely self-glorifying declaration:

> *"Hear, one and all:*
> *My truth as I declare it,*
> *I breathe a strong breath like the wind and the tempest,*
> *I hold together all of existence with my power.*
> *Beyond this wide earth and beyond the heavens*
> *I have become mighty in the grandeur of my Self."*

> *RIG-VEDA*, 10.125

I honor the example of this female spiritual leader. Her embrace of her own truth inspired the many empowered, soulful beings who raised me with the lived wisdom of dharma and moksha in my Vedic family so I can uphold my own sovereignty today and share it with you, my world family.

Tomorrow, your own grandeur shall spread on this earthly plane of consciousness and beyond. This is my deep conviction for you.

Boundless inner freedom and bliss is your destiny. Nothing in your life is random, not even the darkness that led you on the quest for inner light. Everything that you encounter in your life is a gift of the highest order. There is a great reason why you are reading this book, too.

It will awaken you to your Sovereign Self.

With sovereign love,
Acharya Shunya

GLOSSARY OF SANSKRIT WORDS

abhilasha: To desire.

acharya: Spiritual preceptor, master teacher.

adambhitvam: Non-conceit, unpretentiousness, naturalness.

adharma: Absence of dharma, violation of intrinsic human values.

advaita: Not two; points to the essential one-ness of life.

Advaita Vedanta: Nondual Self-knowledge tradition of the Vedic Upanishads.

ahamkara: The mind's identification with ourselves as separate and limited rather than One with the greater whole, giving us the sense of "I" and "mine."

ahara-vihara: Conscious food and lifestyle recommendations from Ayurveda and yoga traditions.

ahimsa: Not causing pain to any living being at any time through the actions of one's mind, speech, or body.

amaanitvam: Value of humility, opposite of self-conceit.

ananda: Unalloyed and uninterrupted bliss of the Self that is independent of any external factors.

anitya: Non-eternal, transient, mortal.

apaurusheya: Having no human author.

arjavam: Straightforwardness, uprightness, cultivated consistency in thought, word, and action.

Arjuna: Student of Krishna in the Bhagavad Gita.

artha: Pursuit of material and emotional security, such as material wealth and relationships.

asana: Seat.

asteya: Non-stealing.

Atma or Atman: The boundless one, our deepest Self, the soul, pure consciousness within.

atmabodha: Knowledge, realization, recognition of the Self.

atma-sankalpa: Decision taken by our true Self; a soul-level decision.

Atma-Stuti: Hymn in celebration of the Self.

atma-tushti: Sense of self-approval that arises from within when we follow dharma.

Atma vasana: Longing for the Self.

Atma vidya: Knowledge of the nature of one's own boundless soul, typically provided by Vedic teachers from Vedic scriptures like Upanishads and Bhagavad Gita.

atmavaan: Mindfulness; consciously aware of Atma.

atmavinigraha: A mastered mind, a mind that is not enslaved by the ego.

avidya: Ignorance of the Self, a screen of spiritual self-ignorance.

Ayodhya: A city on the banks of the Sarayu River in Uttar Pradesh, India, where Acharya Shunya was raised.

Ayurveda: Science of holistic well-being and medicine from ancient India.

bhati: Light, shine.

bhawa: The feeling and emotive aspect of the mind.

bhawashuddhi: Purification or enlightening of our feelings, thoughts, and attitudes with Vedic wisdom.

bheda: Separation, distancing.

brahmacharya: Path or dharmic practices that lead to the ultimate reality of the Self; also voluntary regulation of sexual desires.

Brahmarishi: Seer who knows the Ultimate Reality (Brahman) as Atman (Self) within.

buddhi: The faculty of illumined reasoning, the "higher mind," where resolution, decision, and our will function. The mind when facing inward toward the Self and capable of choosing our thoughts.

buddhimatta: Illumined cognitive faculty suffused with sattva.

buddhi nasha: Chronic corruption of our ability to discern right from wrong.

chaitanyam: Consciousness, awareness.

chakras: Energetic centers of the body.

dama: Sense-control.

dambhitvam: Superficial behavior from false pride.

dana: Giving with gratitude.

danda: Punishment.

deva yajna: Cosmic debit God, Universe, or Brahman.

dharma: Intrinsic moral human values of mindfulness in all interactions toward not only humans, but all beings, even plants, trees, and inanimate nature.

dharma yuddha: Battle between dharma and non-dharma within the mind.

dhi: Wisdom, capacity to discern.

dhyanam: Meditation.

dukkha: Suffering, sorrow.

dwesha: Aversion.

grihastha sadhu: A householder sage.

gunas: A trio of divine qualities (sattva, rajas, and tamas) through which maya acts on the mind.

guru: Spiritual guide.

guru-shishya parampara: Denotes the tradition of succession of teachers and disciples in traditional Vedic culture and religions such as Hinduism, Jainism and Sikhism. Each tradition belongs to a specific lineage with its own head (Acharya).

hamsa: Swan.

himsa: Violence.

hri: Remorse.

ishvara pranidhanam: Devotion to the divine in form or formlessness.

jagat: The external, commonly shared world of objects in which we all transact.

jiva: The ego-based personality made up of the body, mind, and intellect (but is forgetful of the soul).

jivana mukta: The sovereign one, a person who is living their daily life in full awareness of the boundless Self within.

jnana: Knowledge of Self from Vedic scriptures.

jnana mudra: "Wisdom seal," a gesture of fingers associated with meditation jnana yoga—a path of knowledge to spiritual liberation.

jnanam: Refers to knowledge (jnana).

kama: Using senses to enjoy sensorial delight, one of the four universal goals of human life.

Kama Sutra: Text imparting teachings on sex.

karma: Action.

karma yoga: Path of ego-less action to spiritual liberation.

karuna: Compassion.

Krishna: Incarnation of God who instructs Arjuna in knowledge of the Self through the Bhagavad Gita.

krodha: Anger, which often comes out of the grief of not getting something that we desire or the obstacles in the way of us getting something we desire.

kshanti: Cheerful forbearance, willing tolerance, and accommodation.

kshaya: Dissolution, destruction, depletion, end.

loka vasana: World-based unconscious desires that compel us to seek our happiness and sense of self in the world.

lolupa: Eager or intensified desire.

mananam: Contemplation.

mandukya: Frog.

manoshuddhi: Mind purification.

Manu: Hindu sage who codified the law of dharma.

maryada: Boundaries.

maya: The cosmic veil of forgetfulness that blinds us to our deepest Self and allows us to believe we are the mind and body alone.

mithya: Myth-reality beliefs that do not correspond with objective reality but do carry subjective reality in our private samsara until we see through them and discard those beliefs.

moha: Delusional state of mind that arises from being blinded by attachments and aversions.

moksha: Spiritual liberation from the delusions of our own mind.

muchyate: To free, let go, liberate, or release.

mudra: A special gesture of the fingers that forms a kind of "seal" that holds energy.

mukta: Ever free, a state of spiritual freedom.

mukti: A being in a state of moksha.

mumukshutvam: The intense and compelling desire to know the Self.

natya shastra: Teachings on theater.

nidhidhyasanam: The spiritual practice of internalizing the knowledge that has been previously heard and contemplated.

nitya: Eternal.

nitya mukta: A being who is ever free of the colorings of the mind because they have recognized their eternally sovereign nature.

niyama: Dharmic impulses we should cultivate that build sattva in us.

nritya shastra: Teachings on dance.

param-samatvam: Ultimate tranquility, another word for the experience of moksha.

prakasha: "Light of the Self," the special trait of luminosity.

pramana: That which is not contradicted.

pranayama: Breathing practices from classical yoga.

prasada: "Grace of the Self." Root Sanskrit word refers to tranquility, calmness, satisfaction of the mind.

pratipaksha bhavana: Method of deliberate opposite thoughts.

priyam: Love, pleasure.

purna: Radical wholeness that remains ever whole, self-fulfillment.

purnam: Fullness, wholeness.

purushartha: Four legitimate universal human desires worth pursuing in life.

raga: "Becoming colored," meaning excessive or obsessive attachments that color and confuse the mind.

rajas: One of the three qualities (gunas) of the mind; causes agitation and projections of samsara in the mind.

rishi/rishika: Male/female seer.

Rishika Vagambhrini: Woman sage and contributor to the *Rig-Veda*.

sadhana: Conscious spiritual discpline taken up voluntarily by seeker of Self.

sadhana chatushtayam: Fourfold path to becoming a qualified seeker of self-knowledge.

Sage Patanjali: Yogic seer who compiled the *Yoga Sutras*.

sakshi, sakshi-chaitanyam: Another name for the Self, the inner witness that observes all the modifications in the body and mind, but itself remains unmodified.

sakshi bhava: Witness awareness.

samadhi: Super-conscious state of mind that is absolutely sans thought where the underlying spirit or pure consciousness previously covered by thoughts is revealed.

samatvam: Tranquility that arises out of dharmic behavior.

Samhita: First section of each book of the Vedas that deals with the laws of karma and dharma.

samsara: The unwanted subjective mental state filled with sorrow-causing attachments and delusions that blocks awareness of the deepest Self.

sankalpa shakti: Manifesting power of the mind that can be applied positively or negatively.

santosha: Objectless contentment, inner peace with what comes to us and what is taken away as part of a universal flow.

Sarayu: River in northern India.

satsanga: Spending time in the company of spiritual teachers and scriptures.

sattva/sattvic: One of three qualities of the mind; brings clarity to the mind.

satyam: Universally applicable spiritual truth.

shadsampat: Six virtues that prevent spiritual bypassing.

shama: Mind management.

shanta: Inner nature of Self which is peaceful for no reason.

sharira vasana: Ignorant fusion with the body as our identity (rather than the soul) that causes us to be obsessed over our body appearance, pleasures, etc.

sharvanam: Listening to teacher or reading the knowledge.

shastra vasana: Ignorant identification with what we intellectually know, which causes us to blindly chase more degrees, knowledge, expertise, etc.

shaucham: Cleanliness in body, mind, and environment.

shilpa shastra: Teachings on sculpture.

shoka: The grief, anxiety, or self-pity that arises when our desires are not met.

shraddha: Cultivated open-mindedness and trust in a spiritual teacher and the teachings.

smriti-nasha: Spiritual forgetfulness where we can forget our values, our prior learning, our prior resolutions.

spriha: Existential greed for life situations to go the way we want.

soundarya shastra: Teachings on beauty.

sthairyam: Steadfastness, firm inner resolve.

swadharma: An individual's unique inner calling to a personalized life duty.

tamas: One of the three gunas, the veiling power of maya.

Tantra: A spiritual philosophy from the Vedas.

tapas: Spiritual disciplines.

titiksha: Forbearance, mental resilience in the face of life challenges.

trikanataka: Three thorns.

tushta: Self-satisfaction, divinely full without effort to acquire externally.

upadhi: Limitation.

Upanishads: The later portion of the Vedas containing nondual and mystical teachings on the Self beyond the body and mind.

uparama: Stablizing mind in reference to chosen lifestyle, profession, and so forth.

vaak: Speech.

vaaktapas: Voluntary disciplines of the speech (dharmic).

vairagyam: Cultivated nonattachment that follows discernment of what is eternal and noneternal, deliberately letting go of attachments that once colored the mind with myths.

vasana: A mental compulsion or obsession; uncontrollable mental desires related to world, body, or seeking knowledge.

Vedas: Universal, timeless, sacred spiritual teachings of ancient India.

vidya: Knowledge.

vinay: Cultivated attitude of mindfulness and gratefulness in the student as they approach the teacher with respectful behavior.

viveka: The faculty or practice of being able to discern between thoughts and choose our thoughts at will.

viyoga: Emotional (not physical) detachment within relationships.

vrittis: Thoughts or mental modifications.

yad bhavam tad bhavati: From the Vedas, "You become what you believe."

yajna: Universal law of relationships expecting that everything is a giver and also a receiver.

yama: Dharmic restraint, unethical behaviors we should not engage in.

yoga: Union.

Bibliography of Vedic Texts

Amrita Bindu Upanishad

Ashtanga Hridayam

Ashtavakra Gita

Atharva-Veda

Atmabodha

Bhagavad Gita

Brihadaranyaka Upanishad

Chandogya Upanishad

Dhammapada

Hamsa Upanishad

Hatha Yoga Pradipika

Isha Upanishad

Kaivalya Upanishad

Katha Upanishad

Kautilya's Arthashastra

Kena Upanishad

Mahabharata

Mahanarayana Upanishad

Maitri Upanishad

Mandukya Upanishad

Manu Smriti

Mundaka Upanishad

Nirvana Shatakam

Prashna Upanishad

Rig-Veda

Sama-Veda

Shandilya Upanishad

Shvetashvatara Upanishad

Taittiriya Upanishad

Tattva Bodha

Tirumantiram of Sage Tirumular

Varuha Upanishad

Vivekachudamani

Upadesha Sahasri

Yajur-Veda

Yoga Sutras of Patanjali

NOTES

Introduction: An Invitation to the Sovereign Self

1. *Brihadaranyaka Upanishad*, 2.4.5.

2. Mahatma Gandhi, *The Bhagavad Gita According to Gandhi* (New York: Penguin Random House, 2009); Rudolf Steiner, *The Bhagavad Gita and the West: The Esoteric Significance of the Bhagavad Gita and Its Relation to the Epistles of Paul* (Barrington, MA: SteinerBooks, 2009), 43; Harold Coward, *Jung and Eastern Thought* (New York: SUNY Press, 1985); Silvia Nagy-Zekmi, ed., *Paradoxical Citizenship: Essays on Edward Said* (Lanham, MD: Lexington Books, 2006); Dana Sawyer, *Huston Smith: Wisdom Keeper: Living the World's Religions: The Authorized Biography of a 21st Century Spiritual Giant* (Louisville, KY: Fons Vitae, 2014); Joseph Campbell, *Baksheesh and Brahmin: Asian Journals—India (The Collected Works of Joseph Campbell)* (Novato, CA: New World Library, 2002); Denise Cush, Catherine Robinson, and Michael York, *Encyclopedia of Hinduism* (New York: Routledge, 2007).

3. Henry David Thoreau, *The Writings of Henry David Thoreau, Journal II: 1850–September 15, 1851* (Boston: Houghton Mifflin & Co., 1906), 4.

4. S. Radhakrishnan, *The Philosophy of the Upanishads* (London: George Allen & Unwin, Ltd., 1924).

5. Merton M. Sealts Jr., ed., *Journals and Miscellaneous Notebooks of Ralph Waldo Emerson, Volume X: 1847–1848, October 1, 1848* (Cambridge, MA: Belknap Press of Harvard University Press, 1973), 360.

6. Erwin Schrödinger, *My View of the World* (Woodbridge, CT: Ox Bow Press, 1983), chapter 4.

7. Stephen Prothero, *God Is Not One: The Eight Rival Religions That Run the World* (New York: HarperOne, 2011), 144.

8. Paul Deussen, *Outline of the Vedanta System of Philosophy According to Shankara* (New York: Grafton Press, 1906; Cornell University Library, 2009), preface.

9   James H. Hijiya, "The *Gita* of J. Robert Oppenheimer," *Proceedings of the American Philosophical Society* 144, no. 2 (2000): 123–167.

10. Ram Dass, *Paths to God: Living the Bhagavad Gita* (New York: Harmony Books, 2005); Eckart Tolle, "Four Types of Spiritual Seekers," eckharttollenow.com/new-home-video /default.aspx?shortcode=nyi1b1, accessed April 7, 2020; Deepak Chopra, *Sacred Verses, Healing Sounds, Volumes I and II: The Bhagavad Gita, Hymns of the Rig Veda* (New World Library, 2004), audio CD.

Chapter 1. Atman: The Self Awaits Your Discovery

1. *Chandogya Upanishad*, 4.12.1–3.

2. Bhagavad Gita, 5.24.

3. *Taittiriya Upanishad*, 1.4.1.

4. Bhagavad Gita, 6.28.

Chapter 2. Maya: The Illusion That Conceals Your True Self

1. Bhagavad Gita, 5.15.

2. Ralph Waldo Emerson, "Maia," American Verse Project, accessed April 22, 2020, quod.lib.umich.edu/a/amverse/BAD1982.0001.001/1:9.2.11?rgn=div3;view=fulltext.

3. Sue Mehrtens, "The Ten Pillars of the Bridge of the Spirit," The Jungian Center for Spiritual Sciences, accessed March 16, 2018, jungiancenter.org/ten-pillars-bridge-spirit/.

4. Adi Shankaracharya, *Vivekachudamani*, 143.

5. *Vivekachudamani*, 47.

6. David Frawley, "Misconceptions About Advaita," American Institute of Vedic Studies, accessed May 26, 2020, vedanet.com/misconceptions-about-advaita/.

7. Robert Augustus Masters, *Spiritual Bypassing: When Spirituality Disconnects Us from What Really Matters* (Berkeley, CA: North Atlantic Books, 2010), 2.

Chapter 4. Raga: Breaking the Cycle of Attachment

1. Bhagavad Gita, 2.62–63.

2. *Ashtavakra Gita*, 15.5.

Chapter 5. Vasana: Healing Our Restless Relationship with Desire

1. Bhagavad Gita, 5.22.
2. Bhagavad Gita, 5.21.
3. *Amrita Bindu Upanishad*, 18.
4. Adi Shankaracharya, *Vivekachudamani*, 162.
5. *Vivekachudamani*, 60.
6. *Vivekachudamani*, 54.
7. *Vivekachudamani*, 272.

Chapter 6. Manoshuddhi: Shining the Light of Consciousness

1. These teachers and religious figures may not use the word "Hindu" per se but give out Hindu mantras.
2. *Mundaka Upanishad*, 2.2.1–2.
3. *Shvetashvatara Upanishad*, 1.16.

Chapter 7. Viyoga: Cultivating Detachment from Possessions and People

1. *Brihadaranyaka Upanishad*, 2.4.5.
2. Bhagavad Gita, 3.39.

Chapter 8. Guru: Recognizing a True Teacher

1. Adi Shankaracharya, *Vivekachudamani*, 33.5.
2. *Katha Upanishad*, 1.3.14.
3. *Dhammapada*, 76.
4. *Katha Upanishad*, 1.2.9.
5. *Vivekachudamani*, 42–43, 45, 47.
6. Bhagavad Gita, 2.56.
7. *Vivekachudamani*, 272.
8. *Shvetashvatara Upanishad*, 3.8.

Chapter 11. Viveka: Walking the Path of Discernment

1. *Vivekachudamani*, 174.
2. Bhagavad Gita, 18.30.
3. *Katha Upanishad*, 2.3.9.
4. Bhagavad Gita, 14.17.

Chapter 12. Vairagyam: Practicing Nonattachment

1. *Vivekachudamani*, 82.

Chapter 13. Shama: Managing Your Thoughts—Really

1. Chapter 5, on vasanas, will help you become alert to the presence of compulsive self-shaming, grief-inflicting thoughts and be better prepared to effectively edit them or switch channels to a preferred thought.
2. Bhagavad Gita, 16.1–3.

Chapter 14. Bhawashuddhi: Cultivating Emotional Intelligence

1. Bhagavad Gita, 17.16.
2. *Isha Upanishad*, 7.

Chapter 15. Nitya-Anitya: Meeting Impermanence and Death

1. Bhagavad Gita, 2.22, 2.13, 2.18, 2.20, 2.23–2.25.
2. Bhagavad Gita, 6.7.
3. *Charaka Samhita*, "Sutrasthanam," 7.25.

Chapter 16. Advaita: Recognizing the Truth of Unity Consciousness

1. *Shvetashvatara Upanishad*, 1.12.
2. *Shvetashvatara Upanishad*, 3.7.
3. *Shvetashvatara Upanishad*, 3.16.
4. Don't confuse "Brahman" with the term "Brahmin." While the former denotes Absolute Reality of Pure Consciousness, the latter is a collective term for any seeker of this

higher truth. With the march of time, "Brahmin" came to be associated with a specific Hindu caste dedicated to Vedic studies and religious pursuit.

5. *Isha Upanishad,* 6.

6. Tarka the Duck, reply to "Advaita and Neo-Advaita," The Project Avalon Forum, February 29, 2012, projectavalon.net/forum4/showthread.php?41687-Advaita-and -Neo-Advaita; Tom Huston, introduction to Jessica Roemischer, "Who's Transforming Anyway?," What Is Enlightenment?, January 1, 2006.

7. Sacred Matters, "American Gurus: Seven Questions for Arthur Versluis," accessed May 12, 2020, web.archive.org/web/20160417164207/https:/scholarblogs.emory.edu /sacredmatters/2015/01/12/seven-questions-for-arthur-versluis/.

8. Arthur Versluis, *American Gurus: From Transcendentalism to New Age Religion* (Oxford: Oxford University Press, 2014), 1–3.

9. Douglas Groothuis, *Unmasking the New Age* (Downers Grove, IL: IVP Books, 1986), 153.

Chapter 17. Dharma: Cultivating a Life of Meaning

1. *Manu Smriti,* 6.92.

2. *Manu Smriti,* 12.35.

3. *Manu Smriti,* 8.15.

Chapter 18. Yamas and Niyamas: Nurturing Higher Values

1. Mahabharata, 12.109.9–11.

2. *Katha Upanishad,* 2.3.10.

3. Acharya Shunya, *Ayurveda Lifestyle Wisdom* (Boulder, CO: Sounds True, 2017); *Ashtanga Hridayam, Sutrasthanam,* 7.75.

4. *Yajur-Veda,* 36.18.

5. Bhagavad Gita, 17.15.

6. There are three types of suffering that can be overcome with mindful endurance: a) self-created—there is some control over such suffering; b) created by surroundings—one has only partial control over these; and c) created by unknown factors—one has no control over these.

7. *Maha Upanishad,* 6.71–75.

8. *Katha Upanishad,* 1.3.14.

9. Bhagavad Gita, 6.9.

Chapter 19. Swadharma: Embracing Your Innate Purpose with Integrity

1. Bhagavad Gita, 3.35.
2. Bhagavad Gita, 3.33, 35.
3. Mahabharata, 5.29.48.
4. Arjavam as a value is mentioned as a single word in the Bhagavad Gita (like all other values). These teachings are my free interpretation.

Chapter 20. Atmashakti: Bringing Soul Power to Relationships

1. *Isha Upanishad*, 8.
2. Bhagavad Gita, 4.36.

Chapter 21. Vaaktapas: Employing Ancient Communication Protocols

1. This statement is often attributed to Rumi, Socrates, and the Buddha (Vaca Sutta or the Subhasita Sutta). It also appears in *Miscellaneous Poems* by Mary Ann Pietzker (London: Griffith and Farran, 1872). See also Bodhipaksa's Fake Buddha Quotes blog entry from August 15, 2012, fakebuddhaquotes.com/if-you-propose-to-speak-always -ask-yourself-is-it-true-is-it-necessary-is-it-kind/.
2. Inspired from *Taittriya Aranyaka*, 1.23.1 of *Yajur-Veda*.
3. *Brihadaranyaka Upanishad*, 4.4.5.

Chapter 22. Samatvam: Cultivating Equanimity by Accepting What Is Arising

1. Bhagavad Gita, 6.31.
2. *Yajur-Veda*, 16.42–43.
3. Bhagavad Gita, 2.38.
4. Bhagavad Gita, 18.59.
5. Bhagavad Gita, 8.7.
6. Bhagavad Gita, 2.65.

Chapter 23. Moksha: Making Awakening Your Supreme Goal

1. Bhagavad Gita, 5.16.
2. Bhagavad Gita, 5.28.
3. Michael W. Taft, "Nonduality and Mindfulness—Two Great Traditions That Go Great Together," *Science & Nonduality*, accessed May 1, 2020, scienceandnonduality.com/article/nonduality-and-mindfulness-two-great-traditions-that-go-great-together.
4. Taft, "Nonduality and Mindfulness."
5. Bhagavad Gita, 5.26.
6. Bhagavad Gita, 2.72.
7. Bhagavad Gita, 6.20–23.
8. Ram Dass, (@BabaRamDass) "If you think you are enlightened, go spend a week with your family," Twitter, November 24, 2016, twitter.com/babaramdass/status/801830478319861760?lang=en.
9. *Vivekachudamani*, 13.

INDEX

Note: Italicized page numbers indicated figures and tables.

Index

nonduality (*continued*)
    preparation for teachings on, 257–58
    reality, three levels of, 259
    Shankaracharya on, 260–61
    spiritual bypassing and, 256–57
    Vishwamitra, example of, 269–71
    world is not an illusion, 260–61
nonharm. *See* nonviolence
nonviolence, 294
    in speech, 339–40
nritya shastra (dance), 277

O

objective world, 37–38, 259
objects
    chronic dissatisfaction, thorn of, 115–16
    emotional bondage to, 111–13
    emotional dependence on, 195–96
    karma and, 116–17
    mental dependence, thorn of, 114–15
    possessing versus needing, 111–13
    three thorns, 113–16
    unavoidable sorrow, thorn of, 116
observances and restraints. *See* yamas and
    niyamas
obsessions, 66
    body obsession, 73–75
    knowledge obsession, 75–78
    unconscious, 68, 84
    See also desire(s); vasanas
oneness, 109, 253–72
    advaita, 2, 30, 109, 253–72
    example of Vishwamitra, 269–71
    genuine awakening to, 272
    maintaining, 258
    See also nonduality
Oppenheimer, Robert, 5
opposite thoughts, 206–7, 294

P

param-samatvam, 370
parents, 197
    forgetfulness manifestations in, 43
    gratitude to, 262
    viyoga (detachment) in parenting, 108
Patanjali, Sage, 85, 153–54, 290–91

yamas and niyamas of, 290–93, *293*, 296
    Yoga Sutras, 85, 154, 290–92, 296
pause, cognitive, 186–88
peace, 161–62
permanence, 246–47
    See also death; impermanence
personal reality, 259
pity. *See* self-pity
pleasant speech, 342–44
pleasure, 276–77
    of the body, 73–74
    dependence on, 114, 116
    dharma and, 279
    healthy, 63
    kama (sex) and, 63, 194, 276–77
    materialistic, 90, 93, 109
    pleasure-seeking propensity, 311–12, 313
    priyam (loving pleasure), 313
    transitory, 28, 35, 48, 115–16
    See also ananda; happiness
pop spirituality, 85–88
    going beyond, 85–88
    gurus in, 123
power, 325–37
    atmashakti vs. ahamshakti, 327–28,
        327–28
    boundaries and, 326
    dharmic power, 327–28, *327–28*
    personal power, 325–26
    silence and, 347–50
    soul power (atmashakti), 325–37
powerlessness, 23–24
prakasha, 183
pramana, 6
prasada (grace), 183
pratipaksha bhavana, 206–7
predetermination, 116–17
pride, 318–20
priyam, 313, 342
priyam vaak (pleasant speech), 339, 342
problem solving, 362–63
projections, 20, 21, 216
psychological sovereignty, 283
purification
    of ego, 31–33, 96–98, 216
    mental (manoshuddhi), 83–104
    of motivations, 86, 96–98

420

ACKNOWLEDGMENTS

Every book is initially a dream, no more than a seed sleeping in the soil. For the seed to germinate and become a sapling, then a plant, then a tree, and one fine day a fruit-bearing tree, it needs, besides the fertile soil of the author's consciousness, a consistent supply of water, air, sunshine, and warmth. I offer heartfelt gratitude to all the people who became air, water, warmth, and sunshine to my book and helped me bring it from inspiration to manifestation.

I want to first thank my brilliant team at Sounds True: Tami Simon, Jennifer Brown, Gretel Hakanson, Jade Lascelles, Rebecca Job, Laurel Kallenbach, Jennifer Miles, Happenstance Type-O-Rama, Christine Day, and Nick Small. After chatting with publisher Tami Simon about my former book *Ayurveda Lifestyle Wisdom* on her podcast, she said, "I am waiting for your spiritual book, Shunya." I feel like Tami first watered my seed that day, and she expedited this book's emergence from the depths of my being sooner rather than later.

Deep bows to Jennifer Y. Brown, my book's acquisition and chief editor. Jennifer, you not only believed in my writing from the get-go, but you suggested the theme of sovereignty! Your support has been unfailing, and your judgments unerring. My work is better because of you. A big thanks to my copyeditor Gretel Hakanson. It was a pleasure to work with you again after we teamed up for *Ayurveda Lifestyle Wisdom*. You did a masterful job with my completed manuscript (as usual)!

A special shout out for my literary agent Stephany Evans. You are not only a terrific agent but also a friend and wise mentor to me. I can't say enough good things about you. I treasure your wisdom, guidance, industry knowledge, and (most especially) your unwavering belief that *truth matters*.

I have no words to express my gratitude to my life partner Chef Sanjai. You have this book in your hands because of him and his loving support of my two-and-half-years-long writer's sojurn. Thank you for your unending patience with my process and tender care of my being, Sanjai. You make me laugh every day, and you make me ginger chai to die for! I must add a line about our beloved labradoodle Noddy, whose love of walks, tug-of-war, and backyard squirrel missions became cheerful distractions amidst the writing.

I want to express appreciation for my students who read initial chapters and gave me their suggestions; many contributed their heartfelt stories, too. I honor your open hearts and acclaim your journey to sovereignty. Specifically, I want to recognize Ishani Naidu, my student of eleven-plus years and author of children's book *The Song at the Heart of the River*, who provided critical feedback, prepared the initial glossary, and proofread not once but several times.

Finally, I express my profound gratitude to my teachers, including my beloved father and living mentor Padmashri Daya Prakash Sinha; my Guru Baba Ayodhya Nath, who is God incarnate to me; and his teacher, my great-grandfather Paramatma Shanti Prakash. I have tried to let their teachings live in me, guide me, and speak through me through this book.

ABOUT THE AUTHOR

Acharya Shunya is a wisdom teacher and catalyst for empowering health and elevating consciousness worldwide. As an internationally recognized author and sought-after spiritual teacher of Vedic nondual wisdom, she is committed to sharing authentic knowledge, illuminating the way forward.

Shunya's unique gift to humanity is her deeply personal and authentic understanding of the ancient Vedic disciplines of nondual Adwaita, Yoga, and Ayurveda, and their classic scriptures, which she expertly demystifies and adapts into contemporary language and meaningful practices for the Western student. Her ability to translate wisdom from sacred Sanskrit texts into deep insights leaves students experiencing profound shifts from within.

As a teacher who has herself walked this path from darkness to light, from emotional bondage to spiritual freedom, Shunya is uniquely able to communicate these ancient subtle truths to modern seekers. She encourages her students to embrace their humanity and abide in their greater Self simultaneously, creating an *enlightened vulnerability*, bringing forth an authentic and empowered whole person into the world, every day.

The first woman lineage holder in a 2,000-year-old line of Vedic spiritual teachers, and the first to teach in the West, Acharya Shunya spent fourteen years training under her paternal grandfather and Guru, "Baba" Ayodhya Nath from the holy city of Ayodhya, in northern India. Baba tasked Shunya to bring these teachings to the modern world.

Acharya Shunya is the president of The Awakened Self Foundation, with its international headquarters in California, and founder of the spiritual and philanthropic nonprofit Vedika Global. Her spiritual discourse Global Satsangs, top-rated podcast *Shadow to Self*, award-winning *Alchemy with Ayurveda* online program, and signature offerings currently unfolding on the theme of *Sovereign Life*—including e-courses, retreats, and corporate workshops—are creating shifts in consciousness and improving health and well-being on a global scale.

Acharya Shunya is also the author of Amazon's #1 bestseller *Ayurveda Lifestyle Wisdom: A Complete Prescription to Optimize Your Health, Prevent Disease, and Live with Vitality and Joy*, which was acclaimed among the top ten books in Alternative Medicine by Healthline. This book has been translated into seven languages and is taught in various Yoga and Ayurveda programs worldwide.

A sought-after speaker, Acharya Shunya delivers keynote addresses at universities and conferences and leads workshops and global retreats. She is an advisor to many noteworthy national and was recognized as one of the Top 100 Trailblazers of Ayurveda and Yoga in America by *Spirituality & Health Magazine*.

Acharya Shunya lives in Northern California with her partner Chef Sanjai, who is an Ayurvedic culinary expert. She enjoys sunrises, walks in nature, and planting and nurturing her bountiful garden. She delights in decoding scriptures, continuing to write books, and nurturing her global student community.

To find out more, visit acharyashunya.com or awakenedself.com.

ABOUT SOUNDS TRUE

Sounds True is a multimedia publisher whose mission is to inspire and support personal transformation and spiritual awakening. Founded in 1985 and located in Boulder, Colorado, we work with many of the leading spiritual teachers, thinkers, healers, and visionary artists of our time. We strive with every title to preserve the essential "living wisdom" of the author or artist. It is our goal to create products that not only provide information to a reader or listener but also embody the quality of a wisdom transmission.

For those seeking genuine transformation, Sounds True is your trusted partner. At SoundsTrue.com you will find a wealth of free resources to support your journey, including exclusive weekly audio interviews, free downloads, interactive learning tools, and other special savings on all our titles.

To learn more, please visit SoundsTrue.com/freegifts or call us toll-free at 800.333.9185.

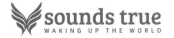